Quantitative Methods
for
HIV/AIDS Research

Chapman & Hall/CRC Biostatistics Series

Editor-in-Chief

Shein-Chung Chow, Ph.D., Professor, Department of Biostatistics and Bioinformatics, Duke University School of Medicine, Durham, North Carolina

Series Editors

Byron Jones, Biometrical Fellow, Statistical Methodology, Integrated Information Sciences, Novartis Pharma AG, Basel, Switzerland

Jen-pei Liu, Professor, Division of Biometry, Department of Agronomy, National Taiwan University, Taipei, Taiwan

Karl E. Peace, Georgia Cancer Coalition, Distinguished Cancer Scholar, Senior Research Scientist and Professor of Biostatistics, Jiann-Ping Hsu College of Public Health, Georgia Southern University, Statesboro, Georgia

Bruce W. Turnbull, Professor, School of Operations Research and Industrial Engineering, Cornell University, Ithaca, New York

Published Titles

Published Titles

Bayesian Modeling in Bioinformatics
Dipak K. Dey, Samiran Ghosh,
and Bani K. Mallick

**Benefit-Risk Assessment in
Pharmaceutical Research and
Development**
Andreas Sashegyi, James Felli,
and Rebecca Noel

**Benefit-Risk Assessment Methods in
Medical Product Development: Bridging
Qualitative and Quantitative Assessments**
Qi Jiang and Weili He

**Bioequivalence and Statistics in Clinical
Pharmacology, Second Edition**
Scott Patterson and Byron Jones

**Biosimilar Clinical Development:
Scientific Considerations and New
Methodologies**
Kerry B. Barker, Sandeep M. Menon,
Ralph B. D'Agostino, Sr., Siyan Xu, and Bo Jin

**Biosimilars: Design and Analysis of
Follow-on Biologics**
Shein-Chung Chow

Biostatistics: A Computing Approach
Stewart J. Anderson

**Cancer Clinical Trials: Current and
Controversial Issues in Design and
Analysis**
Stephen L. George, Xiaofei Wang,
and Herbert Pang

**Causal Analysis in Biomedicine and
Epidemiology: Based on Minimal
Sufficient Causation**
Mikel Aickin

**Clinical and Statistical Considerations in
Personalized Medicine**
Claudio Carini, Sandeep Menon, and Mark Chang

Clinical Trial Data Analysis Using R
Ding-Geng (Din) Chen and Karl E. Peace

**Clinical Trial Data Analysis Using R and SAS,
Second Edition**
Ding-Geng (Din) Chen, Karl E. Peace,
and Pinggao Zhang

Clinical Trial Methodology
Karl E. Peace and Ding-Geng (Din) Chen

Clinical Trial Optimization Using R
Alex Dmitrienko and Erik Pulkstenis

**Cluster Randomised Trials:
Second Edition**
Richard J. Hayes and Lawrence H. Moulton

**Computational Methods in Biomedical
Research**
Ravindra Khattree and Dayanand N. Naik

Computational Pharmacokinetics
Anders Källén

**Confidence Intervals for Proportions
and Related Measures of Effect Size**
Robert G. Newcombe

**Controversial Statistical Issues in
Clinical Trials**
Shein-Chung Chow

**Data Analysis with Competing Risks
and Intermediate States**
Ronald B. Geskus

**Data and Safety Monitoring Committees
in Clinical Trials, Second Edition**
Jay Herson

**Design and Analysis of Animal Studies
in Pharmaceutical Development**
Shein-Chung Chow and Jen-pei Liu

**Design and Analysis of Bioavailability
and Bioequivalence Studies, Third Edition**
Shein-Chung Chow and Jen-pei Liu

Design and Analysis of Bridging Studies
Jen-pei Liu, Shein-Chung Chow,
and Chin-Fu Hsiao

**Design & Analysis of Clinical Trials for
Economic Evaluation & Reimbursement:
An Applied Approach Using SAS & STATA**
Iftekhar Khan

**Design and Analysis of Clinical Trials
for Predictive Medicine**
Shigeyuki Matsui, Marc Buyse,
and Richard Simon

**Design and Analysis of Clinical Trials with
Time-to-Event Endpoints**
Karl E. Peace

Design and Analysis of Non-Inferiority Trials
Mark D. Rothmann, Brian L. Wiens,
and Ivan S. F. Chan

Published Titles

Difference Equations with Public Health Applications
Lemuel A. Moyé and Asha Seth Kapadia

DNA Methylation Microarrays: Experimental Design and Statistical Analysis
Sun-Chong Wang and Arturas Petronis

DNA Microarrays and Related Genomics Techniques: Design, Analysis, and Interpretation of Experiments
David B. Allison, Grier P. Page, T. Mark Beasley, and Jode W. Edwards

Dose Finding by the Continual Reassessment Method
Ying Kuen Cheung

Dynamical Biostatistical Models
Daniel Commenges and Hélène Jacqmin-Gadda

Elementary Bayesian Biostatistics
Lemuel A. Moyé

Emerging Non-Clinical Biostatistics in Biopharmaceutical Development and Manufacturing
Harry Yang

Empirical Likelihood Method in Survival Analysis
Mai Zhou

Essentials of a Successful Biostatistical Collaboration
Arul Earnest

Exposure–Response Modeling: Methods and Practical Implementation
Jixian Wang

Frailty Models in Survival Analysis
Andreas Wienke

Fundamental Concepts for New Clinical Trialists
Scott Evans and Naitee Ting

Generalized Linear Models: A Bayesian Perspective
Dipak K. Dey, Sujit K. Ghosh, and Bani K. Mallick

Handbook of Regression and Modeling: Applications for the Clinical and Pharmaceutical Industries
Daryl S. Paulson

Inference Principles for Biostatisticians
Ian C. Marschner

Interval-Censored Time-to-Event Data: Methods and Applications
Ding-Geng (Din) Chen, Jianguo Sun, and Karl E. Peace

Introductory Adaptive Trial Designs: A Practical Guide with R
Mark Chang

Joint Models for Longitudinal and Time-to-Event Data: With Applications in R
Dimitris Rizopoulos

Measures of Interobserver Agreement and Reliability, Second Edition
Mohamed M. Shoukri

Medical Biostatistics, Third Edition
A. Indrayan

Meta-Analysis in Medicine and Health Policy
Dalene Stangl and Donald A. Berry

Methods in Comparative Effectiveness Research
Constantine Gatsonis and Sally C. Morton

Mixed Effects Models for the Population Approach: Models, Tasks, Methods and Tools
Marc Lavielle

Modeling to Inform Infectious Disease Control
Niels G. Becker

Modern Adaptive Randomized Clinical Trials: Statistical and Practical Aspects
Oleksandr Sverdlov

Monte Carlo Simulation for the Pharmaceutical Industry: Concepts, Algorithms, and Case Studies
Mark Chang

Multiregional Clinical Trials for Simultaneous Global New Drug Development
Joshua Chen and Hui Quan

Multiple Testing Problems in Pharmaceutical Statistics
Alex Dmitrienko, Ajit C. Tamhane, and Frank Bretz

Published Titles

Noninferiority Testing in Clinical Trials: Issues and Challenges
Tie-Hua Ng

Optimal Design for Nonlinear Response Models
Valerii V. Fedorov and Sergei L. Leonov

Patient-Reported Outcomes: Measurement, Implementation and Interpretation
Joseph C. Cappelleri, Kelly H. Zou, Andrew G. Bushmakin, Jose Ma. J. Alvir, Demissie Alemayehu, and Tara Symonds

Quantitative Evaluation of Safety in Drug Development: Design, Analysis and Reporting
Qi Jiang and H. Amy Xia

Quantitative Methods for HIV/AIDS Research
Cliburn Chan, Michael G. Hudgens, and Shein-Chung Chow

Quantitative Methods for Traditional Chinese Medicine Development
Shein-Chung Chow

Randomized Clinical Trials of Nonpharmacological Treatments
Isabelle Boutron, Philippe Ravaud, and David Moher

Randomized Phase II Cancer Clinical Trials
Sin-Ho Jung

Repeated Measures Design with Generalized Linear Mixed Models for Randomized Controlled Trials
Toshiro Tango

Sample Size Calculations for Clustered and Longitudinal Outcomes in Clinical Research
Chul Ahn, Moonseong Heo, and Song Zhang

Sample Size Calculations in Clinical Research, Second Edition
Shein-Chung Chow, Jun Shao, and Hansheng Wang

Statistical Analysis of Human Growth and Development
Yin Bun Cheung

Statistical Design and Analysis of Clinical Trials: Principles and Methods
Weichung Joe Shih and Joseph Aisner

Statistical Design and Analysis of Stability Studies
Shein-Chung Chow

Statistical Evaluation of Diagnostic Performance: Topics in ROC Analysis
Kelly H. Zou, Aiyi Liu, Andriy Bandos, Lucila Ohno-Machado, and Howard Rockette

Statistical Methods for Clinical Trials
Mark X. Norleans

Statistical Methods for Drug Safety
Robert D. Gibbons and Anup K. Amatya

Statistical Methods for Healthcare Performance Monitoring
Alex Bottle and Paul Aylin

Statistical Methods for Immunogenicity Assessment
Harry Yang, Jianchun Zhang, Binbing Yu, and Wei Zhao

Statistical Methods in Drug Combination Studies
Wei Zhao and Harry Yang

Statistical Testing Strategies in the Health Sciences
Albert Vexler, Alan D. Hutson, and Xiwei Chen

Statistics in Drug Research: Methodologies and Recent Developments
Shein-Chung Chow and Jun Shao

Statistics in the Pharmaceutical Industry, Third Edition
Ralph Buncher and Jia-Yeong Tsay

Survival Analysis in Medicine and Genetics
Jialiang Li and Shuangge Ma

Theory of Drug Development
Eric B. Holmgren

Translational Medicine: Strategies and Statistical Methods
Dennis Cosmatos and Shein-Chung Chow

Quantitative Methods for HIV/AIDS Research

Edited by
Cliburn Chan
Michael G. Hudgens
Shein-Chung Chow

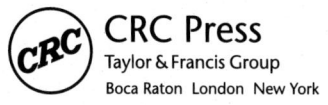

CRC Press
Taylor & Francis Group
Boca Raton London New York

CRC Press is an imprint of the
Taylor & Francis Group, an **informa** business

A CHAPMAN & HALL BOOK

Cover credit: Peter Hraber, Thomas B. Kepler, Hua-Xin Liao, Barton F. Haynes. Adapted from Liao et al. (2013) *Nature* 496: 469.

CRC Press
Taylor & Francis Group
6000 Broken Sound Parkway NW, Suite 300
Boca Raton, FL 33487-2742

International Standard Book Number-13: 978-1-4987-3423-3 (Hardback)

Library of Congress Cataloging-in-Publication Data

Title: Quantitative methods for HIV/AIDS research / Cliburn Chan, Michael G. Hudgens, Shein-Chung Chow.
Description: Boca Raton : Taylor & Francis, 2017. | "A CRC title, part of the Taylor & Francis imprint, a member of the Taylor & Francis Group, the academic division of T&F Informa plc." | Includes bibliographical references and index.
Identifiers: LCCN 2017008215| ISBN 9781498734233 (hardback) | ISBN 9781315120805 (e-book)
Subjects: LCSH: HIV infections Research--Methodology--Popular works. | AIDS (Disease)--Research--Methodology--Popular works.
Classification: LCC RC606.64 .Q36 2017 | DDC 616.97/920072--dc23 LC record available at https://lccn.loc.gov/2017008215

Visit the Taylor & Francis Web site at
http://www.taylorandfrancis.com

and the CRC Press Web site at
http://www.crcpress.com

Contents

**Section III   Quantitative Methods for Dynamical Models
and Computer Simulations**

Preface

Acquired immune deficiency syndrome (AIDS) was first defined by the Centers for Disease Control and Prevention (CDC) in 1982, following unprecedented outbreaks of *Pneumocystis carinii* pneumonia and Kaposi's sarcoma in young men in California and New York. It was soon recognized that AIDS was a pandemic infectious disease, and human immunodeficiency virus (HIV) (then known as *HTLV-III/LAV*) was identified as the causal agent in 1984. The Centers for AIDS Research (CFAR) program was established in 1988 to support a multidisciplinary environment that promotes basic, clinical, epidemiological, behavioral, and translational research in the prevention, detection, and treatment of HIV infection and AIDS. Although sponsored by the Division of AIDS, the CFAR program is supported by multiple NIH institutes and centers, including NIAID, NCI, NICHD, NHLBI, NIDA, NIMH, NIA, NIDDK, NIGMS, NIMHD, FIC, and OAR.

An essential aspect of the multidisciplinary support is the collaboration with and mentoring of biomedical researchers by the statisticians, mathematicians, and computational biologists associated with CFAR quantitative cores. CFAR quantitative core faculty are deeply involved in the cutting edge of statistical and mathematical analysis of HIV/AIDS laboratory tests, clinical trials, vaccine development, and epidemiological surveys across the CFAR. Although many of these analyses are statistical in nature, mathematical modeling and computational simulation play a more important role in HIV/AIDS research compared with many other research fields. HIV/AIDS research has stimulated many innovative statistical, mathematical, and computational developments, but these advances have been dispersed over specialized publications, limiting the ability to see common themes and cross-fertilization of ideas.

This book provides a compilation of statistical and mathematical methods for HIV/AIDS research. Many of the chapter contributors are current or previous directors of the quantitative cores in their institutional CFAR. This book is divided into three sections. The first section focuses on statistical issues in clinical trials and epidemiology that are unique to or particularly challenging in HIV/AIDS research. The second section focuses on the analysis of laboratory data used for immune monitoring, biomarker discovery, and vaccine development. The final section focuses on issues in the mathematical modeling of HIV/AIDS pathogenesis, treatment, and epidemiology.

The first chapter (Statistical Issues in HIV Non-Inferiority Trials) in the clinical trials and epidemiology section discusses how to design, conduct, and analyze HIV non-inferiority trials. The remarkable efficiency of the existing antiretroviral therapy in suppressing HIV makes it difficult to prove the superiority of a new drug. Consequently, establishing non-inferiority has become the more common objective in HIV trials and serves an essential role in finding cheaper, safer, and more convenient drugs. However, a recent survey of published non-inferiority HIV trials shows many methodological flaws including lack of justification for the magnitude of the non-inferiority margin, incorrect sample size determination, and failure to perform the appropriate analyses. This chapter describes the best practices for the design, conduct, and analysis of HIV non-inferiority trials, using the TITAN, ARROW, and CIPRA-SA clinical trials to illustrate concepts and how to handle practical issues such as noncompliance, missing data, and classification or measurement error.

The next chapter (Sample Size for HIV-1 Vaccine Clinical Trials with Extremely Low Incidence Rate) explores the problem of determining sample sizes when HIV incidence rates are very low—for example, when evaluating the efficacy of preventive vaccines. In such cases, power-based calculations, based on detecting absolute differences in incidence rate, often require infeasibly large sample sizes. In contrast, precision-based calculations based on relative changes in incidence rate with a specified maximum error margin can require smaller sample sizes. Frequentist and Bayesian sample size calculations based on precision are described, and a detailed step-by-step example for an HIV vaccine trial is provided. Finally, guidelines for monitoring safety in trials using precision-based sample size calculations are provided.

Adaptive design is a clinical trial design that uses accumulating data to decide how to modify aspects of the study as it continues, without undermining the validity and integrity of the trial. As adaptive designs are more flexible than the traditional randomized clinical trials, they have the potential to shorten the drug or vaccine development process. Interest in adaptive designs has been growing since 2006, when the FDA published the *Critical Path Opportunities List* (https://www.fda.gov/downloads/scienceresearch/specialtopics/CriticalPathinitiative/CriticalPathOpportunitiesreports/UCM077258.pdf) to accelerate the process for introducing new therapeutics, which encouraged the use of prior experience or accumulated information in trial design. Chapter 3 (Adaptive Clinical Trial Design) provides a classification of adaptive trial designs and reviews the advantages, limitations, and feasibility of each design. Suggestions for the use of adaptive designs in HIV vaccine efficacy trials are provided, with discussion of the potential benefits in more rapid assessment and elimination of ineffective vaccines, as well as greater sensitivity in discovering virological or immunological predictors of infection.

The fourth chapter (Generalizing Evidence from HIV Trials Using Inverse Probability of Sampling Weights) in this section investigates how to generalize results from HIV trials that may have a participant distribution that is not representative of the larger population of HIV-positive individuals. The chapter compares existing quantitative approaches for generalizing results from a randomized trial to a specified target population and proposes a novel inverse probability of sampling weighted (IPSW) estimator for generalizing trial results with a time-to-event outcome. Results of using the IPSW estimator to generalize results from two AIDS Clinical Trials Group

(ACTG 320 and ACTG A5202) randomized trials to all people living with HIV in the United States are discussed.

To evaluate whether CDC-recommended screening regimens for HIV testing are being followed, especially in high-risk groups, it is necessary to evaluate the regularity of testing. The challenge for evaluating HIV self-testing is that the testing times are not observed, and whether a testing event occurred during some interval may be the only information available. The final chapter (Statistical Tests of Regularity among Groups with HIV Self-Test Data) in this section reviews the challenges of evaluating the regularity of HIV self-testing. It proposes a statistical model based on the homogeneous Poisson process and defines a likelihood ratio test based on this model for evaluating regularity. This model is applied to a CDC study of text messaging to increase retention in a cohort of HIV-negative men who have sex with men.

The next section deals with new statistical approaches to critical laboratory tests for immune monitoring, biomarker discovery, vaccine development, and population screening in HIV/AIDS clinical research.

The first chapter in this section, "Estimating Partial Correlations between Logged HIV RNA Measurements Subject to Detection Limits," reviews the challenge of nondetection in viral load (VL) or other biomarker measurements, with a focus on estimating the correlation between bivariate measurements from different time points or different reservoirs, when one or both biomarkers may be left censored. Two extensions of likelihood-based methods are proposed for paired or multiple VL measurements that naturally account for covariates. The methods are utilized to analyze sequential RNA levels across two visits of HIV-positive subjects in the HIV Epidemiology Research Study.

The second chapter in this section, "Quantitative Methods and Bayesian Models for Flow Cytometry Analysis in HIV/AIDS Research," reviews Bayesian approaches to flow cytometry data analysis with two applications of multilevel models. The first application shows how hierarchical statistical mixture models can improve the robustness of automated cell subset identification by information sharing across samples; and the second application uses Bayesian modeling to identify novel antigen-specific immune correlates predictive of outcome from intracellular staining assays in the RV144 HIV vaccine trial.

The third chapter in this section, "The Immunoglobulin Variable-Region Gene Repertoire and Its Analysis," describes new methods for analyzing the antibody variable-region gene repertoire for HIV vaccine development. The authors explain the biology of how immunoglobulin diversity is generated and immunoglobulin sequencing assays, as well as how statistical models can be used to infer immunoglobulin clonal phylogenies that may provide insights into the microscale evolution of broadly neutralizing antibodies. Generative Bayesian models are presented for immunoglobulin assembly from germline sequences, somatic mutation, inference of immunoglobulin ancestry from sequenced clonal sequences, and the partitioning of sequences into clonal families.

Chapter 9, "Probability-Scale Residuals in HIV/AIDS Research: Diagnostics and Inference," addresses the challenge of analyzing multiple highly different data types in HIV research, including clinical and demographic data, laboratory results, and viral and host genomics, for predictive modeling. The authors introduce a novel probability-scale residual (PSR), the expectation of the sign function of the contrast between an observed value and its prediction given some fitted distribution, which is useful across a variety of data, outcomes, and regression models. The application of the PSR for model diagnostics and inference is illustrated with a range of HIV studies, including cervical cancer staging, metabolomics, and a genome-wide association study.

The final section is devoted to the mathematical modeling of HIV infection and treatment, with a focus on the integration of statistical methods with mechanistic dynamical systems models. Mathematical models based on ordinary differential equations were originally applied in the HIV context to characterize viral and infected cell decay and have since been extensively used to model viral and immune response dynamics as well as HIV transmission.

Chapter 10, "Simulation Modeling of HIV Infection—From Individuals to Risk Groups and Entire Populations." provides an expansive overview of the role of modeling HIV in human populations, including statistical models, stochastic process models, deterministic mathematical models, discrete event microsimulations, and agent-based models. The discussion of the trade-offs between these model classes, as well as the challenges of model validation and their application to inform clinical and public health decision-making, sets the stage for the final two chapters, which present statistical frameworks for parameterizing and comparing these mathematical and computational simulation models.

Chapter 11, "Review of Statistical Methods for Within-Host HIV Dynamics in AIDS Studies," focuses on the use of nonlinear differential equation host–pathogen models in the context of HIV infection and treatment and reviews the statistical issues with model identifiability, calibration, and comparison. A survey of statistical methods for mathematical models is provided, including the determination of model identifiability based on sensitivity analysis, model fitting based on least squares, mixed effects models, and nonparametric smoothing.

The final chapter in this section, "Precision in the Specification of Ordinary Differential Equations and Parameter Estimation in Modeling Biological Processes," continues the theme of statistical issues with model identifiability, calibration, and comparison. A statistical approach is employed to compare the exponential decay of the standard viral model with a parameterized density-dependent decay model, allowing rejection of the standard model for data on HIV dynamics in a study of six children. The authors also show how the sensitivity matrix of the ordinary differential equations system can be related to the Fisher information matrix to evaluate parameter identifiability. Moreover, the authors provide practical suggestions for how to improve the precision of parameter estimates by combining parameters for identifiability and the utility of using observations from multiple compartments (viral and cellular) to characterize viral decay as compared with increasing the sampling from a single compartment.

This book brings together a broad perspective of new quantitative methods in HIV/AIDS research, contributed by statisticians and mathematicians immersed in HIV research. It is our hope that the work described herein will inspire more statisticians, mathematicians, and computer scientists to collaborate and contribute to the interdisciplinary challenges of understanding and addressing the AIDS pandemic.

This book would not have been possible without the support of the Duke and University of North Carolina Chapel Hill CFAR. We would especially like to thank Ms. Kelly Plonk from the Duke CFAR for her invaluable help with administration and logistics.

Cliburn Chan
Duke University
Michael G. Hudgens
University of North Carolina at Chapel Hill
Shein-Chung Chow
Duke University

Contributors

Georgiy Bobashev
Center for Data Science
RTI International
Research Triangle Park,
    North Carolina

Ashley L. Buchanan
Department of Pharmacy Practice
College of Pharmacy
University of Rhode Island,
Kingston, Rhode Island

Cliburn Chan
Department of Biostatistics and
    Bioinformatics
Duke University
Durham, North Carolina

Shih-Ting Chiu
Providence St. Vincent Medical
    Center
Portland, Oregon

Shein-Chung Chow
Department of Biostatistics and
    Bioinformatics
Duke University School of Medicine
Durham, North Carolina

Stephen R. Cole
Department of Epidemiology
Gillings School of Global Public Health
University of North Carolina
Chapel Hill, North Carolina

Sarah E. Holte
Division of Public Health Sciences
Fred Hutchinson Cancer Research
    Center
Seattle, Washington

Michael G. Hudgens
Department of Biostatistics
Gillings School of Global
    Public Health
University of North Carolina
Chapel Hill, North Carolina

Brent A. Johnson
Department of Biostatistics and
    Computational Biology
University of Rochester
Rochester, New York

Thomas B. Kepler
Department of Microbiology
Boston University School
    of Medicine

and

Department of Mathematics and
    Statistics
Boston University
Boston, Massachusetts

Mimi Kim
Division of Biostatistics
Department of Epidemiology
and Population Health
Albert Einstein College of Medicine
Bronx, New York

Yuanyuan Kong
Clinical Epidemiology and EBM Unit
Beijing Friendship Hospital
Capital Medical University

and

National Clinical Research Center
    for Digestive Disease
Beijing, People's Republic of China

Chun Li
Department of Epidemiology and
  Biostatistics
Case Western Reserve University
Cleveland, Ohio

Lin Lin
Department of Statistics
Pennsylvania State University
State College, Pennsylvania

Qi Liu
Late Development Statistics
Merck & Co.
Rahway, New Jersey

Robert H. Lyles
Department of Biostatistics and
  Bioinformatics
The Rollins School of Public Health
  of Emory University
Atlanta, Georgia

Yajun Mei
H. Milton Stewart School of Industrial
  and Systems Engineering
College of Engineering
Georgia Institute of Technology
Atlanta, Georgia

John Rice
Department of Biostatistics and
Computational Biology
University of Rochester
Rochester, New York

Kaitlin Sawatzki
Department of Microbiology
Boston University School of Medicine
Boston, Massachusetts

Bryan E. Shepherd
Department of Biostatistics
Vanderbilt University School of
  Medicine
Nashville, Tennessee

Fuyu Song
Center for Food and Drug Inspection
China Food and Drug
  Administration
Beijing, People's Republic of China

Robert L. Strawderman
Department of Biostatistics and
  Computational Biology
University of Rochester
Rochester, New York

Ningtao Wang
Department of Biostatistics and
  Data Science
School of Public Health
University of Texas Health Science
  Center at Houston
Houston, Texas

Valentine Wanga
Departments of Epidemiology and
  Global Health
University of Washington
Seattle, Washington

Hulin Wu
Department of Biostatistics and
  Data Science
School of Public Health
University of Texas Health Science
  Center at Houston
Houston, Texas

Section I

Quantitative Methods for Clinical Trials and Epidemiology

1

Statistical Issues in HIV Non-Inferiority Trials

Mimi Kim

Albert Einstein College of Medicine, Bronx, NY

CONTENTS

1.1 Introduction

One of the most common study designs currently used to evaluate new treatments for patients infected with the human immunodeficiency virus (HIV) is the non-inferiority (NI) clinical trial. While the goal in a conventional randomized superiority trial is to demonstrate that the new therapy is more efficacious than the control, the objective in an NI trial is to establish that the new treatment is not worse by more than a prespecified margin than the comparator, which is usually a standard therapy. This goal is of interest when the new treatment offers benefits such as improved safety, increased tolerability, lower cost, or greater convenience that make it a desirable alternative even if it is not necessarily more efficacious than the standard. An NI trial is also conducted to evaluate an experimental therapy when the use of a placebo is unethical due to the availability of existing effective regimens. In this case, the efficacy of the new drug is demonstrated by showing that it is non-inferior to an approved treatment.

Because of the high level of HIV RNA suppression with current antiretroviral (ARV) therapies, there is growing use of the NI trial design for the evaluation of new HIV drugs in both ARV-experienced and -naïve patients (Flandre 2013). In HIV patients who have not previously been treated with ARV regimens, it is difficult for experimental therapies to yield viral suppression rates that surpass the rates in excess of 90% that have been observed with potent, approved first-line treatments (Mani et al. 2012). Likewise, in treatment-experienced HIV patients, the benefit of adding a new ARV to an existing regimen is not easy to demonstrate statistically, given that optimized background therapies have become so effective. As such, establishing non-inferiority rather than superiority of new regimens has become the more common objective in HIV trials. Hernandez et al. (2013), however, found that the methodological quality, reporting, and interpretation of HIV NI trials is generally poor, based on a survey of over 40 studies of this type. Major weaknesses identified by the authors included lack of justification for the magnitude of the NI margin, incorrect sample size determination, and failure to perform the appropriate analyses. The goal of this chapter is to provide an overview of the basic principles for designing, conducting, and analyzing HIV NI trials. We begin by describing three recent examples.

Example 1.1: TMC114/r In Treatment-Experienced Patients Naïve to Lopinavir Trial (Madruga et al. 2007)

Despite the availability of highly active antiretroviral therapy (HAART), there remains a need to develop safe ARV treatments that can maintain virological suppression in a broad range of HIV-infected patients from diverse clinical settings. The TMC114/r In Treatment-Experienced Patients Naïve to Lopinavir (TITAN) trial was conducted in 159 centers across 26 countries to compare the safety and efficacy of darunavir–ritonavir with lopinavir–ritonavir in treatment-experienced, lopinavir-naïve, HIV-1–infected patients who had a plasma HIV-1 RNA concentration of greater than 1,000 copies/mL. The main goal was to show that the rate of virological response, defined as confirmed HIV-1 RNA of less than 400 copies/mL in plasma at Week 48, with darunavir–ritonavir 600/100 mg twice daily, was not lower by more than 12% than the response rate with lopinavir–ritonavir 400/100 mg twice daily.

Example 1.2: ARROW Trial (Bwakura-Dangarembizi et al. 2014)

In children infected with HIV, administering co-trimoxazole prophylactically before ARV therapy can reduce morbidity. Bwakura-Dangarembizi et al. performed the Antiretroviral Research for Watoto (ARROW) trial to investigate whether pediatric patients receiving long-term ARV therapy in Uganda and Zimbabwe could safely discontinue co-trimoxazole. This study was designed as an NI trial to compare the effects of stopping versus continuing daily open-label co-trimoxazole with a primary endpoint of hospitalization or death. The investigators aimed to demonstrate that the between-group difference in the rate of hospitalization or death was no more than three events per 100 participant-years, assuming a rate of five events per 100 participant-years among participants continuing to receive co-trimoxazole.

Example 1.3: CIPRA-SA Trial (Sanne et al. 2010)

Studies in industrialized countries have shown that ARV management of HIV outpatients results in better outcomes when physicians with HIV expertise provide the medical care rather than nonphysicians. However, there is a shortage of medical practitioners in sub-Saharan countries like South Africa. As part of the Comprehensive International Program for Research in AIDS in South Africa (CIPRA-SA), Sanne et al. conducted a randomized clinical trial in two South African primary care clinics to evaluate whether nurse-monitored ARV care of HIV patients is non-inferior to doctor-monitored care. The primary endpoint was a composite endpoint of treatment-limiting events, incorporating mortality, viral failure, treatment-limiting toxic effects, and adherence to visit schedule. Non-inferiority of nurse care to physician care was defined as a hazard ratio (nurse vs. physician care) for the primary outcome of less than 1.40.

1.2 Margin of Non-Inferiority

As illustrated in the above three examples, the general strategy for establishing non-inferiority of an experimental therapy to a standard therapy for HIV is to demonstrate that the difference in efficacy between the two treatments is less than some prespecified margin of non-inferiority, Δ. The margin can be expressed in different ways depending on the nature of the outcome variable. Consider a binary outcome, such as achieving HIV RNA levels below the limit of assay detection by 48 weeks, and let p_S and p_E denote the true proportion of patients who achieve this endpoint in the standard and experimental arms, respectively. Then Δ can be formulated in terms of an absolute difference in proportions: $p_S - p_E$, ratio of proportions: p_S/p_E, or odds ratio: $[p_S/(1-p_S)]/[p_E/(1-p_E)]$. There are pros and cons to each formulation; defining the margin as a ratio or relative risk rather than a difference in proportions may be more appropriate and conservative when the event rates are changing or unpredictable (Siegel 2000). However, Hauck and Anderson (1999) point out that the relative risk is difficult to interpret without reference to the rate in the denominator. The odds ratio is frequently used as a measure of association in retrospective designs or case-control studies but less so in clinical trials.

For an outcome that is a continuous variable, such as $\log_{10}$ reduction in viral load, which has been evaluated in some HIV trials (Johnson et al. 2005), Δ can be expressed as the difference between groups in mean levels of the variable, that is, $\mu_S - \mu_E$, where μ_S and μ_E are the means in the standard and experimental groups, respectively. For time-to-event outcomes, Δ is often specified as either a hazard ratio between the two treatments, $\lambda_S(t)/\lambda_E(t)$, or as a difference in the cumulative failure or survival probabilities at a specific point in time. In the CIPRA-SA NI trial comparing nurse versus physician management of HIV patients in South Africa, Δ was specified as the hazard ratio for a treatment-limiting event. However, in the ARROW trial, in which the primary outcome was first hospitalization or death, the NI margin was specified as the absolute difference in event rates because control group event rates were expected to be low. Uno et al. (2015) pointed out that the hazard ratio may be difficult to interpret clinically, especially when the underlying proportional hazards assumption is violated. Therefore, they recommended that investigators in the design stage should consider alternative robust and clinically interpretable model-free measures when defining the NI margin, such as the risk difference or the difference between two restricted mean survival times.

Once the metric for defining Δ has been specified, the next step is determining the magnitude of Δ. The margin is often chosen to be the largest clinically acceptable difference in efficacy between treatment arms, but the magnitude can also depend on statistical, feasibility, and regulatory considerations. For example, in the TITAN trial, the NI margin of 12% for the difference in virological response rate between darunavir–ritonavir and lopinavir–ritonavir was selected taking into consideration findings from earlier studies as well as US Food and Drug Administration (FDA) guidelines for NI margins based on HIV RNA levels (US Food and Drug Administration 2013). In contrast, the NI margin in the ARROW trial was chosen by a consensus of the study investigators.

The size of the margin also varies according to whether the goal of the trial is to evaluate efficacy or safety. In NI trials comparing the efficacy of a new therapy compared to a standard therapy, the margin should be chosen to minimize the possibility that a new therapy that is found to be non-inferior to standard therapy would not at the same time be inferior to placebo had a placebo been included in the trial. A typical approach is to set Δ to be a fraction, f, of the lower limit of the confidence interval (CI) for the standard therapy effect based on prior trials of the standard therapy versus placebo. In oncology and thrombolytic trials where mortality is the endpoint, the FDA has suggested $f = 0.5$ (Kaul and Diamond 2006).

Parienti et al. (2006) reviewed NI AIDS clinical trials published after HAART became available and reported that the NI margin generally ranged from 10% to 15% for trials that used a composite outcome that included virologic failure, clinical progression to AIDS, or death. In the FDA *Guidance for Industry for Human Immunodeficiency Virus-1 Infection* (2013), the recommended margin varies according to whether the specific HIV study population is (1) treatment naïve, (2) treatment experienced with available approved treatment options, or (3) treatment experienced with few or no available approved options. For HIV treatment-naïve patients, NI margins of 10%–12% when the outcome is viral response are recommended, which was based on a desired amount of the active control treatment effect that should be preserved by the experimental therapy. Determining the margin in ARV-experienced patients, however, is especially complicated since prior trials of the active control that are used to justify the margin may have used different background medications or may have included patients with different characteristics compared to patients in the current trial. In addition, ARV-experienced patients are more likely to develop virological failure and resistance to ARV drugs. Flandre (2013) argued that the NI margin in ARV-naïve patients should be at least as large as the margin in ARV-experienced patients. In treatment-experienced patients with few or no available approved treatment options, also referred to as *heavily treatment-experienced patients*, non-inferiority studies are generally not feasible because there usually is no appropriate active control with a sufficiently well-characterized effect that can be used to define an NI margin.

As response rates with standard drugs increase, the acceptable margin should correspondingly get smaller (Hill and Sabine 2008). Another key factor that influences Δ is the severity of the outcome of interest; the margin for an endpoint such as mortality would be expected to be smaller than the margin for an intermediate endpoint like viral suppression. However, the smaller the margin, the more difficult it is to establish non-inferiority. As discussed further below, the size of the margin has a significant impact on the sample size requirements of the trial, so cost and feasibility considerations may also dictate the lower limit of Δ. Regardless, the rationale for choosing the margin should always be clearly stated when reporting the results of the NI trial.

1.3 Analysis of NI Trials

A common inferential mistake is to assume that failure to observe a statistically significant difference in a conventional superiority trial is evidence that the two treatments being compared are similar. It should be emphasized that proving non-inferiority of one treatment to another requires an alternative formulation of the null and alternative hypotheses. Assume again that the outcome of interest is reducing the viral load to below the assay limit of detection and that p_S and p_E are the true proportions of patients who achieve this outcome with the standard and experimental therapies, respectively. If Δ is defined as the maximum clinically acceptable difference in these proportions, the relevant null and alternative hypotheses for testing non-inferiority of the experimental therapy to the standard can be expressed as

$$H_0^*: p_S - p_E \geq \Delta \qquad H_A^*: p_S - p_E < \Delta$$

Thus, the null hypothesis, H_0^*, specifies the situation when the decrease in efficacy in the experimental group is unacceptably large, and the alternative hypothesis, H_A^*, corresponds to the case where the difference in efficacy is smaller than the NI margin. In addition, note that in this formulation of the null and alternative hypotheses, the Type I error rate (α-level) is defined as the probability of erroneously concluding that E is non-inferior to S, and the Type II error rate (β-level) is the probability of erroneously *failing* to conclude that E is non-inferior to S.

One way to evaluate the null hypothesis in the NI trial setting is to compute either the two-sided 95% CI or one-sided upper 97.5% CI for the true difference: $p_S - p_E$. If the upper bound of the CI is smaller than Δ, then non-inferiority is declared. Figure 1.1 shows examples of how different conclusions can be reached with the two-sided 95% CI depending on where the values within the CI fall relative to 0 and the margin of non-inferiority: (1) the CI includes both 0 and Δ: inconclusive; (2) the CI includes 0 but the upper bound is less than Δ: the experimental therapy is non-inferior to the standard; (3) the upper bound is less than 0: the experimental therapy is superior to the standard; (4) the lower bound is greater than Δ: the experimental therapy is inferior to the standard.

It is also possible to evaluate the NI null hypothesis by computing a test statistic and the corresponding one-sided p-value. While the CI approach provides information about the range of values for the true treatment difference that are consistent with the data and can also be used to evaluate the null hypothesis, a test statistic provides additional information about the degree of significance of the observed result. For a binary outcome and under the assumption that the sample size is sufficiently large such that the binomial distribution can be approximated by the normal distribution, the general form of the test statistic to evaluate H_0^* is as follows: $Z = \frac{\hat{p}_S - \hat{p}_E - \Delta}{SE(\hat{p}_S - \hat{p}_E)}$, where $\hat{p}_S$ and $\hat{p}_E$ are the estimated proportions of patients who achieved the endpoint in the standard and experimental groups, respectively; Z is

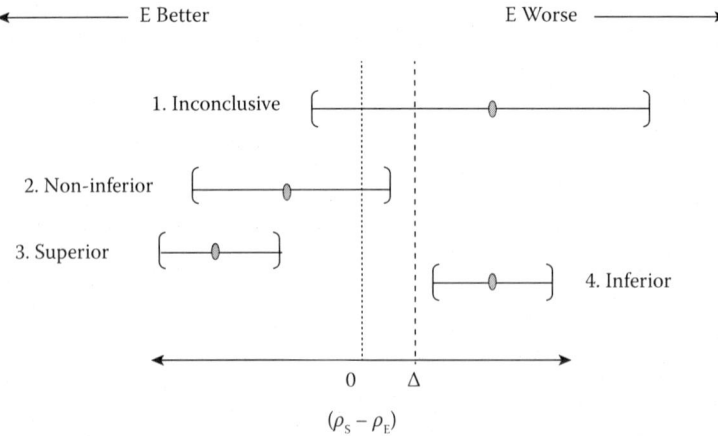

FIGURE 1.1
Examples of two-sided 95% confidence intervals and corresponding conclusions about the non-inferiority of the experimental therapy (E) compared to the standard therapy (S).

assumed to follow a standard normal distribution under H_0^*; and SE denotes the standard error. If z_{obs} is the observed value of Z, then non-inferiority is declared with a one-sided Type I error rate of α if $z_{obs} < z_\alpha$, where z_α is the $100 \times \alpha$ percentile of the standard normal distribution. The one-sided p-value is given by $p = \Phi(z_{obs})$, where $\Phi(\cdot)$ denotes the cumulative distribution function for the standard normal distribution. Different approaches have been suggested for estimating the standard error term in the denominator: (1) the unrestricted maximum likelihood estimator (MLE), in which the observed proportions are used to estimate the standard error, that is,

$SE = \sqrt{\left(\frac{\hat{p}_S(1-\hat{p}_S)}{n}\right) + \left(\frac{\hat{p}_E(1-\hat{p}_E)}{n}\right)}$, where n is the sample size and assumed to

be the same in each arm; (2) the approach of Dunnett and Gent (1977), which estimates the SE conditional on the total number of successes; and (3) the Farrington and Manning (1990) method, which estimates the MLE under the restriction that the between-group difference in success rates is equal to Δ. Simulation results showed that the restricted MLE method performs better than the other approaches, is asymptotically valid, and shown to be accurate even when the expected number of successes in each arm is small. Exact and asymptotic methods of tests for non-inferiority when the margin is specified as a relative risk or odds ratio are addressed by Rothmann et al. (2012).

The above discussion assumes that the primary outcome is binary. Testing NI hypotheses for normally distributed continuous outcomes can be accomplished simply by subtracting Δ from the numerator of the usual test statistic for comparing two means, that is, $Z = \frac{\bar{x}_S - \bar{x}_E - \Delta}{SE(\bar{x}_S - \bar{x}_E)}$, and determining statistical significance by using either the standard Z- or t-distribution, depending on the sample size. For time-to-event outcomes, Com-Nougue et al. (1993) describe extensions of the log–rank test statistic and the Cox proportional hazards regression model to evaluate non-inferiority in survival analysis.

1.4 Sample Size Determination

The sample size software package PASS and other programs make it easy and convenient to compute sample size requirements for a variety of test statistics frequently used in NI trials. When the outcome is a continuous variable and 1:1 randomization is planned, the general formula for the sample size per group required to achieve a power of $100 \times (1 - \beta)$ percent with a one-sided α-significance level to conclude that the true difference in efficacy between the standard and experimental groups is no greater than Δ, assuming the true difference is Δ_A, can be expressed as $N = 2\sigma^2 \left[\frac{Z_\alpha + Z_\beta}{(\Delta_A - \Delta)}\right]^2$, where

z_γ is the $100 \times \gamma$ percentile of the standard normal distribution and σ^2 is the population variance of the outcome, which is assumed to be the same in each arm. The sample size is generally evaluated under the alternative hypothesis that the two treatment groups are exactly the same ($\Delta_A = 0$), in which case the sample size formula reduces to $N = 2\sigma^2 \left[\frac{Z_\alpha + Z_\beta}{\Delta} \right]^2$.

For binary outcomes, Blackwelder (1982) and Makuch and Simon (1978) proposed the following approach for computing the required sample size per group for an NI trial: $N = \frac{[(p_S(1-p_S) + p_E(1-p_E))](z_\alpha + z_\beta)^2}{(p_S - p_E - \Delta)^2}$, which is derived by assuming the unrestricted MLE method is used to estimate the variance of the test statistic under the null hypothesis. Farrington and Manning (1990), however, found that this approach may yield incorrect sample sizes and proposed instead that the restricted maximum likelihood approach discussed earlier be used for the null variance when computing the sample size.

NI trials are viewed as requiring larger sample sizes than traditional superiority trials, but this is because the margin of non-inferiority is typically smaller than the effect size of interest in a superiority trial. Small changes in Δ can have a marked impact on the sample size requirements in NI trials. For example, suppose the expected success rate in both the standard and experimental arms is 70% so that the true difference between treatments is $\Delta_A = 0$. Then if the NI margin is $\Delta = 15\%$, the study would require 150 subjects per arm to achieve 80% power at a one-sided $\alpha = 0.025$ level. However, for a smaller margin of $\Delta = 10\%$, the required sample size is 330 subjects per arm, more than double the sample size required for the larger margin. In a superiority trial, if $\Delta = 10\%$ now corresponds to the minimum effect size of interest, then the sample size requirement is also about 300 subjects per arm for 80% power.

As in the example above, the sample size is generally evaluated under the alternative hypothesis that the event rates in the two treatment groups are exactly the same ($\Delta_A = 0$). If it can be assumed under the alternative hypothesis that the experimental therapy is in fact more efficacious than the standard but the goal is still to show non-inferiority, then the sample size requirements are considerably reduced. To illustrate, suppose the expected success rates are 70% for the standard therapy and 75% for the experimental therapy so that $\Delta_A = -5\%$ and $\Delta = 15\%$. Under these assumptions, the required sample size is 78 subjects per arm to achieve 80% power, about half that required when the expected success rate on both arms is assumed to be 70%.

1.5 Other Considerations in NI Trials

NI trials need to be executed especially rigorously to preserve assay sensitivity, that is, the ability of the trial to detect between-group differences of a specific size and to minimize sources of bias that may make it easier to show non-inferiority. The general perception is that extra noise introduced into the data—from factors such as poor study conduct, patient nonadherence to the treatment protocol, missing data, and misclassification and measurement error in the primary outcome—tends to diminish true treatment differences and therefore favors the goal of demonstrating non-inferiority. As discussed further below, however, the effects of such factors on the NI trial are actually more complicated than this and resulting biases may be in either direction.

1.5.1 Noncompliance

In the conventional clinical trial, noncompliance is handled using the intent-to-treat (ITT) approach, in which subjects are analyzed according to the treatment group to which they were originally randomized, regardless of protocol adherence. The ITT method maintains balance in patient characteristics across treatment groups and yields an estimate of the "pragmatic" effect of the treatment. This approach is viewed as conservative in a superiority trial, the rationale being that noncompliance in both groups will tend to make treatment groups more similar and hence the observed difference will be smaller than the true difference. However, in an NI trial since the ITT approach may make it easier to show non-inferiority, the per-protocol (PP) analysis, which excludes protocol violators, is usually also performed. The European Medicines Agency publication, *Points to Consider on Switching between Superiority and Non-inferiority* (2000), requires that to claim non-inferiority in an NI trial, non-inferiority must be demonstrated with both the ITT and the PP approaches. The USFDA-issued draft *Guidance for industry: Noninferiority clinical trials* (2010) advises that investigators conduct both types of analyses and examine closely any findings that are discrepant.

Sheng and Kim (2006) and Sanchez and Chen (2006) showed that in an ITT analysis, noncompliance can make it easier or harder to demonstrate non-inferiority: the direction and magnitude of the effect depend on the patterns of noncompliance, event probabilities, margin of non-inferiority, missing data, and other factors. By contrast, performing a PP analysis and excluding subjects who are noncompliant may introduce selection bias. In addition, when the degree of noncompliance is high, the proportion of subjects who are included in the PP analysis will be small; this compromises both the power of the trial to detect non-inferiority and the generalizability of results. The lower the proportion of nonadherers, the more likely it is that ITT and PP results will be consistent. Yet even if non-inferiority is demonstrated with both approaches, Sanchez has shown that this does not guarantee the validity of a non-inferiority conclusion.

Alternative approaches for addressing noncompliance in NI trials have been explored. Sanchez proposed a hybrid ITT/PP approach that excludes noncompliant patients as in the PP analysis and uses a maximum-likelihood–based approach to address missing data in the ITT analysis. Kim (2010) considered an instrumental variables (IV) approach to estimate the complier average causal effect, but this method applies mainly to NI trials in which the control group is a true placebo, such as in an NI safety trial, or when the comparison group is a wait-list control or assigned to a watch-and-wait approach. Fischer et al. (2011) proposed a structural mean modelling approach to adjust for differential noncompliance and obtain unbiased estimates of treatment efficacy. This method, however, requires the availability of baseline variables that predict adherence in the two arms but are assumed not to influence the causal effect of treatment.

It should be noted that all of these methods for addressing noncompliance are based on underlying assumptions that are difficult to verify or, like the IV approach, have low power when the proportion of noncompliers is not trivial. Therefore, the best way to increase the likelihood of reaching the correct conclusion is to incorporate ways to minimize the number of noncompliers into the study design, a principle that is important for any clinical trial, not just NI trials.

1.5.2 Missing Data

Missing data is difficult to avoid in most clinical trials and can complicate the analysis, results, and interpretation of the study. The bias resulting from some missing data patterns may diminish treatment differences and make it easier to demonstrate non-inferiority, whereas other patterns can make it more difficult. For example, suppose a higher proportion of patients randomized to the standard arm drop out and are lost to follow-up because of lack of efficacy. The response rate in the remaining patients in the standard arm will be biased upward, and therefore it will be harder to demonstrate non-inferiority of the experimental arm if the analysis is based only on the observed data. A number of approaches have been proposed for addressing missing data, including complete case analysis (also referred to as *listwise deletion*); simple imputation methods such as last observation carried forward (LOCF), assuming all missing values are failures, or assuming missing values are failures in the experimental group and successes in the standard group (worst-case scenario); and multiple imputation. The complete case analysis includes only those subjects with nonmissing data and is therefore inconsistent with the ITT principle, in which all randomized subjects are analyzed. Because results from the complete case analysis may be biased, this approach is not recommended for the primary analysis but could be performed in sensitivity analyses. LOCF, in which a patient's last observed value is used to impute any subsequent missing values, may also lead to bias unless the patient's underlying disease state does not change after dropout. Alternatively, if all missing outcomes are treated as failures and missing data rates are comparable in the two groups, then this would clearly tend to equalize the two groups and make it easier to demonstrate non-inferiority.

Koch (2008) proposed imputing values under the NI null hypothesis, that is, a penalized imputation approach. For example, for a continuous outcome, one might subtract Δ from the imputed value for each patient in the experimental arm. Wiens and Rosenkranz (2012) performed a simulation study of different strategies for assessing non-inferiority in the presence of missing data and found that the single imputation procedure and observed case analyses resulted in reduced power and occasional inflation in the Type I error rate as well as bias in treatment effect estimates. Mixed effects models performed better, but they require that data be missing at random. Multiple imputation is a more complicated approach that takes into consideration the uncertainty in the imputed values, but this method also requires the missing at random assumption. Rothmann et al. (2012) proposed combining a penalized imputation approach with multiple imputation in an NI analysis.

Regardless, sensitivity analyses are important in evaluating the robustness of conclusions to different missing data approaches and are routinely recommended by regulatory agencies. Most importantly, strategies for preventing the occurrence of missing data should be incorporated into the trial from the beginning. For example, in a longitudinal study of mother-to-child HIV transmission conducted by Jackson et al. (2003) in Kampala, Uganda, many of the families lived far away from the study clinic. The dropout rate was minimized by using "health visitors" to provide support to the mothers and encourage their continued participation in the study.

1.5.3 Misclassification and Measurement Error in Outcome Variables

Sloppiness in the study conduct, inconsistent measurements, and inadequate diagnostic criteria have been cited as factors that may mask true treatment differences (Cooper 1990). If these sources of noise result in nondifferential misclassification (i.e., equal across treatment groups) of a dichotomous outcome, estimates of between-group differences in proportions will be reduced and estimates of relative risks will be biased toward unity (Bross 1954). In a standard superiority trial, such errors would lead to conservative estimates of efficacy, whereas in an NI trial the resulting bias would be in the anticonservative direction. The well-known attenuating effects of nondifferential misclassification may lead one to expect that this type of error consequently increases the ability to establish non-inferiority. However, because misclassification potentially affects not only the estimates of between-group differences but also the Type I error rate and power of statistical tests, demonstrating non-inferiority may not always be more easily achieved in the presence of outcome misclassification.

Kim and Goldberg (2001) formally investigated the effects of outcome misclassification and measurement error on the estimates of treatment effects, Type I error rate, and power of NI trials. They found that the magnitude and direction of the effects depend on a number of factors, including the nature of the outcome variable, formulation of the NI margin (i.e., difference or ratio of proportions), size of the error rates, and assumptions regarding the true treatment effect. Specifically, when true treatment differences exist, nondifferential misclassification increases the probability of erroneously declaring non-inferiority in trials where the margin is defined as a difference in proportions or where the margin is specified as a ratio and the false positive misclassification rate (probability of misclassifying the absence of the outcome) is nonzero. For the scenarios considered by Kim and Goldberg where the margin is specified as a difference in proportions, the Type I error rate can be as high as 15% when the nominal rate is 5%. If the margin is specified as a ratio and the false positive rate is zero, then there is no inflation of the Type I error rate in an NI trial regardless of the magnitude of the false negative misclassification rate (probability of misclassifying the presence of the outcome). When the outcome is a continuous variable, nondifferential error will also not inflate the Type I error rate when the margin is specified as a difference in means, but the power of the study will be diminished.

Whether the objective is to demonstrate superiority or non-inferiority, outcome variables need to be evaluated carefully. The consequences of nondifferential error are potentially greater in an NI trial, however, given that both the Type I and Type II errors may be increased, whereas in a superiority trial it is mainly the power that is affected.

1.6 Summary

Determining the NI margin is one of the primary challenges in designing an NI trial. Multiple factors need to be considered, including the goal of the study, the primary outcome, the expected rate in the control group, feasibility issues, regulatory perspectives, and the study population. Most importantly, the margin should be determined prior to initiation of the study and clearly justified in the reporting of trial results. In addition, aspects of study conduct and treatment adherence that may compromise NI trial results need to be carefully considered. Strategies for minimizing the occurrence of losses to follow-up, other protocol violations, and measurement error should be devised prior to initiation of the trial. In the data analysis phase, sensitivity analyses are especially important to demonstrate that conclusions of non-inferiority are robust to different ways of handling noncompliance and missing data. Additional guidelines for the proper reporting of NI trials are available in the CONSORT statement on NI trials (Piaggio et al. 2012). The reader is also referred to the FDA guidance document for developing ARV drugs for treatment of HIV (US Food and Drug Administration 2010).

References

Blackwelder, W. Proving the null hypothesis in clinical trials. *Controlled Clinical Trials* 1982; 3: 345–353.

Bross, I. Misclassification in 2 × 2 tables. *Biometrics* 1954; 10: 478–486.

Bwakura-Dangarembizi, M., Kendall, L., Bakeera-Kitaka, S., Nahirya-Ntege, P., Keishanyu, R., Nathoo, K., Spyer, M., et al. Randomized trial of co-trimoxazole in HIV-infected children in Africa. *New England Journal of Medicine* 2014; 370: 41–53.

Committee for Proprietary Medicinal Products (CPMP). *Points to Consider on Switching between Superiority and Non-Inferiority.* European Medicines Agency: London, 2000.

Com-Nougue, C., Rodary, C., and Patte, C. How to establish equivalence when data are censored: A randomized trial of treatments for B non-Hodgkin lymphoma. *Statistics in Medicine* 1993; 12: 1353–1364.

Cooper, E. Designs of clinical trials: Active control (equivalence trials). *Journal of Acquired Immune Deficiency Syndromes* 1990; 3: S77–S81.

Dunnett, C. and Gent, M. Significance testing to establish equivalence between treatments with special reference to data in the form of 2 x 2 tables. *Biometrics* 1977; 33: 593–602.

Farrington, C.P. and Manning, G. Test statistics and sample size formulae for comparative binomial trials with null hypothesis of non-zero risk difference or non-unity relative risk. *Statistics in Medicine* 1990; 9: 1447–1454.

Fischer, K., Goetghebeur, E., Vrijens, B., and White, I.R. A structural mean model to allow for noncompliance in a randomized trial comparing 2 active treatments. *Biostatistics* 2011; 12: 247–257.

Flandre, P. Design of HIV noninferiority trials: Where are we going? *AIDS* 2013; 27: 653–657.

Hauck, W. and Anderson, S. Some issues in the design and analysis of equivalence trials. *Drug Information Journal* 1999; 33: 109–118.

Hernandez, A.V., Pasupuleti, V., Deshpande, A., Thota, P., Collins, J.A., and Vidal, J.E. Deficient reporting and interpretation of non-inferiority randomized clinical trials in HIV patients: A systematic review. *PLoS One* 2013; 8: e63272.

Hill, A. and Sabin, C. Designing and interpreting HIV noninferiority trials in naïve and experienced patients. *AIDS* 2008; 22: 913–921.

Jackson, J.B., Musoke, P., Fleming, T., Guay, L.A., Bagenda, D., Allen, M., Nakabiito, C., et al. Intrapartum and neonatal single-dose nevirapine compared with zidovudine for prevention of mother-to-child transmission of HIV-1 in Kampala, Uganda: 18-month follow-up of the HIVNET 012 randomised trial. *The Lancet* 2003; 362: 859–868.

Johnson, M., Grinsztejn, B., Rodriguez, C., Coco, J., DeJesus, E., Lazzarin, A., Lichtenstein, K., Rightmire, A., Sankoh, S., and Wilber, R. Atazanavir plus ritonavir or saquinavir, and lopinavir/ritonavir in patients experiencing multiple virological failures. *AIDS* 2005; 19: 685–694.

Kaul, S. and Diamond, G. Good enough: A primer on the analysis and interpretation of non-inferiority trials. *Annals of Internal Medicine* 2006; 4: 62–69.

Kim, M.Y. Using the instrumental variables estimator to analyze non-inferiority trials with non-compliance. *Journal of Biopharmaceutical Statistics* 2010; 20: 745–758.

Kim, M.Y. and Goldberg, J.D. The effects of outcome misclassification and measurement error on the design and analysis of therapeutic equivalence trials. *Statistics in Medicine* 2001; 20: 2065–2078.

Koch, G.G. Comments on 'current issues in non-inferiority trials' by Thomas R. Fleming. *Statistics in Medicine* 2008; 27: 333–342.

Madruga, J., Berger, D., McMurchie, M., Suter, F., Banhegyi, D., Ruxrungtham, K., Norris, D., et al. Efficacy and safety of darunavir-ritonavir compared with that of lopinavir-ritonavir at 48 weeks in treatment-experienced, HIV-infected patients in TITAN: A randomised controlled phase III trial. *The Lancet* 2007; 370: 49–58.

Makuch, R. and Simon, R. Sample size requirements for evaluating a conservative therapy. *Cancer Treatment Reports* 1978; 62: 1037–1040.

Mani, N., Murray, J., Gulick, R., Josephson, F., Miller, V., Miele, P., Strobos, J., and Struble, K. Novel clinical trial designs for the development of new antiretroviral agents. *AIDS* 2012; 26: 899–907.

Parienti, J., Verdon, R., and Massari, V. Methodological standards in non-inferiority AIDS trials: Moving from adherence to compliance. *BMC Medical Research Methodology* 2006; 6: 46.

Piaggio, G., Elbourne, D.R., Pocock, S.J., Evans, S.J.W., Altman, D.G., and CONSORT Group. Reporting of non-inferiority and equivalence randomized trials. Extension of the CONSORT 2010 statement. *JAMA* 2012; 308(24): 2594–2604.

Rothmann, M., Wiens, B., and Chan, I. *Design and Analysis of Non-Inferiority trials.* Chapman and Hall, Boca Raton, FL, 2012.

Sanchez, M. and Chen, X. Choosing the analysis population in non-inferiority studies: Per protocol or intent-to-treat. *Statistics in Medicine* 2006; 25: 1169–1181.

Sanne, I., Orrell, C., Fox, M., Conradie, F., Ive, P., Zeinecker, J., Cornell, M., et al. Nurse versus doctor management of HIV-infected patients receiving antiretroviral therapy (CIPRA-SA): A randomised non-inferiority trial. *The Lancet* 2010; 376: 33–40.

Sheng, D. and Kim, M.Y. The effects of non-compliance on intent-to-treat analysis of equivalence trials. *Statistics in Medicine* 2006; 25: 1183–1199.

Siegel, J. Equivalence and non-inferiority trials. *American Heart Journal* 2000; 139: S166–S170.

Uno, H., Wittes, J., Fu, H., Solomon, S., Claggett, B., Tian, L., Cai, T., Pfeffer, M., Evans, R., and Wei, L.J. Alternatives to hazard ratios for comparing the efficacy or safety of therapies in non-inferiority studies. *Annals of Internal Medicine* 2015; 163(2): 127–134.

US Food and Drug Administration. *Guidance for Industry: Noninferiority Clinical Trials.* FDA: Rockville, MD, 2010.

US Food and Drug Administration. *Guidance for Industry: Human Immunodeficiency Virus-1 Infection: Developing Antiretroviral Drugs for Treatment.* FDA: Rockville, MD, 2013.

Wiens, B. and Rosenkranz, G. Missing data in non-inferiority trials. *Statistics in Biopharmaceutical Research* 2013; 5: 383–393.

2

Sample Size for HIV-1 Vaccine Clinical Trials with Extremely Low Incidence Rate

Shein-Chung Chow

Duke University School of Medicine, Durham, NC

Yuanyuan Kong

Beijing Friendship Hospital, Capital Medical University, Beijing, People's Republic of China
National Clinical Research Center for Digestive Disease, Beijing, People's Republic of China

Shih-Ting Chiu

Providence St. Vincent Medical Center, Portland, OR

CONTENTS

2.1 Introduction

One of the major challenges when conducting a clinical trial for investigation of treatments or drugs for rare disease is probably endpoint selection and power analysis for sample size based on the selected study endpoint

(Gaddipati 2012). In some clinical trials, the incidence rate of certain events such as adverse events, immune responses, and infections are commonly considered clinical study endpoints for evaluation of safety and efficacy of the test treatment under investigation (O'Neill 1988; Rerks-Ngarm et al. 2009). In epidemiological/clinical studies, incidence rate expresses the number of new cases of disease that occur in a defined population of disease-free individuals. The observed incidence rate provides a direct estimate of the probability or risk of illness. Boyle and Parkin (1991) introduced the methods required for using incidence rates in comparative studies. For example, one may compare incidence rates from different time periods or from different geographical areas in the studies. In contrast, one may compare incidence rates (e.g., adverse events, infections postsurgery, or immune responses for immunogenicity) in clinical trials (Chow and Liu 2004; FDA 2002). In practice, however, there are only a few references available in the literature regarding the sample size required for achieving certain statistical inference (e.g., in terms of power or precision) for the studies with extremely low incidence rates (Chow and Chiu 2013).

In clinical trials, a prestudy power analysis for sample size calculation (power calculation) is usually performed for determining an appropriate sample size (usually the minimum sample size required) to achieve a desired power (e.g., 80% or 90%) for detecting a clinically meaningful difference at a prespecified level of significance (e.g., 1% or 5%) (see, e.g., Chow and Liu 2004; Chow et al. 2007). The power of a statistical test is the probability of correctly detecting a clinically meaningful difference if such a difference truly exists. In practice, a much larger sample size is expected for detecting a relatively smaller difference, especially for clinical trials with an extremely low incidence rate. For example, the incidence rate for hemoglobin A_{1C} ($H_b A_{1C}$) in diabetic studies and the immune responses for immunogenicity in biosimilar studies and/or vaccine clinical trials are usually extremely low.

As an example, consider clinical trials for preventive HIV vaccine development. In 2008, it was estimated that the total number of people living with HIV was 33.4 million people, with 97% living in low- and middle-income countries (UNAIDS 2009). As a result, the development of a safe and efficacious preventive HIV vaccine had become the top priority in global health for the control of HIV-1 in the long term. In their excellent review article, Kim et al. (2010) indicated that the immune response elicited by a successful vaccine likely will require both antibodies and T cells that recognize, neutralize, and/or inactivate diverse strains of HIV and that reach the site of infection before the infection becomes irreversibly established (see also Haynes and Shattock 2008). Basically, the development of an HIV vaccine focuses on evaluating vaccines capable of reducing viral replication after infection, as the control of viral replication could prevent transmission of HIV in the heterosexual population (Excler et al. 2013) and/or conceivably slow the rate of disease progression as suggested by nonhuman primate challenge studies (see e.g., Gupta et al. 2007; Mattapallil et al. 2006; Watkins et al. 2008).

The goal of a preventive HIV vaccine is to induce cell-mediated immune (CMI) responses and subsequently to reduce the plasma viral load at set point and preserve memory CD4+ lymphocytes. As a result, clinical efforts have mainly focused on CMI-inducing vaccines such as DNA and vectors alone or in prime-boost regimens (Belyakov et al. 2008; Esteban 2009). In a recent Thai efficacy trial (RV144), the data revealed the first evidence that HIV-1 vaccine protection against HIV-1 acquisition could be achieved. The results of RV144 indicated that patients with the lowest risk (yearly incidence of 0.23/100 person-years) had an apparent efficacy of 40%, whereas those with the highest risk (incidence of 0.36/100 person-years) had an efficacy of 3.7%. This finding suggested that clinical meaningful difference in vaccine efficacy can be detected by means of the difference in the incidence of risk rate. In addition, the vaccine efficacy appeared to decrease with time (e.g., at 12 months, the vaccine efficacy was about 60% and fell to 29% by 42 months). As a result, at a specific time point, the sample size required for achieving a desired vaccine efficacy can be obtained by detecting a clinically meaningful difference in the incidence of the risk rate at baseline.

Thus, in vaccine clinical trials with extremely low incidence rates, sample size calculation based on a prestudy power analysis may not be feasible. Alternatively, as indicated by Chow et al. (2007), sample size may be justified based on a precision analysis for achieving certain statistical assurance (inference). Chow and Chiu (2013) proposed a procedure based on precision analysis for sample size calculation for clinical studies with an extremely low incidence rate. Chow and Chiu's method is to justify a selected sample size based on a precision analysis and a sensitivity analysis in conjunction with a power analysis. They recommended a step-by-step procedure for sample size determination in clinical trials with extremely low incidence rate. In addition, a statistical procedure for data safety monitoring based on a probability statement during the conduct of the clinical trial was discussed.

In the next section, statistical methods for sample size calculation/justification including power analysis and precision analysis are outlined. Also included in this section is the application of a Bayesian approach with a non-informative uniform prior. A sensitivity analysis for the proposed method is studied in Section 2.3. An example concerning a clinical trial for evaluating extremely low incidence rate is presented in Section 2.4. Section 2.5 gives a statistical procedure for data safety monitoring based on a probability statement during the conduct of a clinical trial with an extremely low incidence rate. Brief concluding remarks are given in the last section.

2.2 Sample Size Determination

In clinical trials, a prestudy power analysis for sample size calculation is often performed to ensure that an intended clinical trial will achieve the desired power in order to correctly detect a clinically meaningful treatment effect at a prespecified level of significance. For clinical trials with extremely low incidence rate, sample size calculation based on a power analysis may not be feasible. Alternatively, it is suggested that sample size calculation be done based on precision analysis. In this section, prestudy power analysis and precision analysis for sample size calculation are briefly described.

2.2.1 Power Analysis

Under a two-sample parallel group design, let x_{ij} be a binary response (e.g., adverse events immune responses, or infection rate postsurgery) from the jth subject in the ith group, $j = 1, \ldots, n$, $I = T$ (test), R (reference or control). Then,

$$\hat{p}_i = \frac{1}{n} \sum_{i=1}^{n} x_{ij}$$

are the infection rates for the test group and the control group, respectively. Let $\delta = p_R - p_T$ be the difference in response rate between the test group and the control group. For simplicity, consider the following hypotheses for testing equality between p_R and p_T:

$$H_0: \delta = 0 \quad \text{vs.} \quad H_a: \delta \neq 0$$

Thus, under the alternative hypothesis, the power of $1 - \beta$ can be approximately obtained by the following equation (see, e.g., Chow et al. 2007):

$$\Phi \left(\frac{|\delta|}{\sqrt{\dfrac{\hat{p}_R(1 - \hat{p}_R) + \hat{p}_T(1 - \hat{p}_T)}{n}}} - Z_{1-\alpha/2} \right),$$

where Φ is the cumulative standard normal distribution function and $Z_{1-\alpha/2}$ is the upper $\frac{\alpha}{2}$th quantile of the standard normal distribution. As a result, the sample size needed for achieving a desired power of $1 - \beta$ at the α level of significance can be obtained by the following equation:

$$n_{power} = \frac{(Z_{1-\alpha/2} + Z_\beta)^2}{\delta^2} \hat{\sigma}^2 \tag{2.1}$$

where $\delta = p_R - p_T$ and $\hat{\sigma}^2 = \hat{p}_R(1 - \hat{p}_R) + \hat{p}_T(1 - \hat{p}_T)$.

2.2.2 Precision Analysis

In contrast, the $(1-\alpha) \times 100\%$ confidence interval for $\delta = p_R - p_T$ based on large sample normal approximation is given by

$$\hat{\delta} \pm Z_{1-\alpha/2} \frac{\hat{\sigma}}{\sqrt{n}}$$

where $\hat{\delta} = \hat{p}_R - \hat{p}_T$, $\hat{\sigma} = \sqrt{\hat{\sigma}_R^2 + \hat{\sigma}_T^2}$, $\hat{\sigma}_R^2 = \hat{p}_R(1-\hat{p}_R)$, $\hat{\sigma}_T^2 = \hat{p}_T(1-\hat{p}_T)$, and $Z_{1-\alpha/2}$ is the upper $\frac{\alpha}{2}$th quantile of the standard normal distribution.

Denote half of the width of the confidence interval by $w = Z_{1-\alpha/2} \frac{\hat{\sigma}}{\sqrt{n}}$, which is usually referred to as the *maximum error margin allowed* for a given sample size n. In practice, the maximum error margin allowed represents the precision that one would expect for the selected sample size. The precision analysis for sample size determination is to consider the maximum error margin allowed. In other words, we are confident that the true difference $\delta = p_R - p_T$ would fall within the margin of $w = Z_{1-\alpha/2}\hat{\sigma}$ for a given sample size of n. Thus, the sample size required for achieving the desired precision can be chosen as

$$n_{precision} = \frac{Z_{1-\alpha/2}^2 \hat{\sigma}^2}{w^2} \tag{2.2}$$

where $\hat{\sigma}^2 = \hat{p}_R(1-\hat{p}_R) + \hat{p}_T(1-\hat{p}_T)$.

This approach, based on the interest of a type I error only, is to specify the precision while estimating the true δ for selecting n.

With Equations 2.1 and 2.2, we can also get the relationship between the sample size based on power analysis and precision analysis:

$$R = \frac{n_{power}}{n_{precision}} = \left(1 + \frac{z_\beta}{z_{1-\alpha/2}}\right)^2 \frac{w^2}{\delta^2}.$$

Thus, R is proportional to $\frac{1}{\delta^2}$ or w^2.

Under a fixed power and significance level, the sample size based on a power analysis is much larger than the sample size based on a precision analysis, with an extremely low infection rate difference or large error margin allowed. Without loss of generality, $\left(1 + \frac{z_\beta}{z_{1-\alpha/2}}\right)$ is always much larger than 1 (e.g., power = 80%, significance level = 5%, then $\left(1 + \frac{z_\beta}{z_{1-\alpha/2}}\right)^2 = 2.04$). It means that if $\frac{w}{\delta} > 0.7$, the proposed sample size based on power analysis will be

TABLE 2.1

Sample Size Based on Power Analysis and Precision Analysis

ω		δ		n_{power}	$n_{precision}$	R
0.08$\hat{\sigma}$	1.37%	0.04$\hat{\sigma}$	0.69%	4906	600	8.2
	1.37%	0.05$\hat{\sigma}$	0.86%	3140	600	5.2
	1.37%	0.06$\hat{\sigma}$	1.03%	2180	600	3.6
	1.37%	0.07$\hat{\sigma}$	1.20%	1602	600	2.7
	1.37%	0.08$\hat{\sigma}$	1.37%	1226	600	2.0
0.10$\hat{\sigma}$	1.72%	0.04$\hat{\sigma}$	0.69%	4906	384	12.8
	1.72%	0.05$\hat{\sigma}$	0.86%	3140	384	8.2
	1.72%	0.06$\hat{\sigma}$	1.03%	2180	384	5.7
	1.72%	0.07$\hat{\sigma}$	1.20%	1602	384	4.2
	1.72%	0.08$\hat{\sigma}$	1.37%	1226	384	3.2
0.12$\hat{\sigma}$	2.06%	0.04$\hat{\sigma}$	0.69%	4906	267	18.4
	2.06%	0.05$\hat{\sigma}$	0.86%	3140	267	11.8
	2.06%	0.06$\hat{\sigma}$	1.03%	2180	267	8.2
	2.06%	0.07$\hat{\sigma}$	1.20%	1602	267	6.0
	2.06%	0.08$\hat{\sigma}$	1.37%	1226	267	4.6

larger than one based on precision analysis. The sample size determined by power analysis will be large when the difference between the test group and the control group is extremely small. Table 2.1 shows the comparison of sample sizes determined by power analysis and precision analysis. The power is fixed at 80% and the significance level is 5%. When $(\hat{p}_R, \hat{p}_R) = (2\%, 1\%)$, compare the sample size calculated by the two methods. The sample sizes determined by precision analysis are much smaller than the sample sizes determined by power analysis.

2.2.3 Remarks

In the previous sections, the formulas for sample size calculation were derived based on the concept of frequentist probability. Information obtained from previous studies or small pilot studies is often used to estimate the parameters required for sample size calculation. In practice, the sample size required for achieving a desired precision may be further improved by taking the Bayesian approach into consideration. For the purpose of illustration, sample size calculation based on precision analysis in conjunction with the Bayesian approach with a non-informative uniform prior is performed based on the following assumptions:

1. Because the primary endpoint x_{ij} is a binary response, it follows the Bernoulli distribution.

2. $p_R > p_T$.
3. Let $\delta_i | \theta, \sigma^2 \sim N(\theta, \sigma^2)$ and $\sigma^2 \sim Uniform(0, 1)$.

We would like to estimate the likelihood of the data. Assuming that the treatment effect δ is normally distributed with a known mean θ and unknown variance σ^2, that is, $\delta_i \sim N(\theta, \sigma^2)$. Thus, we have

$$f(\delta_i | \theta, \sigma^2) = \frac{1}{\sqrt{2\pi\sigma^2}} \exp\left\{ \frac{-(\delta_i - \theta)^2}{2\sigma^2} \right\} \quad \text{and} \quad \pi(\sigma^2) \equiv 1$$

$$L(\delta_i | \theta, \sigma^2) = \prod_{i=1}^{n} f(\delta_i | \theta, \sigma^2) = [2\pi\sigma^2]^{-\frac{n}{2}} \exp\left\{ \frac{-\sum_{i=1}^{n}(\delta_i - \theta)^2}{2\sigma^2} \right\}$$

As a result, the posterior distribution can be obtained as follows:

$$\pi(\sigma^2 | \theta, \delta_i) \propto (\sigma^2)^{-\frac{n}{2}} \exp\left\{ \frac{-\sum_{i=1}^{n}(\delta_i - \theta)^2}{2\sigma^2} \right\}$$

$$\pi(\sigma^2 | \theta, \delta_i) \sim IG\left(\alpha = \frac{n}{2} - 1, \ \beta = \frac{-\sum_{i=1}^{n}(\delta_i - \theta)^2}{2} \right)$$

where IG stands for an inverse gamma distribution with parameters α and β.
As a result, the sample size required for achieving a desired precision can be obtained by the following iterative steps:

Step 1: Start with an initial guess for n_0.

Step 2: Generate σ^2 from $IG\left(\alpha = \frac{n}{2} - 1, \ \beta = \frac{-\sum_{i=1}^{n}(\delta_i - \theta)^2}{2} \right)$.

Step 3: Calculate the required sample size n with σ^2 (generated from Step 2) by Equation 2.2.

Step 4: If $n \neq n_0$, then let $n_0 = n$ and repeat Steps 1–4. If $n = n_0$, then let $n_0 = n$.

The sample size based on the Bayesian approach n_b can be obtained; it will converge in probability to n after several iterations.

2.2.4 Chow and Chiu's Procedure for Sample Size Estimation

As indicated earlier, for clinical trials with extremely low incidence rates, the sample size required for achieving a desired power to detect a small difference may not be feasible. Sample size justification based on a small difference (absolute change) may not be of practical interest. Alternatively, sample size justification based on relative change is often considered. For example, suppose the postsurgery infection rate for the control group is 2% and the incidence rate for the test group is 1%. The absolute change in infection rate is 1% = 2% − 1%. This small difference may not have any clinical or practical meaning. However, if we consider the relative change, then the difference becomes appealing. In other words, there is a 50% relative reduction in the infection rate from 2% to 1%. In this section, we propose a procedure based on precision analysis for selecting an appropriate sample size for clinical trials with an extremely low incidence rate.

Suppose p_R and p_T are the infection rate for the control group and the test group, respectively. Define the relative improvement (or percent improvement) as follows:

$$\% \text{ improvement} = \frac{p_R - p_T}{p_R} \times 100\%$$

Note that in cases where $p_R < p_T$, the above measurement becomes a measure of percent worsening. Based on the precision analysis and considering the relative improvement at the same time, the following step-by-step procedure for choosing an appropriate sample size is recommended:

Step 1: Determine the maximum error margin allowed.

We first choose the maximum error margin that we feel comfortable with. In other words, we are 95% confident that the true difference in incidence rate between the two groups is within the maximum error margin.

Step 2: Select the highest percentage (%) of relative improvement.

Because it is expected that the relative improvement in infection rate is somewhere within the range, we may choose the combination of incidence rates that gives the highest percentage of relative improvement.

Step 3: Select a sample size that reaches statistical significance.

We then select a sample size for achieving statistical significance (i.e., those confidence intervals that don't cover 0). In other words, the observed difference is not by chance above and is reproducible if we repeat the study under similar experimental conditions.

Note that with a selected sample size (based on the above procedure), we can also evaluate the corresponding power. If we feel uncomfortable, we may increase the sample size. In practice, it is suggested that the selected sample size have at least 50% power at a prespecified level of significance.

2.3 Sensitivity Analysis

The value of $n_{precision}$ in Equation 2.2 is very sensitive to a small change in p_R and p_T. The following sensitivity analysis study evaluates the impact of the small deviations from the true incidence rates. The true infection rates for the reference and control group have a small shift:

$$p'_R = p_R + \varepsilon_R \text{ and } p'_T = p_T + \varepsilon_T$$

Thus, the sample size required can be chosen as

$$n_s = \frac{Z^2_{1-\alpha/2}\hat{\sigma}'^2}{w^2} \tag{2.3}$$

where

$$\hat{\sigma}' = \sqrt{\sigma'^2_R + \sigma'^2_T}, \quad \sigma'^2_R = (\hat{p}_R + \varepsilon_R)(1 - \hat{p}_R - \varepsilon_R), \quad \sigma'^2_T = (\hat{p}_T + \varepsilon_T)(1 - \hat{p}_T - \varepsilon_T)$$

and $Z_{1-\alpha/2}$ is the upper $(\alpha/2)$th quantile of the standard normal distribution.

If we let the shift $\varepsilon_R = \varepsilon_T = \varepsilon$, with Equations 2.2 and 2.3, we can also get the relationship between the sample size based on precision analysis and the sample size adjusted by sensitivity analysis.

$$\frac{n_s}{n_{precision}} = \frac{(p_R + \varepsilon)(1 - p_R - \varepsilon) + (p_T + \varepsilon)(1 - p_T - \varepsilon)}{p_R(1 - p_R) + p_T(1 - p_T)}$$

$$= \frac{p_R + p_T - p_R^2 - p_T^2 - 2(p_R + p_T)\varepsilon + 2\varepsilon - \varepsilon^2}{p_R + p_T - p_R^2 - p_T^2}$$

Obviously the ratio above is independent of $Z_{1-\alpha/2}$ and w. It becomes a ratio of variances before and after shift. Moreover,

$$\frac{n_s}{n_{precision}} < 1 \text{ if } \varepsilon > 0$$

$$\frac{n_s}{n_{precision}} > 1 \ \ if \ \ \varepsilon < 0$$

and

$$\frac{n_s}{n_{precision}} = 1 \ \ if \ \ \varepsilon = 0$$

This means that when $\varepsilon > 0$, the sample size adjusted by sensitivity analysis n_s will be smaller than the one $n_{precision}$ proposed by precision analysis. On the contrary, n_s will be larger than $n_{precision}$ if $\varepsilon < 0$.

2.4 An Example

A pharmaceutical company is conducting a clinical trial for developing a preventive vaccine for HIV. The incidence rate for immune responses is extremely low, ranging from 1.7% to 2.1% with a mean incidence rate of 1.9%. The sponsor expects the incidence rate for the vaccine candidate (test) to be about 1.0% and is targeting at least a 50% improvement in the incidence rate postvaccination. Based on the prestudy power analysis for sample size calculation, a total sample size of 6,532 (3,266 per group) is required for achieving 90% power for detecting a difference in the incidence rate of 0.95%, if such a difference truly exists at the 5% level of significance, assuming that the true incidence rate for the control group is 1.9%. With this huge sample size, not only can the sponsor not afford to support the study, but it may not be of any practical use. Alternatively, Chow and Chiu (2013) suggested the following steps (as described in Section 2.2.4) for choosing an appropriate sample size for the proposed vaccine clinical trial:

Step 1: Assume that the true incidence rate for the control group is 1.9%, and we expect there to be a 50% relative reduction for the test group. In other words, the true incidence rate for the test group is 0.95%. Now suppose the sponsor is willing to tolerate a 0.5% error margin. Thus, we choose 0.05% as the maximum error margin allowed.

Step 2: We then use Table 2.2 to select the combination of (p_R, p_T) with the highest possible percentage improvement. Table 2.2 suggests that the third column with 50% relative improvement be considered.

TABLE 2.2

Ninety-Five Percent Confidence Intervals ($p_R = 1.90\%$)

p_T	0.85%			0.90%			0.95%			1.00%			1.05%		
% of Improvement	55%			53%			50%			47%			45%		
n	Lower	Upper	Power	Lower	Upper	Power	Lower	Upper	Power	Lower	Upper	Power	Lower	Upper	Power
200	-1.23%	3.33%	14.52%	-1.30%	3.30%	13.39%	-1.37%	3.27%	12.35%	-1.44%	3.24%	11.38%	-1.51%	3.21%	10.48%
300	-0.81%	2.91%	19.64%	-0.88%	2.88%	17.97%	-0.95%	2.85%	16.42%	-1.01%	2.81%	14.98%	-1.08%	2.78%	13.66%
400	-0.56%	2.66%	24.71%	-0.63%	2.63%	22.51%	-0.69%	2.59%	20.45%	-0.76%	2.56%	18.55%	-0.82%	2.52%	16.80%
500	-0.39%	2.49%	29.71%	-0.46%	2.46%	26.99%	-0.52%	2.42%	24.46%	-0.58%	2.38%	22.10%	-0.64%	2.34%	19.92%
600	-0.27%	2.37%	34.58%	-0.33%	2.33%	31.40%	-0.39%	2.29%	28.42%	-0.45%	2.25%	25.62%	-0.51%	2.21%	23.03%
700	-0.17%	2.27%	39.30%	-0.23%	2.23%	35.71%	-0.29%	2.19%	32.30%	-0.35%	2.15%	29.10%	-0.41%	2.11%	26.11%
800	-0.09%	2.19%	43.85%	-0.15%	2.15%	39.89%	-0.21%	2.11%	36.11%	-0.27%	2.07%	32.52%	-0.33%	2.03%	29.15%
900	-0.02%	2.12%	48.19%	-0.08%	2.08%	43.93%	-0.14%	2.04%	39.81%	-0.20%	2.00%	35.88%	-0.26%	1.96%	32.16%
1000	0.03%	2.07%	52.32%	-0.03%	2.03%	47.81%	-0.09%	1.99%	43.40%	-0.15%	1.95%	39.16%	-0.21%	1.91%	35.11%
1100	0.08%	2.02%	56.23%	0.02%	1.98%	51.51%	-0.04%	1.94%	46.87%	-0.10%	1.90%	42.35%	-0.16%	1.86%	38.01%

(Continued)

TABLE 2.2 *(Continued)*

Ninety-Five Percent Confidence Intervals ($p_R = 1.90\%$)

p_T	0.85%		0.90%		0.95%		1.00%		1.05%	
% of Improvement	55%		53%		50%		47%		45%	
n	Lower	Upper Power	Lower	Upper Power	Lower	Upper Power	Lower	Upper Power	Lower	Upper Power
1200	0.12%	1.98% 59.91%	0.06%	1.94% 55.04%	0.00%	1.90% 50.20%	−0.06%	1.86% 45.44%	−0.11%	1.81% 40.84%
1300	0.16%	1.94% 63.35%	0.10%	1.90% 58.39%	0.04%	1.86% 53.40%	−0.02%	1.82% 48.44%	−0.08%	1.78% 43.60%
1400	0.19%	1.91% 66.57%	0.13%	1.87% 61.56%	0.07%	1.83% 56.45%	0.02%	1.78% 51.33%	−0.04%	1.74% 46.28%
1500	0.22%	1.88% 69.56%	0.16%	1.84% 64.55%	0.10%	1.80% 59.37%	0.05%	1.75% 54.12%	−0.01%	1.71% 48.89%

Step 3: We then select a sample size that reaches statistical significance. It is evident from Table 2.2 that $n = 1{,}300$ per group will reach statistical significance (i.e., the observed difference is *not* by chance alone and it is reproducible).

Thus, total sample size required for the proposed vaccine trial for achieving the desired precision (i.e., the maximum error margin allowed) and the relative improvement of 50% is 2,600 (1,300 per group), assuming that the true incidence rate for the control group is 1.9%. With the selected sample size of $N = 2n = 2{,}600$, the corresponding power for correctly detecting a difference of $\delta = p_R - p_T = 1.9\% - 0.95\% = 0.95\%$ is 53.40%. Note that the selected sample size does not account for possible dropout of the proposed study.

2.5 Data Safety Monitoring Procedure

For vaccine clinical trials with an extremely low incidence rate, it will take a large sample to observe a few responses. The time and cost is a great concern to the sponsor of the trial. In practice, it is then of particular interest to stop the trial early if the candidate vaccine will not achieve the study objectives. In this section, a statistical data safety monitoring procedure based on a probability statement is developed to assist the sponsor in making a decision as to whether the trial should stop at interim (Table 2.3).

Assume that an interim analysis is to take place when we reach a sample size of $N' = N/2 = n$, where $N = 2n$ is the total sample size for the trial. At interim, suppose $p\%$ (where $p = \frac{p_R + p_T}{2}$ incidences are expected to be observed from the N' samples. Then we can follow the procedure described below for data safety monitoring (Figure 2.1).

For the purpose of illustration, consider the example described in Section 2.4. Assuming that the incidence rate is 1.9% for the control group and 0.95% for the test group. Thus, the blinded expected total incidence rate will be 1.425% and the expected mean is $15.68 \approx 16$. We can also find the 95% upper and lower limit of the expected observed number for the whole trial, which is (8, 23). If the observed incidence number is 23 ($\hat{\mu} = 23$, which is within the 95% confidence interval) at interim, we can consider continuing the trial by calculating the probability for each case. The expected incidence numbers for each case are shown in Table 2.4 for reference. For the whole trial, the estimated expected mean and 95% confidence interval in the reference group are 28 and (16, 40), respectively; in the test group, these values are 14 and (6, 23), respectively, if $\hat{\mu} = \mu_U$. For the possible combination of sample sizes, we provide the probabilities $P(\sum_{i=1}^{n} x_{Rj} | p_R) \times P(\sum_{i=1}^{n} x_{Tj} | p_T)$ in each case in Table 2.5.

TABLE 2.3

Ninety-Five Percent Confidence Intervals (p$_R$ = 2.00%)

p$_T$	0.90%			0.95%			1.00%			1.05%			1.10%		
% of improvement	55%			53%			50%			48%			45%		
n	Lower	Upper	Power	Lower	Upper	Power	Lower	Upper	Power	Lower	Upper	Power	Lower	Upper	Power
200	−1.24%	3.44%	14.95%	−1.31%	3.41%	13.83%	−1.38%	3.38%	12.79%	−1.45%	3.35%	11.82%	−1.52%	3.32%	10.92%
300	−0.81%	3.01%	20.28%	−0.88%	2.98%	18.61%	−0.94%	2.94%	17.07%	−1.01%	2.91%	15.63%	−1.08%	2.88%	14.30%
400	−0.55%	2.75%	25.55%	−0.62%	2.72%	23.36%	−0.68%	2.68%	21.32%	−0.75%	2.65%	19.41%	−0.81%	2.61%	17.65%
500	−0.38%	2.58%	30.73%	−0.44%	2.54%	28.05%	−0.51%	2.51%	25.52%	−0.57%	2.47%	23.17%	−0.63%	2.43%	20.98%
600	−0.25%	2.45%	35.78%	−0.31%	2.41%	32.64%	−0.37%	2.37%	29.67%	−0.44%	2.34%	26.89%	−0.50%	2.30%	24.28%
700	−0.15%	2.35%	40.65%	−0.21%	2.31%	37.11%	−0.27%	2.27%	33.74%	−0.33%	2.23%	30.55%	−0.39%	2.19%	27.56%
800	−0.07%	2.27%	45.32%	−0.13%	2.23%	41.44%	−0.19%	2.19%	37.71%	−0.25%	2.15%	34.15%	−0.31%	2.11%	30.79%
900	0.00%	2.20%	49.77%	−0.06%	2.16%	45.60%	−0.12%	2.12%	41.55%	−0.18%	2.08%	37.67%	−0.24%	2.04%	33.97%
1000	0.05%	2.15%	53.98%	−0.01%	2.11%	49.58%	−0.06%	2.06%	45.27%	−0.12%	2.02%	41.09%	−0.18%	1.98%	37.08%

(Continued)

TABLE 2.3 *(Continued)*

Ninety-Five Percent Confidence Intervals ($p_R = 2.00\%$)

| p_T | 0.90% | | | 0.95% | | | 1.00% | | | 1.05% | | | 1.10% | | |
| % of improvement | 55% | | | 53% | | | 50% | | | 48% | | | 45% | | |
n	Lower	Upper	Power	Lower	Upper	Power	Lower	Upper	Power	Lower	Upper	Power	Lower	Upper	Power
1100	0.10%	2.10%	57.94%	0.04%	2.06%	53.37%	-0.01%	2.01%	48.85%	-0.07%	1.97%	44.41%	-0.13%	1.93%	40.12%
1200	0.14%	2.06%	61.66%	0.09%	2.01%	56.97%	0.03%	1.97%	52.27%	-0.03%	1.93%	47.62%	-0.09%	1.89%	43.09%
1300	0.18%	2.02%	65.12%	0.12%	1.98%	60.36%	0.07%	1.93%	55.54%	0.01%	1.89%	50.72%	-0.05%	1.85%	45.97%
1400	0.22%	1.98%	68.34%	0.16%	1.94%	63.56%	0.10%	1.90%	58.65%	0.04%	1.86%	53.69%	-0.01%	1.81%	48.76%
1500	0.25%	1.95%	71.32%	0.19%	1.91%	66.55%	0.13%	1.87%	61.60%	0.07%	1.83%	56.54%	0.02%	1.78%	51.46%

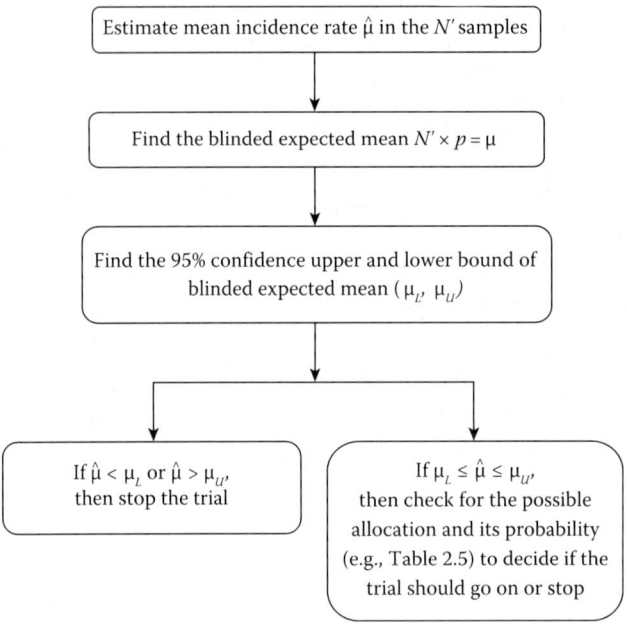

FIGURE 2.1

Data safety monitoring procedure.

TABLE 2.4

Expected Incidence Numbers and Corresponding 95% Confidence Intervals of Each Group for the Whole Trial at Interim

	Intern	Target	Reference			Test		
Sample Size	$N' = 1100$	$N = 2200$	$n_R = 1100$			$n_T = 1100$		
	Expected Incidence Numbers		Lower	Mean	Upper	Lower	Mean	Upper
Upper	23	47	16	28	40	6	14	23
Mean	16	31	12	21	30	4	10	17
Lower	8	16	8	14	19	3	7	11

TABLE 2.5

Probability of Each Sample Size Combination Occurring

Incidence Numbers		Probabilities (%)	Incidence Numbers		Probabilities (%)	Incidence Numbers		Probabilities (%)	Incidence Numbers		Probabilities (%)	Incidence Numbers		Probabilities (%)
Reference	Test		Reference	Test		Reference	Test		Reference	Test		Reference	Test	
16	6	1.71	21	6	5.84	26	6	9.17	31	6	10.17	36	6	10.30
16	7	3.00	21	7	10.26	26	7	16.10	31	7	17.87	36	7	18.10
16	8	4.69	21	8	16.05	26	8	25.19	31	8	27.95	36	8	28.31
16	9	6.66	21	9	22.78	26	9	35.76	31	9	39.68	36	9	40.19
16	10	8.73	21	10	29.83	26	10	46.83	31	10	51.96	36	10	52.62
16	11	10.68	21	11	36.53	26	11	57.34	31	11	63.62	36	11	64.44
16	12	12.39	21	12	42.36	26	12	66.50	31	12	73.78	36	12	74.73
16	13	13.76	21	13	47.04	26	13	73.84	31	13	81.93	36	13	82.98
16	14	14.78	21	14	50.53	26	14	79.31	31	14	88.00	36	14	89.13
16	15	15.49	21	15	52.95	26	15	83.11	31	15	92.22	36	15	93.40
16	16	15.95	21	16	54.52	26	16	85.58	31	16	94.96	36	16	96.18
16	17	16.23	21	17	55.49	26	17	87.10	31	17	96.63	36	17	97.87
16	18	16.39	21	18	56.04	26	18	87.97	31	18	97.60	36	18	98.85
16	19	16.48	21	19	56.34	26	19	88.44	31	19	98.13	36	19	99.39
16	20	16.53	21	20	56.50	26	20	88.69	31	20	98.40	36	20	99.67
16	21	16.55	21	21	56.58	26	21	88.81	31	21	98.54	36	21	99.80
16	22	16.56	21	22	56.62	26	22	88.87	31	22	98.60	36	22	99.87
16	23	16.56	21	23	56.63	26	23	88.90	31	23	98.63	36	23	99.90
17	6	2.38	22	6	6.70	27	6	9.52	32	6	10.23	37	6	10.31
17	7	4.18	22	7	11.76	27	7	16.71	32	7	17.96	37	7	18.10
17	8	6.54	22	8	18.40	27	8	26.14	32	8	28.10	37	8	28.32

(Continued)

TABLE 2.5 (Continued)

Probability of Each Sample Size Combination Occurring

| Incidence Numbers | | Probabilities | Incidence Numbers | | Probabilities | Incidence Numbers | | Probabilities | Incidence Numbers | | Probabilities | Incidence Numbers | | Probabilities |
Reference	Test	(%)	Reference	Test	(%)	Reference	Test	(%)	Reference	Test	(%)	Reference	Test	(%)
17	9	9.29	22	9	26.13	27	9	37.12	32	9	39.90	37	9	40.20
17	10	12.17	22	10	34.21	27	10	48.60	32	10	52.24	37	10	52.64
17	11	14.90	22	11	41.89	27	11	59.52	32	11	63.97	37	11	64.47
17	12	17.27	22	12	48.58	27	12	69.02	32	12	74.18	37	12	74.75
17	13	19.18	22	13	53.95	27	13	76.64	32	13	82.38	37	13	83.01
17	14	20.60	22	14	57.95	27	14	82.32	32	14	88.48	37	14	89.16
17	15	21.59	22	15	60.72	27	15	86.27	32	15	92.72	37	15	93.44
17	16	22.23	22	16	62.53	27	16	88.83	32	16	95.47	37	16	96.21
17	17	22.63	22	17	63.63	27	17	90.40	32	17	97.16	37	17	97.91
17	18	22.85	22	18	64.27	27	18	91.31	32	18	98.13	37	18	98.89
17	19	22.98	22	19	64.62	27	19	91.80	32	19	98.66	37	19	99.43
17	20	23.04	22	20	64.80	27	20	92.06	32	20	98.94	37	20	99.71
17	21	23.07	22	21	64.88	27	21	92.18	32	21	99.08	37	21	99.84
17	22	23.09	22	22	64.93	27	22	92.24	32	22	99.14	37	22	99.91
17	23	23.09	22	23	64.95	27	23	92.27	32	23	99.17	37	23	99.94
18	6	3.17	23	6	7.48	28	6	9.77	33	6	10.26	38	6	10.31
18	7	5.56	23	7	13.13	28	7	17.17	33	7	18.02	38	7	18.11
18	8	8.70	23	8	20.54	28	8	26.85	33	8	28.19	38	8	28.32
18	9	12.35	23	9	29.16	28	9	38.13	33	9	40.03	38	9	40.21
18	10	16.17	23	10	38.19	28	10	49.92	33	10	52.42	38	10	52.65
18	11	19.81	23	11	46.76	28	11	61.13	33	11	64.19	38	11	64.48
18	12	22.97	23	12	54.23	28	12	70.89	33	12	74.43	38	12	74.77

(Continued)

TABLE 2.5 (Continued)
Probability of Each Sample Size Combination Occurring

Incidence Numbers Reference	Test	Probabilities (%)	Incidence Numbers Reference	Test	Probabilities (%)	Incidence Numbers Reference	Test	Probabilities (%)	Incidence Numbers Reference	Test	Probabilities (%)	Incidence Numbers Reference	Test	Probabilities (%)
18	13	25.50	23	13	60.22	28	13	78.72	33	13	82.66	38	13	83.03
18	14	27.39	23	14	64.68	28	14	84.56	33	14	88.78	38	14	89.18
18	15	28.71	23	15	67.78	28	15	88.61	33	15	93.03	38	15	93.46
18	16	29.56	23	16	69.79	28	16	91.24	33	16	95.80	38	16	96.23
18	17	30.08	23	17	71.02	28	17	92.85	33	17	97.49	38	17	97.93
18	18	30.38	23	18	71.73	28	18	93.78	33	18	98.47	38	18	98.91
18	19	30.55	23	19	72.12	28	19	94.29	33	19	99.00	38	19	99.45
18	20	30.63	23	20	72.32	28	20	94.55	33	20	99.27	38	20	99.73
18	21	30.67	23	21	72.42	28	21	94.68	33	21	99.41	38	21	99.86
18	22	30.69	23	22	72.47	28	22	94.74	33	22	99.48	38	22	99.93
18	23	30.70	23	23	72.49	28	23	94.77	33	23	99.50	38	23	99.96
19	6	4.03	24	6	8.15	29	6	9.96	34	6	10.28	39	6	10.31
19	7	7.08	24	7	14.32	29	7	17.49	34	7	18.06	39	7	18.11
19	8	11.08	24	8	22.40	29	8	27.36	34	8	28.25	39	8	28.33
19	9	15.73	24	9	31.80	29	9	38.85	34	9	40.11	39	9	40.22
19	10	20.59	24	10	41.64	29	10	50.87	34	10	52.52	39	10	52.66
19	11	25.22	24	11	50.99	29	11	62.29	34	11	64.32	39	11	64.49
19	12	29.24	24	12	59.13	29	12	72.23	34	12	74.58	39	12	74.78
19	13	32.48	24	13	65.66	29	13	80.21	34	13	82.82	39	13	83.04
19	14	34.88	24	14	70.53	29	14	86.16	34	14	88.96	39	14	89.19
19	15	36.55	24	15	73.91	29	15	90.28	34	15	93.22	39	15	93.47
19	16	37.64	24	16	76.11	29	16	92.97	34	16	95.99	39	16	96.24

(Continued)

TABLE 2.5 (Continued)

Probability of Each Sample Size Combination Occurring

| Incidence Numbers | | Probabilities | Incidence Numbers | | Probabilities | Incidence Numbers | | Probabilities | Incidence Numbers | | Probabilities | Incidence Numbers | | Probabilities |
Reference	Test	(%)	Reference	Test	(%)	Reference	Test	(%)	Reference	Test	(%)	Reference	Test	(%)
19	17	38.30	24	17	77.45	29	17	94.61	34	17	97.69	39	17	97.94
19	18	38.69	24	18	78.22	29	18	95.56	34	18	98.67	39	18	98.92
19	19	38.90	24	19	78.65	29	19	96.07	34	19	99.20	39	19	99.46
19	20	39.01	24	20	78.87	29	20	96.34	34	20	99.48	39	20	99.74
19	21	39.06	24	21	78.98	29	21	96.47	34	21	99.62	39	21	99.87
19	22	39.08	24	22	79.03	29	22	96.54	34	22	99.68	39	22	99.94
19	23	39.10	24	23	79.05	29	23	96.56	34	23	99.71	39	23	99.97
20	6	4.94	25	6	8.72	30	6	10.09	35	6	10.30	40	6	10.31
20	7	8.67	25	7	15.31	30	7	17.72	35	7	18.08	40	7	18.11
20	8	13.57	25	8	23.95	30	8	27.71	35	8	28.29	40	8	28.33
20	9	19.26	25	9	34.00	30	9	39.35	35	9	40.16	40	9	40.22
20	10	25.22	25	10	44.52	30	10	51.52	35	10	52.59	40	10	52.66
20	11	30.89	25	11	54.52	30	11	63.09	35	11	64.40	40	11	64.49
20	12	35.82	25	12	63.22	30	12	73.16	35	12	74.67	40	12	74.78
20	13	39.77	25	13	70.21	30	13	81.24	35	13	82.92	40	13	83.05
20	14	42.72	25	14	75.41	30	14	87.26	35	14	89.07	40	14	89.20
20	15	44.77	25	15	79.02	30	15	91.44	35	15	93.34	40	15	93.47
20	16	46.10	25	16	81.37	30	16	94.16	35	16	96.11	40	16	96.25
20	17	46.91	25	17	82.81	30	17	95.82	35	17	97.81	40	17	97.95
20	18	47.38	25	18	83.63	30	18	96.78	35	18	98.79	40	18	98.93

(Continued)

TABLE 2.5 (Continued)

Probability of Each Sample Size Combination Occurring

Incidence Numbers		Probabilities	Incidence Numbers		Probabilities	Incidence Numbers		Probabilities	Incidence Numbers		Probabilities	Incidence Numbers		Probabilities
Reference	Test	(%)	Reference	Test	(%)	Reference	Test	(%)	Reference	Test	(%)	Reference	Test	(%)
20	19	47.64	25	19	84.09	30	19	97.31	35	19	99.32	40	19	99.47
20	20	47.77	25	20	84.32	30	20	97.58	35	20	99.60	40	20	99.74
20	21	47.84	25	21	84.44	30	21	97.71	35	21	99.74	40	21	99.88
20	22	47.87	25	22	84.49	30	22	97.78	35	22	99.80	40	22	99.94
20	23	47.88	25	23	84.52	30	23	97.80	35	23	99.83	40	23	99.97

2.6 Concluding Remarks

For vaccine clinical trials with extremely low incidence rates, the sample size required for achieving a desired power to correctly detect a small clinically meaningful difference, if such a difference truly exists, is often huge. This huge sample size may not be of practical use. In this chapter, an alternative approach proposed by Chow and Chiu (2013) based on precision analysis and sensitivity analysis in conjunction with power analysis was discussed. Chow and Chiu's proposed method reduces the sample size required for achieving a desired precision with certain statistical assurance.

Most importantly, the statistical data safety monitoring procedure proposed by Chow and Chiu (2013), which was developed based on a probability statement, is useful in assisting the investigator or sponsor in making a decision as to whether the trial should stop early due to safety, futility, and/or efficacy at interim.

References

Belyakov IM, Ahlers JD, Nabel GJ, et al. (2008). Generation of functionally active HIV-1 specific CD8+ CTL in intestinal mucosa following mucosal, systemic or mixed prime-boost immunization. *Virology* 381, 106–115.

Boyle P and Parkin DM. (1991). Statistical methods for registries. In *Cancer Registration. Principles and Methods. Eds: Jensen OM, Parkin DM, MacLennan R, Muir CS, and Skeet RG*, IARC Scientific, Lyon, France, pp. 126–158.

Chow SC and Chiu ST. (2013). Sample size and data monitoring for clinical trials with extremely low incidence rate. *Ther Innov Regul Sci.* 47, 438–446.

Chow SC and Liu JP. (2004). *Design and Analysis of Clinical Trials.* Wiley, New York, NY.

Chow SC, Shao J, and Wang H. (2007). *Sample Size Calculation in Clinical Research.* 2nd Edition, Chapman and Hall, New York, NY.

Esteban M. (2009). Attenuated poxvirus vectors MVA and NYVAC as promising vaccine candidates against HIV/AIDS. *Hum Vaccin.* 5, 1–5.

Excler JL, Tomaras GD, and Russell ND. (2013). Novel directions in HIV-1 vaccines revealed from clinical trials. *Curr Opin HIV AIDS.* 8(5), 421–431.

FDA. (2002). *Guidance for Industry Immiotoxicology Eevaluation of Investigational New Drugs.* Center for Drug Evaluation and Research, the United States Food and Drug Administration, Rockville, MD.

Gaddipati H, Liu K, Pariser A, and Pazdu R. (2012). Rare cancer trial design: Lessons from FDA approvals. *Clin Cancer Res.* 18(19), 5172–5178. DOI:10.1158/1078-0432.CCR-12-113

Gupta SB, Jacobson LP, Margolick JB, et al. (2007). Estimating the benefit of an HIV-1 vaccine that reduces viral load set point. *J Infect Dis.* 4, 546–550.

Haynes BF and Shattock RJ. (2008). Critical issues in mucosal immunity for HIV-1 vaccine development. *J Allergy Clin Immunol.* 122, 3–9.

Kim JH, Perks-Ngarm S, Excler J-L, and Michael NL. (2010). HIV vaccines: Lessons learned and the way forward. *Curr Opin HIV AIDS*. 5(5), 428–434.

Mattapallil JJ, Douek DC, Buckler-White A, et al. (2006). Vaccination preserves CD4 memory T cells during acute simian immunodeficiency virus challenge. *J Exp Med*. 203, 1533–1541.

O'Neill RT. (1988). On sample sizes to estimate the protective efficacy of a vaccine. *Stat Med*. 7(12), 1279–1288.

Rerks-Ngarm S, Pitisuttithum P, Nitayaphan S, et al. (2009). Vaccination with ALVAC and AIDSVAX to prevent HIV-1 infection in Thailand. *N Engl J Med*. 361, 1–12.

UNAIDS. (2009). *UNAIDS annual report 2009: Uniting the world against AIDS*. UNAIDS, Geneva, Switzerland.

Watkins DI, Burton DR, Kallas EG, et al. (2008). Nonhuman primate models and the failure of the Merck HIV-1 vaccine in humans. *Nat Med*. 14, 617–621.

3

Adaptive Clinical Trial Design

Shein-Chung Chow

Duke University School of Medicine, Durham, NC

Fuyu Song

China Food and Drug Administration, Beijing, People's Republic of China

CONTENTS

3.1 Introduction

In the past decade, it has been recognized that increasing spending on biomedical research has not resulted in an increase in the success rate of pharmaceutical and clinical development. Moreover, many drug products have been withdrawn after regulatory approval due to safety concerns. Woodcock (2005) made an attempt to diagnose the possible causes of the discrepancy between the increased spending and low success rate. She found that the low success rate of clinical development could be due to the following factors: (1) there exists a diminished margin for improvement that escalates the level of difficulty for proving drug benefits; (2) genomics and other new fields of science have not yet reached their full potential; (3) mergers and other business arrangements have decreased candidates; (4) easy targets are the focus, as chronic diseases are harder to study; (5) failure rates have not improved; and (6) rapidly escalating costs and complexity have decreased the willingness/ability to bring many candidates forward into the clinic. As a result, the US Food and Drug Administration (FDA) kicked off the Critical Path Initiative to identify possible causes of the discrepancy between increasing spending and low success rate (FDA 2004).

The ultimate goal of the Critical Path Initiative is to provide possible solutions and to increase the probability of success in pharmaceutical and clinical development in a more efficient and cost-effective way. In 2006, the FDA released a *Critical Path Opportunities Report* that outlines six broad topic areas to bridge the gap between the quick pace of new biomedical discoveries and the slower pace at which those discoveries are currently developed into therapies. Among the six broad topic areas, the FDA calls for advancing innovative trial designs and especially for the use of prior experience or accumulated information in trial design. Many researchers have interpreted this report as encouraging the use of adaptive design methods in clinical trials or a Bayesian approach utilizing accumulated data at interim in clinical development. At the same time, the European Medicines Agency (EMA) of the European Union published a draft reflection paper on flexible designs used in confirmatory clinical trials (EMA 2006). Thus, in many cases, an adaptive design is also known as a flexible design (EMEA 2002; EMA 2006). The potential use of adaptive design methods in clinical trials has attracted much attention and led to tremendous discussion among the pharmaceutical industry, the FDA, and academia since then (see e.g., Chow 2006; Chow and Chang 2008, 2011; Chow and Corey 2011; Chow et al. 2005; FDA 2010a; Gallo et al. 2006).

The concept of adaptive design methods in clinical trials is to provide the principal investigator certain flexibility for identifying any signal, possible pattern/trend, and/or optimal clinical benefits of a test drug or therapy under investigation in a more efficient way. *Flexibility* refers to the ability to accommodate changing trial/statistical procedures and/or conditions, whereas *efficiency* is the ability to achieve study objectives in less than the usual development time. In addition, Chow and Chang (2011) indicated that adaptive design methods are attractive to investigators and/or sponsors because (1) they reflect real medical/clinical practice; (2) they may be ethical with respect to both the efficacy and safety (toxicity) of the test treatment under investigation; and (3) they help increase the probability of success not only in early-phase clinical development but consequently also in late-phase clinical development.

A typical example of clinical development utilizing adaptive methods in clinical trials is probably the development of Velcade by Millennium Pharmaceuticals in the early 2000s. Velcade is intended for treating patients with multiple myeloma. Velcade was on the FDA accelerated track for orphan drugs, which was established specifically for unmet medical needs and/or rare diseases. It took the company about 2 years and 4 months (from the first patient in to the last patient out) to receive an approvable letter from the FDA based on a limited phase II study. During the development process, the sponsor utilized the concept of adaptive design methods in clinical trials by modifying the trial design as it continued, such as changing the primary study endpoint of response rate to a co-primary endpoint of response rate and time-to-disease progression and changing the superiority hypothesis to a non-inferiority hypothesis. Velcade was subsequently approved by the FDA on June 23, 2008. Velcade's successful example indicates that if the study drug is promising and/or no alternative treatments are available, the FDA is willing to help the sponsor to identify the clinical benefits of the drug under investigation. Moreover, new methodology is acceptable to the FDA as long as the sponsor can demonstrate the scientific/statistical validity of the proposed method and most importantly the integrity of the data collected from the trial.

The purpose of this chapter is not only to introduce the concept of adaptive design but also to review the relative advantages, limitations, feasibility, and acceptability of commonly considered adaptive designs in clinical development. The remainder of this chapter is organized as follows. In the next section, various definitions are given, including the FDA's definition of adaptive trial design. Section 3.3 reviews several types of adaptive designs depending upon the modifications or adaptations employed. Utilization of the Bayesian approach in adaptive design is discussed in Section 3.4. Section 3.5 focuses on the possible benefits and limitations of using adaptive design methods in clinical trials. Section 3.6 expresses regulatory and statistical concerns regarding implementation of adaptive trial designs in clinical trials. An application of adaptive design in HIV-1 vaccine trials is discussed in Section 3.7. Some concluding remarks are provided in the last section of this chapter.

3.2 Definition of *Adaptive Design*

Although the use of adaptive design methods in clinical trials can be traced back to late 1970, when the concept of adaptive randomization was introduced to increase the probability of success in clinical trials (see e.g., Wei 1978), there existed no universal agreement on and formal definition of adaptive trial design in the literature until 2005. In 2005, Chow et al. (2005) defined adaptive design as a study design that allows adaptations (modifications or changes) to trial procedures and/or statistical procedures after initiation of the trial without undermining the validity and integrity of the trial. Chow, Chang, and Pong's definition allows prospective, concurrent (or ad hoc), and retrospective adaptations when conducting a clinical trial. In 2006, the Pharmaceutical Research Manufacturer Association (PhRMA) Working Group on Adaptive Design published a white paper and provided a PhRMA official definition of adaptive design. *Adaptive design* is defined as a clinical trial design that uses accumulating data to decide how to modify aspects of the study as it continues, without undermining the validity and integrity of the trial (Gallo et al. 2006). Unlike Chow, Chang, and Pong's definition, PhRMA's definition emphasizes *design* adaptations. PhRMA's definition has been criticized not reflecting real clinical practices such as protocol amendments for ad hoc adaptations.

In February 2010, the FDA circulated a draft guidance on adaptive design clinical trials, which defined adaptive design as a study that includes a prospectively planned opportunity for modification of one or more specified aspects of the study design and hypotheses based on analysis of (usually interim) data from subjects in the study (FDA 2010a). Analyses of the accumulating study data are performed at prospectively planned time points within the study, with or without formal statistical hypothesis testing. The FDA's definition has been criticized for inflexibility in the sense that it is difficult, if not impossible, to consider all possible scenarios (plan opportunities) ahead of time for clinical investigation of a test treatment, especially when the test treatment has a complicated structure with some uncertainties. The 2010 FDA draft guidance classifies adaptive designs into two categories, namely *well-understood* designs and *less well-understood* designs. According to informal communications with the FDA medical/statistical reviewers, a well-understood design is referred to as a study design that meets the following criteria: (1) it has been in use for years (e.g., group sequential design); (2) under the study design, the corresponding statistical methods are well established; and (3) most importantly the FDA is familiar with the study design through the review of submissions utilizing the study design. For a less well-understood design, in contrast, the relative merits and limitations of the study design have not yet been fully evaluated. Valid statistical methods have not yet been developed or established, and most importantly the FDA does not have sufficient experience with submissions utilizing such a study design.

It should be noted that the term *adaptation* refers to a modification or change made to the study design before, during, or after the conduct of a clinical trial. In practice, there are three types of adaptations, namely, prospective adaptation, concurrent adaptation, and retrospective adaptation. *Prospective adaptations* refer to adaptations *by design* that are usually implemented by study protocol, whereas *concurrent adaptations* are often implemented through protocol amendments. *Retrospective adaptations* are typically incorporated into the statistical analysis plan prior to unblinding or database lock.

3.3 Types of Adaptive Design

Depending on the adaptations employed, Chow and Chang (2011) classified adaptive designs into 10 types: (1) an adaptive randomization design, (2) a group sequential design or an adaptive group sequential design, (3) a flexible sample size re-estimation (SSRE) design, (4) a drop-the-losers design (or pick-the-winner design), (5) an adaptive dose-finding design, (6) a bio-marker-adaptive design (or enrichment design in a target clinical trial), (7) an adaptive treatment-switching design, (8) an adaptive-hypothesis design, (9) a two-stage seamless adaptive design (e.g., a two-stage phase I/II or II/III adaptive design), and (10) a multiple adaptive design. These designs are briefly described below. Detailed information regarding these adaptive designs can be found elsewhere (Chow and Chang 2008, 2011).

3.3.1 Adaptive Randomization Design

Adaptive randomization design allows modification of randomization schedules based on varied and/or unequal probabilities of treatment assignment, both prospectively and after review of the response of previously assigned subjects. The purpose is to assign more subjects to a promising test treatment under investigation and potentially to increase the probability of success of the trial. The commonly used adaptive randomization procedures include treatment-adaptive randomization, covariate-adaptive randomization, and response-adaptive randomization. In practice, adaptive randomization design may be valuable in trials with a relatively small sample size or trials with shorter treatment duration or short-term outcomes (e.g., biomarker or surrogate endpoint), but it may not be feasible for a large trial with a relatively long treatment duration.

Adaptive randomization is considered a less well-understood design according to the FDA draft guidance (FDA 2010a). In practice, it is often difficult, if not impossible, to characterize the probability structure of a clinical trial utilizing adaptive randomization design, especially when varied and/or unequal probabilities of treatment assignment are used. In addition, the balance of patient characteristics between the treatment groups is a concern for this type of design. An imbalance in important characteristics is problematic, especially for confirmatory studies. In practice, an extreme imbalance may be caused by adaptive randomization at a relatively early stage of a trial. A typical example would be the Michigan Extracorporeal Membrane Oxygenation trial, in which only 1 out of 12 infants was enrolled to receive conventional therapy (Bartlett et al. 1985). As a result, Mugford et al. (2008) considered this trial to have a high potential risk for assignment bias.

3.3.2 Adaptive Group Sequential Design

Classic group sequential design is a study design that has the option to (1) review accumulating data (either safety or efficacy or both) at interim, (2) stop the trial early due to safety, futility, or efficacy after review of the interim data, and (3) perform SSRE at interim to determine whether the study will achieve its objective if the observed treatment effect is preserved until the end of the study. Classic group sequential design with the above-described options is considered a well-understood design by the FDA (FDA 2010a) because the corresponding statistical methods and various stopping boundaries based on different boundary functions for controlling an overall type I error rate are well established and available in the literature (see e.g., Chow and Chang 2011).

Adaptive group sequential design, in contrast, is a classical group sequential design with prespecified options for additional adaptations (e.g., modification/deletion/addition of treatment arms, change of study endpoints, modification of dose and/or treatment duration, modification of randomization schedules, etc.) after interim analysis. With additional adaptations, adaptive group sequential design has become a less well-understood design. In this case, standard methods for the classical group sequential design may not be appropriate. For example, they may not be able to control the overall type I error rate at the desired level of 5%, owing to potential issues pertaining to adaptations of a given study design. Appropriate statistical procedures are necessary to avoid the potential increase in the study-wide type I error rate (FDA 2010a).

3.3.3 Flexible Sample Size Re-Estimation Design

Flexible SSRE design allows for sample size adjustment or re-estimation based on the observed data at interim. In general, sample size is determined before the trial formally starts and is based on either pilot estimates of efficacy endpoints and their variability or a best guess for the lowest clinically meaningful effect size between the treatment and control groups. Practically, parameter misspecification may be inevitable, which can lead to an underpowered design if the true variability is much larger than the initial specification (Buchbinder et al. 2008). Thus, it is of interest to adjust sample sizes adaptively based on accrued data from the ongoing trial.

SSRE, however, suffers from the same disadvantage as the original power analysis for sample size calculation prior to the conduct of the study, because it is performed by treating estimates of the study parameters, which are based on data observed at interim, as true values. Note that the observed difference at interim based on a small number of subjects may not be statistically significant. The observed results may be due to chance alone and not reproducible. Thus, standard methods for SSRE based on observed differences with a limited number of subjects may be biased and misleading (FDA 2010a).

Sample size adjustment or re-estimation could be done in either a blinded fashion (e.g., Gould 1992, 1995), which is based on overall data, or an unblinded fashion (e.g., Bauer and Köhne 1996; Cui et al. 1999; Proschan 2005), which is based on the criteria of treatment-effect size, variability, conditional power, and/or reproducibility probability. In the 2010 FDA draft guidance, SSRE methods based on blinded interim analyses of aggregate/ overall data are considered well-understood designs, and they are recommended because they do not introduce bias or impair interpretability. In contrast, statistical methods for SSRE based on knowledge of the unblinded treatment-effect sizes at an interim stage of the study are considered less well-understood designs. Such designs may have the potential of increasing the type I error rate, which is the major regulatory concern for this class of designs. As indicated in the draft guidance, a statistical adjustment is necessary for the final study analysis to protect against such an increase of the type I error rate. Note that sample size in SSRE is a random variable rather than a fixed number.

3.3.4 Drop-the-Losers Design

Drop-the-losers design is a multistage design that allows (1) dropping the inferior treatment groups, (2) modifying treatment arms, and/or (3) adding additional arms after the review of accumulated data at interim. Drop-the-losers design is also known as *selection design* or *pick-the-winner* design. It is useful in phase II trials with the ultimate goal of finding the appropriate dose, such as the minimum effective dose or the maximum tolerable dose (MTD), and the frequency of dosing for later phases of clinical development. In practice, drop-the-losers design is useful in selecting a promising dose moving forward to the later phase of clinical development, especially when there are a number of candidate doses with uncertainties.

Typically, drop-the-losers design is employed at the first stage of a two-stage design (e.g., Cohen and Sackrowitz 1989; Sampson and Sill 2005; Thall et al. 1988, 1989). At the end of the first stage, the inferior arms are dropped according to some prespecified criteria. The winners (promising arms) proceed to the next stage. In practice, such a study is often powered for achieving a desired power at the end of the second stage (or at the end of the study). In other words, there may not be any statistical power at the end of the first stage for the analysis that leads to dropping the losers. In this case, precision analysis is often considered the selection criteria, because effect size based on power analysis may be exaggerated and may consequently have a negative impact on future phase III study design. Other risks are that the investigator may pick the wrong dose group or drop a group that contains valuable information regarding dose response of the treatment under study. Therefore, the selection criteria and decision rules play important roles in drop-the-losers designs.

3.3.5 Adaptive Dose-Finding Design

Adaptive dose-finding design is often used in early-phase clinical development to identify the MTD, which is usually considered the optimal dose for later phases of clinical development. In practice, it is undesirable to have too many subjects exposed to dose-limiting toxicity (DLT), and it is desirable to have a high probability for achieving the MTD with a limited number of subjects. Thus, the selection of initial dose, dose range, and criteria for dose escalation and/or dose de-escalation is important to the success of the adaptive dose-finding design. The commonly considered adaptive dose-finding designs in the early phase of clinical development include (1) algorithm-based designs, such as the traditional dose escalation rule (TER) design (see, e.g., Storer 1989, 1993, 2001; Ting 2006) and (2) model-based designs, such as the continued reassessment method (CRM) design (e.g., Eisenbauer et al. 2000; Iasonos et al. 2008; O'Quigley et al. 1990).

The 3 + 3 TER trial design consists of entering three patients at a new dose level and then entering another three patients when a DLT is observed. The six patients are then assessed to determine whether to stop the trial at that level or to escalate to the next dose level. For CRM, the dose–response relationship is continually reassessed based on accumulative data collected from the trial. The next patient to enter the trial is then assigned to the potential MTD level. However, the model may overestimate the MTD owing to delayed response and/or a constraint on dose-jump (Chow and Chang 2011; Eisenhauer et al. 2000; Iasonos et al. 2008; Song and Chow 2015). It is not uncommon for trial sponsors to propose CRM approaches in their regulatory submissions. In general, CRM approaches are considered more efficient than the commonly used 3 + 3 rule with respect to accuracy and the allocation of the MTD, except when the true dose is among the lower levels (Iasonos et al. 2008). Note that CRM design is also known as *Bayesian sequential design* in dose-finding studies.

Note that both the drop-the-loser design and the adaptive dose-finding design are best left to exploratory or early-phase studies with the goal of obtaining information for designing subsequent studies.

3.3.6 Biomarker-Adaptive Design

Biomarker-adaptive design enables adaptations based on the response of biomarkers. A biomarker is a characteristic that is objectively measured and evaluated as an indicator of normal biologic processes, pathogenic processes, or pharmacologic responses to a therapeutic intervention (BDWG 2001;

Freidlin and Korn 2010). Biomarker-adaptive design involves biomarker qualification, standard optimal screening design, and model selection and validation. Biomarker-adaptive design is useful to (1) identify the patient population most likely to respond to the test treatment under study, (2) identify the natural course of the disease, (3) detect early disease, and (4) help in developing personalized medicine (e.g., Charkravarty 2005; Wang et al. 2007).

It should be noted that correlation between a biomarker and true clinical endpoint, regardless of the treatment given, constitutes a prognostic biomarker (Chow and Chang 2011). A prognostic biomarker informs distinct expected clinical outcomes, independent of treatment (Chow and Chang 2011; Freidlin et al. 2010). It provides information about the natural course of the disease in individuals who have or have not received the treatment under study. Prognostic biomarkers may be used to separate patients with good and poor prognosis at the time of diagnosis. In this case, stratification on prognostic biomarkers often improves design efficiency. However, prognostic biomarkers cannot be used to guide the selection of a particular therapy (Sargent et al. 2005). In contrast, a predictive biomarker informs the treatment effect on the clinical endpoint, that is, it identifies patients who are sensitive or nonsensitive to a given agent. Therefore, predictive markers can guide the choice of treatment methods (Freidlin et al. 2010; Sargent et al. 2005). Correlation between a biomarker and a true clinical endpoint does not make a predictive biomarker.

Biomarker-adaptive designs are typically used in exploratory studies, which are important in selecting the patient population for subsequent trials. However, as indicated in the draft guidance (FDA 2010a), this type of design is considered less well-understood if it is imbedded in a confirmatory trial to modify patient eligibility criteria after the interim look. In such a situation, statistical adjustment is needed to avoid increasing the type I error rate (Simon 2005).

3.3.7 Adaptive Treatment-Switching Design

Adaptive treatment-switching design allows the investigator to switch a patient's treatment from an initial assignment to an alternative treatment if there is evidence of lack of efficacy, disease progression, or safety issues associated with the initial treatment. Adaptive treatment-switching is commonly seen in oncology clinical trials owing to ethical considerations (e.g., Branson and Whitehead 2002; Shao et al. 2005; White 2006).

In a cancer trial, estimation of survival (the clinical endpoint) is a challenge when treatment-switching has occurred in some patients. In practice, it is not uncommon that up to 80% of patients may switch from one treatment to another. Such a high percentage of subjects switching because of disease progression could lead to changes in hypotheses to be tested and cause further challenges in interpreting the results (Shao et al. 2005).

3.3.8 Adaptive-Hypothesis Design

Adaptive-hypothesis design permits changes in hypotheses in response to interim analysis results. Modifications of hypotheses of ongoing clinical trials based on accrued data can certainly have an impact on the type I error rate. A typical example is to switch from a superiority hypothesis to a non-inferiority hypothesis. The purpose is to increase the probability of success of the clinical trial under study. In practice, after adaptation, we can still test for superiority after non-inferiority has been established without paying any statistical penalty due to the nature of the closed test procedure.

Some other examples of adaptive-hypothesis design include a preplanned switch from a single hypothesis to a composite hypothesis or multiple hypotheses, preplanned switching between the null hypothesis and the alternative hypothesis, and preplanned switching between the primary study endpoint and the secondary endpoints. Although adaptive-hypothesis design provides a certain flexibility for changing the hypothesis, the scientific/statistical validity needs to be carefully examined.

3.3.9 Two-Stage Phase I/II (or Phase II/III) Adaptive Design

Adaptive seamless design combines the study objectives, which are traditionally addressed in separate trials, into a single study. Most commonly used adaptive seamless designs include (1) adaptive seamless phase I/II design and (2) adaptive seamless phase II/III design. For example, two-stage phase I/II adaptive seamless design combines a phase I trial, which usually aims to find the MTD for an investigational drug, and a phase II trial, which examines the efficacy of the drug at the identified MTD. For another example, adaptive seamless phase II/III design is a two-stage design consisting of a so-called learning or exploratory stage (phase II) and a confirmatory stage (phase III) (e.g., Chow and Lin 2015).

Adaptive seamless design would use data from patients enrolled before and after the adaptation in the final analysis (Maca 2006). Thus, adaptive seamless design may reduce the study sample size compared to traditional designs. In addition, adaptive seamless design is considered more efficient because there is no lead time between the two stages, that is, the study moves to the second stage without holding the enrollment process. In practice, sponsors often propose using so-called operationally adaptive seamless designs, in which two traditional trials (e.g., phase II and phase III) are conducted under a single study protocol but analyzed separately to address each objective using data from each stage. In this case, the investigators simply enjoy the savings in time.

For adaptive seamless phase II/III design, a typical approach is to power the study for the phase III confirmatory phase and obtain valuable information with a certain assurance at the phase II learning stage. The validity and efficiency of this approach, however, has been challenged. According to the draft guidance (FDA 2010a), adaptive seamless phase II/III design is considered a less well-understood design and may introduce bias. The type I error rate may be higher than stated in this design and could be a cause for concern.

3.3.10 Multiple Adaptive Design

Multiple adaptive design is a combination of the adaptations of the above-mentioned adaptive designs. As a result, a multiple adaptive design is very complicated and its statistical properties are difficult, if not impossible, to characterize and hence are usually not fully understood and/or developed. Thus, multiple adaptive design is the least well-understood design as compared to the known adaptive designs in the literature. Thus, it is suggested that a multiple adaptive design should be used with caution to maintain the validity and integrity of the study.

3.3.11 Remarks

As noted in the draft guidance (FDA 2010a), the main concerns with designs that are less well-understood at this time include (1) control of the study-wide type I error rate, (2) minimization of the impact of any adaptation-associated statistical or operational bias on the estimates of treatment effects, and (3) the interpretability of the results. In addition, it is strongly suggested that an independent data monitoring committee be established for clinical studies utilizing adaptive designs to maintain the validity and integrity of the intended clinical trial.

3.4 Utilization of Bayesian Methods

The use of Bayesian approaches in clinical trials is of great interest in the medical product development community because it may be a valid alternative way to infer treatment effects (see Berry and Eick 1995; Berry and Stangl 1996; Berry et al. 2011; Chow et al. 2012; FDA 2010b; Gelman et al. 2003; Spiegelhalter et al. 2004). In the Bayesian paradigm, initial beliefs concerning a parameter of interest (discrete or continuous) are expressed by a prior distribution. Evidence from subsequently accumulated data is then modeled by a likelihood function for the parameter. The normalized product of the prior and the likelihood forms a so-called posterior distribution. From the Bayesian point of view, conclusions regarding the parameter of interest can then be drawn from the posterior distribution.

There is no doubt that Bayesian approaches are attractive to clinical investigators and sponsors because they provide the opportunity to continue updating information regarding the test treatment under study. An example is the ongoing I-SPY 2 breast cancer trial. In this phase II study, a Bayesian approach is employed to drive the adaptive randomization of patients with prespecified biomarker signatures to treatment arms.

Adaptive designs based on Bayesian methods have been extensively studied in recent years (e.g., Berry and Eick 1995; Berry and Stangl 1996; Berry et al. 2011; FDA 2010b; Gelman et al. 2003; Spiegelhalter et al. 2004). However, type I and type II error rates may not be controlled under Bayesian designs. Therefore, comprehensive simulations are usually required in order to estimate the type I and II error rates during the planning stage, and these may pose computational challenges if the model is complex.

As noted in the FDA guidance on the use of Bayesian statistics in medical device clinical trials (FDA 2010b), appropriate prior information should be carefully selected. Subjective priors for a confirmatory trial are generally not recommended but may provide insight during the planning stage. In addition, the choice of prior distribution, which is based on previous experience, could introduce bias into the results (Lai et al. 2011). Therefore, the utilization of Bayesian inference has been mainly limited to early-phase trials and exploratory studies. In those settings, the Bayesian framework provides a way to gain preliminary information with more parsimonious allocation of time, resources, and investigational subjects.

3.5 Benefits and Limitations of Adaptive Design

This section describes the relative advantages, limitations, and feasibility of various adaptive designs.

3.5.1 Possible Benefits

As indicated by Chow and Corey (2011), the use of adaptive design methods in clinical trials entails the following possible benefits: (1) they allow the investigator to correct wrong assumptions made at the beginning of the trial; (2) they help the investigator to select the most promising option early; (3) they make use of external information (e.g., recent publications in the literature); (4) they enable the investigator to react earlier to surprises (either positive or negative); and (5) they may shorten the development time and consequently speed up the development process.

The use of adaptive design methods in clinical research and development may provide the investigator a second chance to modify or reevaluate the trial after seeing data from the trial itself at interim. However, despite the flexibility and possible benefits of adaptive design methods in clinical trials, it should be noted that valid statistical inference is often difficult, if not impossible, under complicated adaptive designs.

3.5.2 Limitations

Both Chow et al. (2005) and Gallo et al. (2006) indicated that adaptive design methods must not undermine the validity and integrity of a trial (see also Emerson 2006). *Validity* is defined as (1) minimization of operational biases that may be introduced when applying adaptations to the trial, (2) correct or valid statistical inference, and (3) results that are convincing (e.g., accurate and reliable) to the broader scientific community. *Integrity* is defined as (1) minimizing operational biases, (2) maintaining data confidentiality, and (3) assuring consistency during the conduct of the trial, especially when multistage adaptive design is used. As indicated in the FDA draft guidance (FDA 2010a), bias introduced through adaptive design methods can adversely affect decision-making during the conduct of a trial. However, adaptations based on blinded analyses at interim, if the blinding is strictly maintained, can largely reduce or completely avoid bias.

3.6 Regulatory and Statistical Concerns

From a statistical point of view, major adaptations (significant modifications to trial and/or statistical procedures) could have three kinds of undesired results: they could introduce bias/variation to data collection, result in a shift in the target patient population, and cause inconsistencies between the hypotheses to be tested and the corresponding statistical tests. Chow (2006) indicated that the misuse and/or abuse of adaptive design methods in clinical trials could lead to inconsistencies between hypotheses to be tested and corresponding statistical tests where (1) there are wrong tests for the right hypotheses (i.e., validity is a concern); (2) there are right tests for the wrong hypotheses (evidence of the misuse of certain adaptations); (3) there are wrong tests for the wrong hypotheses (evidence of abuse of adaptive design methods); and (4) there are right tests for the right hypotheses with insufficient power.

Practically, the use of adaptive design methods in clinical trials may introduce operational bias. It may not be possible to preserve the overall type I error rate at the prespecified level of significance owing to multiple adaptation options or biased estimates of the treatment effect at interim. Thus, p-values may not be correct. In addition, adaptive design methods may inflate the type II error rate because of the limited amount of interim data. Therefore, using adaptive designs may result in a totally different trial that cannot address the medical questions that the original study was intended to answer.

The 2010 FDA draft guidance (FDA 2010a) provided sponsors with information on the clinical, statistical, and regulatory aspects of adaptive designs.

As mentioned above, the draft guidance classified adaptive designs as either well-understood or less well-understood. Many statistical issues surrounding the less well-understood designs were discussed in the draft guidance representing the FDA's current thinking. As noted in the section "Types of Adaptive Design," the chief concerns with these designs noted in the draft guidance are control of the study-wide type I error rate, minimization of the impact of any adaptation-associated statistical or operational bias on the estimates of treatment effects, and the interpretability of the results.

3.7 Application of HIV-1 Vaccine Trials

For application of adaptive design methods in vaccine clinical development, without loss of generalizability, we consider the example concerning HIV-1 vaccine development described in Corey et al. (2011).

Corey et al. (2011) pointed out that developing a vaccine against the human immunodeficiency virus (HIV) is a great challenge to an investigator or sponsor especially because there are no documented cases of immune-mediated clearance of HIV from an infected individual and no known correlates of immune protection. Although nonhuman primate models of some infections such as lentivirus have provided valuable data about HIV pathogenesis, it is not clear whether such nonhuman models are predictive of HIV vaccine efficacy in humans. Corey et al. (2011) suggested that vaccines to the pathogen with combined lack of a predictive animal model and undefined biomarkers of immune protection against HIV be tested directly in clinical trials utilizing adaptive designs. The use of adaptive design methods in vaccine clinical trials not only can accelerate vaccine development by rapidly screening out poor vaccines but also extends the evaluation of efficacious ones and consequently improves the characterization of promising vaccine candidates and the identification of correlates of immune protection.

Corey et al. (2011) indicated that four HIV vaccine efficacy trials have been undertaken since the late 1990s, which have provided some insights into host immune protection. Figure 3.1 summarizes the timeline of these vaccine trials during the development process. As indicated in Figure 3.1, the first two phase III clinical trials of an HIV vaccine were initiated in 1998 by VaxGen. The vaccine, which is a gp120 subunit immunogen mixed with alum adjuvant that generated only limited levels of neutralizing antibodies in phase I and II clinical trials, showed no efficacy in men who had sex with men or injecting drug users (Flynn et al. 2005; Gilbert et al. 2005a, 2005b; Pitisuttithum et al. 2006). The next HIV vaccine efficacy trial (the STEP trial) was initiated in 2005 to evaluate a vaccine that

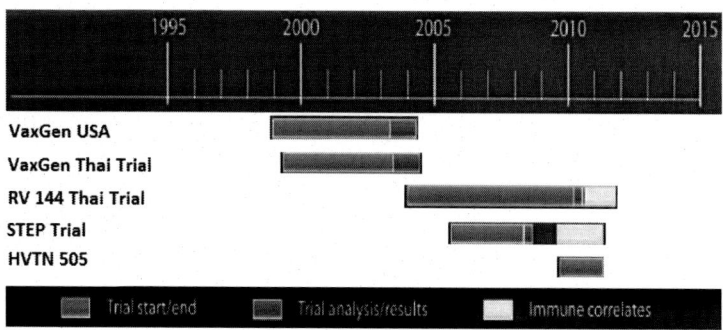

FIGURE 3.1
Milestones of HIV vaccine efficacy trials. (Corey, L., et al., *Sci. Transl. Med.*, 3(79), 79, 2011.)

primarily stimulated T-cell immunity with a recombinant adenovirus (Ad5) vector. This immunogen was found to induce robust T-cell responses to HIV gene products inside the viral particle. Despite the high immunogenicity of this vaccine, there was no reduction in acquisition or long-term control of postinfection viremia (Buchbinder et al. 2008). In addition, a *post hoc* analysis demonstrated an unexpected interaction in those vaccine recipients who were both uncircumcised and immune to Ad5 prior to vaccination (Rolland et al. 2011). Uncircumcised Ad5-seropositive male recipients experienced an increased rate of HIV infection for the first 18 months after the immunization regimen. This effect fortunately waned over time, such that between months 18 and 36 of follow-up the risk of acquisition among these men equaled that of placebo (Buchbinder et al. 2008). The mechanism of these vaccine interactions, however, remains undefined.

Based on the review of the HIV vaccine efficacy trials described above, developing an effective HIV vaccine is possible. The development process, however, is not efficient and painfully slow. Thus, there is a need to accelerate the development process of vaccine clinical research. For this purpose, Corey et al. (2011) suggested adaptive trial designs be used in vaccine clinical trials to provide a sound scientific basis for the following:

1. Developing data on what types of immune responses or signatures, whether they be humoral, adaptive, or innate, are associated with vaccine-induced protection. Such signatures require close collaboration between sophisticated laboratory investigations and human vaccine efficacy trials.

2. Changing the traditional approach to clinical translational research, that is, from sequential human trials that take years to complete to parallel adaptive hypothesis-generating clinical trials evaluated in real time, which can both inform the field with regard to the immunological basis for the prevention of HIV infection and accelerate the path to a highly effective HIV vaccine.

Adaptive trial designs allow modification of the trial in response to the review of interim data acquired during the study. Adaptations to the vaccine trial require access to evolving clinical data earlier (usually at interim) in the process of vaccine development and may accelerate (e.g., go/no-go) decisions about vaccines. Adaptive design can prespecify one or more decision points in the trial, based on the review of interim data. Adaptations may be divided into two major types: those governed by prespecified rules and those that make unplanned changes. FDA (2010) recommends the first type because the second type may lead to bias and reduced statistical power and may complicate the interpretation of results. In practice, it is suggested that close monitoring of the trial utilizing adaptive design methods should be performed, allowing an adaptation of the trial after it has begun. This might mean stopping the trial for lack of efficacy or adapting the trial if efficacy is observed. This adaptation could include vaccinating the placebo group for immune correlate analyses, adding a booster vaccination if vaccine efficacy appears to wane, or expanding the trial design to include a higher risk population. Despite the advantages of adaptive designs, there are certain disadvantages associated with the approach. For example, decisions may sometimes be based on preliminary data with insufficient power. Care must also be taken to preserve the integrity and objectivity of the trial.

As indicated by Corey et al. (2011), in addition to enabling more rapid assessment and elimination of ineffective vaccines, adaptive trial designs may also allow the definition of immunological and virological factors that affect HIV acquisition to be more readily defined. For example, if vaccine efficacy studies are performed in populations with a high incidence of HIV infection, this information can be ascertained more expeditiously, with greater certainty, and possibly with greater cost-efficiency. Additionally, if multiple phase II studies can be conducted in parallel, with the capability of examining efficacy endpoints and immune correlates in real time, the likelihood for advancing a successful vaccine to an efficacy trial in a more rapid time frame will increase greatly (Figure 3.2). Moreover, the ability to see common immunological findings either with different vaccine regimens or the same vaccine regimen in different populations (e.g., men vs. women) provides more than circumstantial evidence that such responses have an underlying biological basis.

3.8 Concluding Remarks

The motivation behind the use of adaptive design methods in clinical trials includes (1) the flexibility of being able to modify trial and statistical procedures for identifying the best clinical benefits of a product under study and (2) the possibility of shortening the development time of the compound. In practice, adaptations or modifications to trial and/or statistical procedures

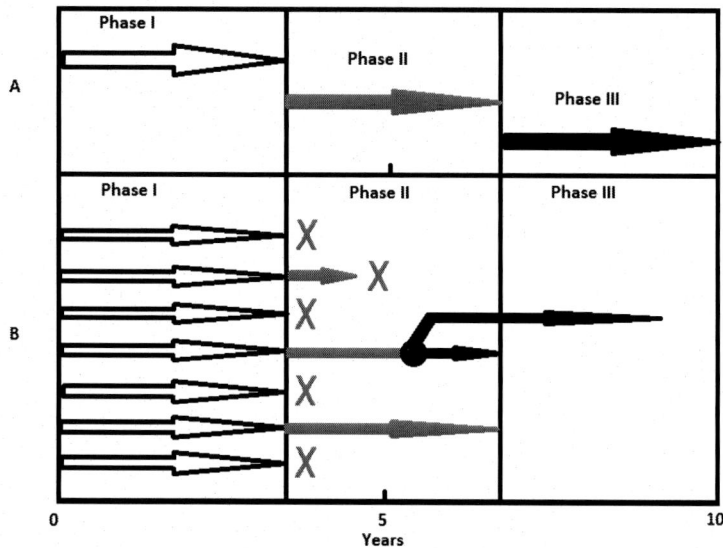

FIGURE 3.2
Adaptive trial designs accelerate vaccine development. (Corey, L., et al., *Sci. Transl. Med.*, 3(79), 79, 2011.)

of ongoing clinical trials may be necessary if the changes reflect real medical practice on the actual patient population with the disease under study; they may therefore increase the probability of successfully identifying the potential clinical benefit of the treatment under investigation. From the clinical point of view, adaptive designs provide the investigator a second chance to evaluate the trial with more relevant data observed at interim. However, adaptations of ongoing clinical trials based on accrued data will certainly have an immediate impact on statistical inference concerning the treatment effect.

As the FDA released the draft guidance on adaptive design clinical trials (FDA 2010a), the use of adaptive design methods in clinical trials was moving in the right direction. However, there is still a long way to go until all of the scientific issues from the clinical, statistical, and regulatory perspectives are addressed properly (see also Coffey and Kairalla 2008). In the draft guidance, sponsors were encouraged to gain experience through the implementation of adaptive design methods in early-phase trials and/or exploratory studies. For confirmatory trials involving a less well-understood adaptive design, communications between sponsors and the regulatory body during the planning stage was recommended. Note that early stops for futility in phase III studies may have an impact on overall type I error. Therefore, comprehensive simulation studies with and without stops for futility should be considered. In addition, the qualifications, composition, role/responsibility, and function/activity of a data-monitoring committee for implementation of adaptive trial design need to be established for an objective and unbiased assessment of the treatment effect of the drug under investigation (Chow et al. 2012; Quinlan and Krams 2006). Thus, Chow and Corey (2011) suggested that, despite escalating momentum, adaptive design methods should be implemented in clinical trials with caution. Meanwhile, valid statistical methods for less well-understood adaptive designs with various adaptations should be developed to prevent the possible misuse and/or abuse of adaptive design methods in clinical trials (Woodcock 2005).

References

Bartlett RH, Roloff DW, Cornell RG, Andrews AF, Dillon PW, and Zwischenberger JB. (1985). Extracorporeal circulation in neonatal respiratory failure: A prospective randomized study. *Pediatrics* 76:479487.

Bauer P, Köhne K. (1996). Evaluation of experiments with adaptive interim analyses. *Biometrics* 52:380.

BDWG. (2001). Biomarkers and surrogate endpoints: Preferred definitions and conceptual framework. *Clin. Pharmacol. Ther.* 69:89–95.

Berry DA and Eick SG. (1995). Adaptive assignment versus balanced randomization in clinical trials: A decision analysis. *Stat. Med.* 14:231–246.

Berry DA and Stangl DK. (1996). *Bayesian Biostatistics*. Marcel Dekker, New York.

Berry SM, Carlin BP, Lee JJ, and Muller P. (2011). *Bayesian Adaptive Methods for Clinical Trials*. Chapman and Hall, Boca Raton, FL.

Branson M and Whitehead J. (2002). Estimating a treatment effect in survival studies in which patients switch treatment. *Stat. Med.* 21:2449–2463.

Buchbinder SP, Mehrotra DV, Duerr A, Fitzgerald DW, Mogg R, Li D, Gilbert PB, et al. (2008). Efficacy assessment of a cell-mediated immunity HIV-1 vaccine (the Step Study): A double-blind, randomized, placebo-controlled, test-of-concept trial. *Lancet* 372:1881–1893.

Charkravarty A. (2005). Regulatory aspects in using surrogate markers in clinical trials. In *The Evaluation of Surrogate Endpoints*, eds. Burzykowski T, Molenberghs G, Buys M. Springer, New York, pp. 13–51.

Chow SC. (2006). Adaptive design methods in clinical trials. *Int. Chin. Stat. Assoc. Bull.* 200:37–41.

Chow SC and Chang M. (2008). Adaptive design methods in clinical trials—A review. *Orphanet J. Rare Dis.* 3:11.

Chow SC and Chang M. (2011). *Adaptive Design Methods in Clinical Trials*. 2nd Edition, Chapman and Hall, New York.

Chow SC, Chang M, and Pong A. (2005). Statistical consideration of adaptive methods in clinical development. *J. Biopharm. Stat.* 15:575–591.

Chow SC and Corey R. (2011). Benefits, challenges and obstacles of adaptive designs in clinical trials. *Orphanet J. Rare Dis.* 6:79.

Chow SC, Corey R, and Lin M. (2012). On the independence of data monitoring committee in adaptive design clinical trials. *J. Biopharm. Stat.* 22:853–867.

Chow SC and Lin M. (2015). Analysis of two-stage adaptive seamless trial design. *Pharm. Anal. Acta* 6:3. doi: http://dx.doi.org/10.4172/2153-2435.1000341

Coffey CS and Kairalla JA. (2008). Adaptive clinical trials: Progress and challenges. *Drugs R D.* 9:229–242.

Cohen A and Sackrowitz HB. (1989). Exact tests that recover interblock information in balanced incomplete block design. *J. Am. Stat. Assoc.* 84:556–559.

Corey L, Nabel GJ, Dieffenbach C, Gilbert P, Haynes BF, Johnston M, Kublin J, et al. (2011). HIV-1 vaccines and adaptive trial designs. *Sci. Transl. Med.* 3(79):79. doi: 10.1126/scitranslmed.3001863

Cui L, Hung HMJ, and Wang SJ. (1999). Modification of sample size in group sequential trials. *Biometrics* 55:853–857.

Eisenhauer EA, O'Dwyer PJ, Christian M, and Humphrey JS. (2000). Phase I clinical trial design in cancer drug development. *J. Clin. Oncol.* 18(3):684–692.

EMA. (2006). *Methodological Issues in Confirmatory Clinical Trials with Flexible Design and Analysis Plan.* Reflection paper, CPMP/EWP/2459/02, European Medicines Agency, London, UK.

EMEA. (2002). *Point to Consider on Methodological Issues in Confirmatory Clinical Trials with Flexible Design and Analysis Plan. European Agency for the Evaluation of Medicinal Products Evaluation of Medicines for Human Use.* CPMP/EWP/2459/02, EMEA, London, UK.

Emerson SS. (2006). Issues in the use of adaptive clinical trial designs. *Stat. Med.* 25:3270–3296.

FDA. (2004). *Innovation or Stagnation: Challenges and Opportunity on the Critical Path to New Medical Products.* United States Food and Drug Administration, Rockville, MD.

FDA. (2010a). *Draft Guidance for Industry—Adaptive Design Clinical Trials for Drugs and Biologics.* US Food and Drug Administration, Rockville, MD.

FDA. (2010b). *Guidance for the Use of Bayesian Statistics in Medical Device Clinical Trials.* US Food and Drug Administration, Rockville, MD.

Flynn NM, Forthal DN, Harro CD, Judson FN, Mayer KH, and Para MF. (2005). Placebo-controlled phase 3 trial of a recombinant glycoprotein 120 vaccine to prevent HIV-1 infection. *J. Infect. Dis.* 191:654–665.

Freidlin B and Korn EL. (2010). Biomarker-adaptive clinical trial designs. *Pharmacogenomics* 11(12):1679–1682.

Freidlin B, McShane L, and Korn EL. (2010). Randomized clinical trials with biomarkers: Design issues. *J. Natl. Cancer Inst.* 102(3):152–160.

Gallo P, Chuang-Stein C, Dragalin V, Gaydos B, Krams M, and Pinheiro J, PhRMA Working Group. (2006). Adaptive design in clinical drug development—An executive summary of the PhRMA Working Group (with discussions). *J. Biopharm. Stat.* 16:275–283.

Gelman A, Carlin JB, Stein H, and Rubin DB. (2003). *Bayesian Data Analysis.* 2nd Edition, Chapman, New York.

Gilbert PB, Ackers ML, Berman PW, Francis DP, Popovic V, Hu DJ, Heyward WL, Sinangil F, Shepherd BE, and Gurwith M. (2005a). HIV-1 virologic and immunologic progression and initiation of antiretroviral therapy among HIV-1-infected subjects in a trial of the efficacy of recombinant glycoprotein 120 vaccine. *J. Infect. Dis.* 192:974–983.

Gilbert PB, Peterson ML, Follmann D, Hudgens MG, Francis DP, Gurwith M, Heyward WL, et al. (2005b). Correlation between immunologic responses to a recombinant glycoprotein 120 vaccine and incidence of HIV-1 infection in a phase 3 HIV-1 preventive vaccine trial. *J. Infect. Dis.* 191:666–677.

Gould AL. (1992). Interim analyses for monitoring clinical trials that do not materially affect the type I error rate. *Stat. Med.* 11:55–66.

Gould AL. (1995). Planning and revising the sample size for a trial. *Stat. Med.* 14: 1039–1051.

Iasonos A, Wilton AS, Riedel ER, Seshan VE, and Spriggs DR. (2008). A comprehensive comparison of the continual reassessment method to the standard 3 + 3 dose escalation scheme in Phase I dose-finding studies. *Clin. Trials* 5(5):465–477.

Lai TL, Lavori PW, and Shih MC. (2011). Adaptive trial designs. *Annu. Rev. Pharmacol. Toxicol.*52:101–110.

Maca J, Bhattacharya S, Dragalin V, Gallo P, and Krams M. (2006). Adaptive seamless phase II/III designs-background, operational aspects, and examples. *Drug Info. J.* 40:463–4674.

Mugford M, Elbourne D, and Field D. (2008). Extracorporeal membrane oxygenation for severe respiratory failure in newborn infants. *Cochrane Database Syst. Rev.* 3:CD001340.

O'Quigley J, Pepe M, and Fisher L. (1990). Continual reassessment method: A practical design for Phase 1 clinical trials in cancer. *Biometrics* 46(1):33–48.

Pitisuttithum P, Gilbert P, Gurwith M, Heyward W, Martin M, van Griensven F, Hu D, Tappero JW, and Choopanya K. (2006). Randomized, double-blind, placebo-controlled efficacy trial of a bivalent recombinant glycoprotein 120 HIV-1 vaccine among injection drug users in Bangkok, Thailand. *J Infect. Dis.* 194:1661–1671.

Proschan MA. (2005). Two-stage sample size re-estimation based on a nuisance parameter: A review. *J. Biopharm. Stat.* 15:539–574.

Quinlan JA and Krams M. (2006). Implementing adaptive designs: Logistical and operational considerations. *Drug Inf. J.* 40(4):437–444.

Rolland M, Tovanabutra S, deCamp AC, Frahm N, Gilbert PB, Sanders-Buell E, Heath L, et al. (2011). Genetic impact of vaccination on breakthrough HIV-1 sequences from the Step trial. *Nat. Med.* 17:366–371.

Sampson AR and Sill MW. (2005). Drop-the-loser design: Normal case (with discussions). *Biom. J.* 47:257–281.

Sargent DJ, Conley BA, Allegra C, and Collette L. (2005). Clinical trial designs for predictive marker validation in cancer treatment trials. *J. Clin. Oncol.* 23:2020–2027.

Shao J, Chang M, and Chow SC. (2005). Statistical inference for cancer trials with treatment switching. *Stat. Med.* 24:1783–1790.

Simon R. (2005). Roadmap for developing and validating therapeutically relevant genomic classifiers. *J. Clin. Oncol.* 23:7332–7341.

Song FY and Chow SC. (2015). A case study for radiation therapy dose finding utilizing Bayesian sequential trial design. *J. Case Stud.* 4(6):78–83.

Spiegelhalter DJ, Abrams KR, and Myles JP. (2004). *Bayesian Approach to Clinical Trials and Health-Care Evaluation.* Wiley, Chichester, UK.

Storer BE. (1989). Design and analysis of phase I clinical trials. *Biometrics* 45:925–937.

Storer BE. (1993). Small-sample confidence sets for the MTD in a phase I clinical trial. *Biometrics* 49:1117–1125.

Storer BE. (2001). An evaluation of phase I clinical trial designs in the continuous dose-response setting. *Stat. Med.* 20:2399–2408.

Thall PF, Simon R, and Ellenberg SS. (1988). Two-stage selection and testing designs for clinical trials. *Biometrika* 75:303–310.

Thall PF, Simon R, and Ellenberg SS. (1989). A two stage design for choosing among several experimental treatments and a control in clinical trials. *Biometrics* 45: 537–547.

Ting NT. (2006). *Dose Finding in Drug Development*. Springer, New York.

Wang SJ, O'Neill RT, and Hung HM. (2007). Approaches to evaluation of treatment effect in randomized clinical trials with genomic subset. *Pharm. Stat.* 6(3):227–244.

Wei LJ. (1978). The adaptive biased-coin design for sequential experiments. *Ann. Stat.* 9:92–100.

White IR. (2006). Letter to the editor: Estimating treatment effects in randomized trials with treatment switching. *Stat. Med.* 25:1619–1622.

Woodcock J. (2005). DFA introduction comments: Clinical studies design and evaluation issues. *Clin. Trials* 2:273–275.

4

Generalizing Evidence from HIV Trials Using Inverse Probability of Sampling Weights

Ashley L. Buchanan
University of Rhode Island, Kingston, RI

Michael G. Hudgens and Stephen R. Cole
University of North Carolina, Chapel Hill, NC

CONTENTS

4.1 Introduction

Generalizability is a concern for many scientific studies, including those in HIV/AIDS research (Cole and Stuart 2010; Hernan and VanderWeele

2011; Stuart et al. 2011, 2015; Tipton 2013). Using information in the study sample, it is often of interest to draw inferences about a specified target population. Therefore, it is important to consider the degree to which an effect estimated from a study sample approximates the true effect in the target population. This is particularly important for HIV because results from trials inform national-level policy for HIV treatment and care. For example, in clinical trials of treatment for HIV-infected individuals, there is often concern that trial participants are not representative of the larger population of HIV-positive individuals. Greenblatt (2011) highlighted the overrepresentation of African-American and Hispanic women among HIV cases in the United States and the limited clinical trial participation of members of these groups. The Women's Interagency HIV Study (WIHS) is a prospective, observational, multicenter study considered to be representative of women living with HIV and women at risk for HIV infection in the United States (Bacon et al. 2005). However, a review of the eligibility criteria of 20 AIDS Clinical Trials Group (ACTG) studies found that 28% to 68% of the HIV-positive women in the WIHS cohort would have been excluded from these trials (Gandhi et al. 2005).

4.1.1 Background

The internal validity of causal effect estimates in randomized controlled trials or observational studies, including the application of methods to minimize the potential for bias due to measurement error, confounding, selection, and model misspecification, is well described (Hernán and Robins 2006).

However, methods to improve external validity have received considerably less attention. For the purposes of this chapter, *external validity* refers to the extent to which an internally valid treatment (or exposure or intervention) effect estimator is consistent for the treatment effect in the target population of interest (Cole and Stuart 2010). External validity encompasses generalizability and transportability. This chapter focuses on generalizability— we refer readers with an interest in transportability to Bareinboim and Pearl (2013). Generalizability is discussed herein using a potential outcomes framework (Neyman 1923).

In public health research, investigators would ideally like to estimate a treatment effect in a target population. In practice, a study sample is typically obtained from a source population that is likely different from the target population, and information from the study sample is used to estimate effects (Rothman et al. 2008). This source population is often chosen instead of the target population due to such reasons as financial or time constraints and ethical considerations. The target population may be defined prior to designing or implementing a specific study, or researchers may be interested in drawing inferences from a published study to a different target population. Once the target population is defined, the question becomes to what extent the sample average treatment effect (i.e., the effect of treatment in the trial/study) approximates the population treatment effect (i.e., the effect of treatment in the target population) (Stuart et al. 2011, 2015).

In an ideal randomized trial (i.e., with full adherence to treatment, no loss to follow-up, and no measurement error) or in an observational study where the treatment effect is identifiable (i.e., assuming exchangeability between the exposed and unexposed conditional on measured covariates, well-defined treatments, and a positive probability of exposure within each strata of covariates), the estimator in the study sample will be unbiased for the sample average treatment effect. Even under these ideal circumstances when our estimator is internally valid, the sample average treatment effect may still not be equal to the population average treatment effect (PATE), that is, the results may not be externally valid. Results obtained in one study may not generalize to target populations due to (i) differences in the distribution of effect modifiers in the study population and target population, (ii) the presence of interference, or (iii) the existence of multiple versions of treatment (Bareinboim and Pearl 2013; Hernan and VanderWeele 2011; Stuart et al. 2011).

Most discussions of generalizability of trial results are limited to considering whether the study sample was representative of the target population. Ensuring a trial is a random sample from the target population yields generalizable results (Stuart et al. 2011). However, this is not always feasible or appropriate. Rothman et al. (2013) notes that a representative sample is not necessary for generalizability if the causal effect is homogeneous across individuals. In many settings, however, assuming the effect of a treatment or exposure is homogeneous is dubious. Therefore, recently methods have been developed for generalizing trial results relying on weaker assumptions (Buchanan et al. 2015; Cole and Stuart 2010; Stuart et al. 2011, 2015; Tipton 2013). These methods can provide externally valid treatment effect estimates in the target population using trial data that is not necessarily based on a random sample, better informing scale-up of interventions and public health policy decisions.

4.1.2 Public Health Examples

We highlight two public health studies in which generalizability issues had an impact on the scientific conclusions and policy decisions. A meta-analysis of trials of antidepressants in adolescents that suggested an increased risk of suicide among the treated (Hammad et al. 2006). However, observational studies did not confirm this increased risk (Simon et al. 2006; Valuck et al. 2004). The majority of these trials excluded participants with the most severe depression who would have experienced the greatest benefits from the therapy and Greenhouse et al. (2008) posited that the exclusion of those at high risk of the event could lead to an upwardly biased rate ratio. In this instance, while the trial effects may have been internally valid, the lack of external validity had serious implications for policy: the Food and Drug Administration justified issuing a black box warning based on the trials advising physicians and patients of this increased suicide risk, limiting potentially beneficial treatment options for depressed adolescent patients.

The Women's Health Initiative randomized trial found an increased risk of coronary heart disease (CHD) among women assigned to estrogen/progestin therapy as compared to those on placebo (Grodstein et al. 1996, 2000). Observational studies, such as the Nurses' Health Study (Manson et al. 2003), had previously reported that hormone use reduced CHD risk. The discrepancies between the conclusions about the effects based on the Women's Health Initiative trial and the Nurses' Health Study could be framed as a generalizability problem if we consider that the age and time-on-exposure stratum-specific effects of hormone replacement therapy estimated in both studies were similar (Hernán et al. 2008), but the distribution of women by age and time on exposure in the target population (young women with no prior exposure) did not match the distribution of women in the study sample from the Nurses' Health Study (older women with substantial prior exposure). In this instance, while lack of internal validity (confounding by some unmeasured factor) was initially blamed for the discrepancy, generalizability of results in this observational study also impacted policy recommendations. Such examples highlight the importance of considering both internal and external validity in study design.

4.1.3 Sampling Score Methods to Generalize Trial Results

There are several methods that provide a quantitative approach for generalizing results from a randomized trial to a specified target population. Some of these methods utilize a model of the probability of trial participation conditional on covariates. Herein, we refer to this conditional probability as the *sampling score*. Generalizability methods employing sampling scores are akin to methods that use treatment propensity scores to adjust for measured confounding (Rubin 1980) and include the use of inverse probability of sampling weights and stratification based on sampling scores. For example, Cole and Stuart (2010) and Buchanan et al. (2015) estimated sampling scores using logistic regression and then employed an inverse probability of sampling weighted (IPSW) method to estimate the treatment effect in the target population. Another approach to generalizing trial results entails an estimator based on stratifying individuals according to their estimated sampling scores (O'Muircheartaigh and Hedges 2013; Tipton 2013; Tipton et al. 2014). To date, there has been a limited number of formal studies or derivations of the large sample statistical properties of these generalizability estimators (i.e., consistency and asymptotic normality) (Buchanan et al. 2015).

In this chapter, we consider extensions of these sampling score methods when a time-to-event outcome is of interest. Time-to-event endpoints are common in HIV/AIDS trials. If the trial is a random sample from the target population, standard time-to-event statistical methods, such as the Kaplan–Meier (KM) estimator and the log rank test (Kalbfleisch and Prentice 2002), will yield valid inferences about the effect of treatment on survival in the target population. However, when the trial sampling mechanism is possibly nonrandom, then standard methods are not guaranteed to provide valid inferences about the survival distribution in the target population.

In this chapter, we focus on the survival distributions in the study sample and target population. Alternatively, the hazard ratio might be considered as the parameter of interest; however, although the hazard ratio is a common summary parameter to compare survival distributions between exposure groups, there are drawbacks to focusing inference on hazard ratios. For instance, the hazard ratio can be difficult to interpret, especially when trying to summarize the effect of a treatment or exposure (Cole and Hernan 2004; Hernan 2010). Presenting estimated survival curves is an alternative to reporting hazard ratios that may be more interpretable because survival curves summarize all information from baseline up to any time t. The IPSW estimator developed below for generalizing trial results is similar to the inverse probability of exposure and inverse probability of censoring weighted KM estimators, which have been proposed to adjust for confounding and selection bias, respectively (Kaufman 2010; Robins and Finkelstein 2000; Xie and Liu 2005).

4.1.4 Overview

In this chapter, we consider estimators based on sampling scores to generalize trial effects to a specified target population. In particular, previously proposed IPSW and stratified estimators for target population effects are extended to the setting where there is right censoring. The outline of the remainder of this chapter is as follows. In Section 4.2, assumptions and notation are discussed. The IPSW and stratified estimators are presented in Section 4.3, and empirical properties of the estimators are investigated in a simulation study in Section 4.4. In Section 4.5, the IPSW and stratified estimators are used to generalize results from two ACTG trials to all people currently living with HIV in the United States. Related work and caveats of this method are discussed in Section 4.6.

4.2 Assumptions and Notation

Suppose we are interested in drawing inferences about a treatment effect (e.g., drug) on a time-to-event outcome (e.g., time to disease onset) in a specified target population. Assume each individual in the target population has two potential outcomes T^0 and T^1, where T^0 is the event time that would have been seen if (possibly contrary to fact) the individual received control, and T^1 is the event time that would have been seen if (possibly contrary to fact) the individual received treatment. Let $\mathfrak{S}^1(t) = P(T^1 > t)$ and $\mathfrak{S}^0(t) = P(T^0 > t)$ denote the survival functions for the potential outcomes in the target population.

Consider a setting where two data sets are available. A random sample (e.g., cohort study) of m individuals is drawn from the target population. A second sample of n individuals participate in a randomized trial. Unlike the cohort study, the trial participants are not necessarily assumed to be a random sample from the target population but rather may be a biased sample. The following random variables are observed for the cohort and trial participants. In general, let uppercase letters denote random variables and lowercase letters denote realizations of those random variables. Define Z as a $1 \times p$ vector of fixed covariates and assume that information on Z is available for those in the trial and those in the cohort. Let $S = 1$ denote trial participation and $S = 0$ otherwise. For those individuals who participate in the trial, define X as the treatment indicator, where $X = 1$ if assigned to treatment and $X = 0$ otherwise. Let $T = XT^1 + (1 - X)T^0$ and C be the censoring time, assuming a single censoring mechanism in the trial; that is, censoring does not differ by treatment assignment. Define $T^* = \min(T, C)$ and let δ be the event indicator with $\delta = 1$ if $T \leq C$ and $\delta = 0$ if $T > C$. Assume (S, Z) is observed for cohort participants and (S, Z, X, T^*) is observed for trial participants. Assume trial participants are randomly assigned to receive treatment or not, such that the treatment assignment mechanism is ignorable, that is, $P(X = x \mid S = 1, Z, T^0, T^1) = P(X = x \mid S = 1)$. Assume an ignorable trial participation mechanism conditional on Z, that is, $P(S = s \mid Z, T^0, T^1) = P(S = s \mid Z)$. In other words, participants in the trial are no different from nonparticipants regarding the treatment–outcome relationship conditional on Z. Trial participation and treatment positivity (Westreich and Cole 2010) are also assumed, that is, $P(S = 1 \mid Z = z) > 0$ for all z such that $P(Z = z) > 0$ and $P(X = x \mid S = 1) > 0$ for $x = 0, 1$. Assume participants in the trial are adherent to their treatment assignment (i.e., there is full compliance). It is assumed throughout that the stable unit treatment value assumption (Rubin 1978) holds, that is, there are no variations of treatment and there is no interference between individuals; that is, the outcome of one individual is assumed to be unaffected by the treatment of others.

Parameters of interest to quantify the treatment effect in the population include the causal risk difference (RD) defined as $RD(t) = \mathfrak{S}^1(t) - \mathfrak{S}^0(t)$ and the causal risk ratio (RR) defined as $RR(t) = \mathfrak{S}^1(t)/\mathfrak{S}^0(t)$ for $t > 0$. The difference in mean survival times defined by $\Delta = \mu_1 - \mu_0$ where $\mu_x = E(T^x)$ for $x = 0, 1$ may also be of interest. The estimand Δ is sometimes referred to as the population average treatment effect (PATE). However, in the presence of administrative censoring typical of biomedical studies, Δ may not be identifiable from the observable data without strong (parametric) assumptions.

4.3 Inference about Population Treatment Effects

4.3.1 No Censoring

First suppose there is no right censoring, such that T is observed for all trial participants. A traditional (i.e., unweighted) approach to estimating treatment effects is a difference in outcome means between the two randomized arms of the trial. Let $i = 1, \ldots, n + m$ index the trial and cohort participants. The within-trial estimator is defined as

$$\hat{\Delta}_T = \frac{\sum_i S_i T_i X_i}{\sum_i S_i X_i} - \frac{\sum_i S_i T_i (1 - X_i)}{\sum_i S_i (1 - X_i)},$$

where here and in the sequel $\sum_i = \sum_{i=1}^{n+m}$. If trial participants are assumed to constitute a random sample from the target population, it is straightforward to show $\hat{\Delta}_T$ is a consistent and asymptotically normal estimator of Δ. By contrast, if we are not willing to assume trial participants are a random sample from the target population, then $\hat{\Delta}_T$ is no longer guaranteed to be consistent.

Below we consider two estimators of Δ that do not assume trial participants are a random sample from the target population. Both estimators utilize sampling scores. Following Cole and Stuart (2010), assume a logistic regression model for the sampling scores such that $P(S = 1 | Z = z) = \{1 + \exp(-z\beta)\}^{-1}$, where β is a $p \times 1$ vector of coefficient parameters. Let $\hat{\beta}$ denote the weighted maximum likelihood estimator of β, where each trial participant has weight $\Pi_{S_i}^{-1} = 1$ and each individual in the cohort has weight $\Pi_{S_i}^{-1} = m/(N-n)$, where N is the size of the target population (Scott and Wild 1986). Because the cohort is assumed to be a representative sample of the target, we inflate the size of the cohort to that of the target population. This allows for consistent estimation of the sampling scores. Let $P(S = 1 | Z = z) = w(z, \beta)$, $w_i = w(Z_i, \beta)$, and $\hat{w}_i = w(Z_i, \hat{\beta})$. The IPSW estimator (Buchanan et al. 2015; Cole and Stuart 2010) of the PATE is

$$\hat{\Delta}_{IPSW} = \hat{\mu}_1 - \hat{\mu}_0 = \frac{\sum_i S_i T_i X_i / \hat{w}_i}{\sum_i S_i X_i / \hat{w}_i} - \frac{\sum_i S_i T_i (1 - X_i) / \hat{w}_i}{\sum_i S_i (1 - X_i) / \hat{w}_i}. \quad (4.1)$$

Another approach for estimating the PATE uses stratification based on the sampling scores (O'Muircheartaigh and Hedges 2013; Tipton 2013; Tipton et al. 2014) and is computed in the following steps. First, β is estimated using a logistic regression model as described above and the estimated sampling scores $\hat{w}_i$ are computed. These estimated sampling scores are used to form L strata. The difference of sample means within each stratum is computed among those in the trial. The PATE is then estimated as a weighted sum of the differences of sample means across strata. The stratum specific weights used in computing this weighted average equal estimates of the proportion of individuals in the target population within the stratum. Specifically, let n_l be the number of individuals in the trial in stratum l and m_l be the number of individuals in the cohort in stratum l. Let $S_{il} = 1$ denote trial participation for individual i in stratum l for $i = 1, \ldots, (n_l + m_l)$ and $l = 1, \ldots, L$ (and $S_{il} = 0$ otherwise). If $S_{il} = 1$, then let X_{il} and T_{il} denote the treatment assignment and outcome for individual i in stratum l; otherwise, if $S_{il} = 0$, then let $X_{il} = T_{il} = 0$. The sampling score stratified estimator is defined as

$$\hat{\Delta}_S = \sum_{l=1}^{L} w_l \left(\frac{\sum_{i=1}^{n_l+m_l} S_{il} T_{il} X_{il}}{\sum_{i=1}^{n_l+m_l} S_{il} X_{il}} - \frac{\sum_{i=1}^{n_l+m_l} S_{il} T_{il}(1-X_{il})}{\sum_{i=1}^{n_l+m_l} S_{il}(1-X_{il})} \right),$$

where $w_l = N_l/N$ where $N_l = \sum_{i=1}^{n_l+m_l} \Pi_{S_{il}}^{-1}$ and $\Pi_{S_{il}}$ is the weight for individual i in stratum l.

4.3.2 Right-Censored Data

Now suppose the survival times T are subject to right censoring such that only some participants are followed to their observed outcome. In this case, $RR(t)$ or $RD(t)$ may be of interest. Suppose the events in the trial occur at D distinct times $t_1 < t_2 < \ldots < t_D$ for $j = 1, \ldots, D$. For $x = 0$ or 1, define $\hat{N}_{jx}$ and $\hat{Y}_{jx}$, where

$$\hat{N}_{jx} = \sum_i I(S_i = 1, X_i = x, T_i = t, \delta_i = 1) \quad \text{and} \quad \hat{Y}_{jx} = \sum_i I(S_i = 1, X_i = x, T_i = t).$$ For treatment group x, the within-trial KM estimator (i.e., unweighted) is defined as

$$\hat{\mathcal{S}}_{KM}^{x}(t) = \prod_{t_j \le t} \left(1 - \frac{\hat{N}_{jx}}{\hat{Y}_{jx}} \right), \tag{4.2}$$

if $\hat{Y}_{jx} > 0$ and $t_1 \le t$. Otherwise, $\hat{S}_{KM}^{x}(t) = 1$ if $t < t_1$. The within-trial estimator of the risk difference at time t is defined as $\widehat{RD}_{KM} = \hat{\mathcal{S}}_{KM}^{1}(t) - \hat{\mathcal{S}}_{KM}^{0}(t)$ and the within-trial estimator of the RR at time t is defined as $\widehat{RR}_{KM} = \hat{\mathcal{S}}_{KM}^{1}(t)/\hat{\mathcal{S}}_{KM}^{0}(t)$.

For $x = 0$ or 1, define $\hat{N}_{jx}^{w}$ and $\hat{Y}_{jx}^{w}$, where $\hat{N}_{jx}^{w} = \sum_i I(S_i = 1, X_i = x, T_i = t, \delta_i = 1)/\hat{w}_i$ and $\hat{Y}_{jx}^{w} = \sum_i I(S_i = 1, X_i = x, T_i = t)/\hat{w}_i$. For treatment group x, the IPSW estimator of the marginal survival function in the target population is defined as

$$\hat{\mathcal{S}}_{IPSW}^{x}(t) = \prod_{t_j \le t} \left(1 - \frac{\hat{N}_{jx}^{w}}{\hat{Y}_{jx}^{w}} \right), \tag{4.3}$$

if $\hat{Y}_{jx}^{w} > 0$ and $t_1 \leq t$. Otherwise, $\hat{S}^x(t) = 1$ if $t < t_1$. The estimation of the sampling weights is described in Section 4.3.1. The IPSW estimator of the RD at time t is defined as $\widehat{RD}_{IPSW}(t) = \hat{\mathcal{S}}_{IPSW}^{1}(t) - \hat{\mathcal{S}}_{IPSW}^{0}(t)$ and the IPSW estimator of RR at time t is defined as $\widehat{RR}_{IPSW}(t) = \hat{\mathcal{S}}_{IPSW}^{1}(t)/\hat{\mathcal{S}}_{IPSW}^{0}(t)$.

An alternative approach for estimating the survival function in the target population uses stratification based on the estimated sampling scores (O'Muircheartaigh and Hedges, 2013; Tipton 2013; Tipton et al., 2014). The steps to compute this estimator are described in Section 4.3.1. For treatment group x, the stratified estimator of the marginal survival function in the target population is defined as

$$\hat{\mathcal{S}}_S^x(t) = \sum_{l=1}^{L} \hat{\omega}_l \hat{\mathcal{S}}_{KM,l}^x(t),$$

where $\hat{\mathcal{S}}_{KM,l}^x(t)$ is the within-trial KM estimator in stratum l. The stratified estimator of the RD at time t is then defined as $\widehat{RD}_S(t) = \hat{\mathcal{S}}_S^{1}(t) - \hat{\mathcal{S}}_S^{0}(t)$ and the stratified estimator of the RR at time t is defined as $\widehat{RR}_S(t) = \hat{\mathcal{S}}_S^{1}(t)/\hat{\mathcal{S}}_S^{0}(t)$.

In the simulations and data analysis below, the standard error for all three estimators is computed using the bootstrap (Efron and Tibshriani 1994) by drawing random samples with replacement from the trial data and random samples with replacement from the cohort data.

4.4 Simulations

A simulation study was conducted to compare the performance of the IPSW and stratified estimators and included scenarios with a continuous or discrete covariate and a right-censored outcome. The following quantities were computed for each scenario: the bias for each estimator, average of the estimated standard errors, empirical standard error, and empirical coverage probability of the 95% Wald-type confidence intervals.

A total of 5,000 datasets were simulated per scenario as follows. There were $N = 10^6$ observations in the target population. In the first four scenarios, one binary covariate $Z_{1i} \sim \text{Bern}(0.2)$ was considered and, for Scenarios 5 to 8, one continuous covariate $Z_i \sim N(0, 1)$ was considered. The covariate Z_i was associated with trial participation and a treatment effect modifier. A Bernoulli trial participation indicator, S_i, was simulated according to the true sampling score w_i and those with $S_i = 1$ were included in the trial. The parameters β_0 and β_1 were set to ensure that the probability of sampling into the trial was a rare event (i.e., the size of the trial was approximately $n \approx 1{,}000$). The cohort was a random sample of size $m = 4{,}000$ from the target population (less those selected into the trial) and S_i was set to zero for those in the cohort. The trial was small compared to the size of the target, so the cohort was essentially a random sample from the target.

For those included in the randomized trial ($S_i = 1$), X_i was generated as Bern(0.5) and the log survival time T was generated according to $T_i = \exp(\nu_0 + \nu_1 Z_i + \xi X_i + \alpha Z_i X_i + \epsilon_i)$, $\epsilon_i \sim N(0, 1)$. Survival times greater than 10 years were administratively censored at that time. For all scenarios, there was an independent censoring mechanism where C_i was the minimum of 10 years and an exponential random variable with mean 2. For Scenarios 1, 2, 5, and 6, $(\nu_0, \nu_1, \xi, \alpha) = (0, 1, \log(2), \log(4))$, and $(\nu_0, \nu_1, \xi, \alpha) = (0, 1, \log(2), \log(6))$ for Scenarios 3, 4, 7 and 8. Two sampling score models were considered: Scenarios 1, 3, 5, and 7 set $\beta = (-7, 0.4)$; Scenarios 2, 4, 6, and 8 set $\beta = (-7, 1)$. The true survival distributions of (T^1, T^0) for each scenario were calculated using the distribution of Z and ϵ in the target population. When Z was binary, $S(t \mid X = 1) = P(T > t \mid X = 1, Z = 1)P(Z = 1) + P(T > t \mid X = 1, Z = 0)P(Z = 0)$ and $S(t \mid X = 0) = P(T > t \mid X = 0, Z = 1)P(Z = 1) + P(T > t \mid X = 0, Z = 0)P(Z = 0)$. When Z was continuous, $S(t \mid X = 1) = \int_z P(T > t \mid X = 1, Z \leq z)P(Z \leq z)dz$ and $S(t \mid X = 0) = \int_z P(T > t \mid X = 0, Z \leq z)P(Z \leq z)dz$.

To estimate the weights, the combined trial ($S_i = 1$) and cohort data ($S_i = 0$) was used to fit a (weighted) logistic regression model with S_i as the outcome and the covariate Z_i as described in Section 4.3.1. The average standard error of all three estimators was computed using a nonparametric bootstrap with 50 random samples with replacement of the trial and 50 random samples with replacement of the cohort data. Wald confidence intervals were computed using the log–log transformation to ensure the confidence interval limits were between 0 and 1.

Comparisons between the IPSW and stratified estimator based on data among those randomized to treatment are summarized in Table 4.1 when the sampling score model was correctly specified. The results based on data among those randomized to control were comparable. The average trial size ranged from $n = 987$ to $n = 1{,}498$. For Scenario 8, the estimated survival curves for each estimator were plotted for the first 100 datasets among those randomized to treatment (Figure 4.1). For all scenarios, the IPSW estimator was less biased than the within-trial KM estimator. The stratified estimator was unbiased when there was a binary covariate in the sampling score model; however, for some scenarios with a continuous covariate, the stratified estimator was biased and its corresponding confidence intervals had coverage below the nominal level. The average of the bootstrap standard error estimates was approximately equal to the empirical standard error, supporting the use of the bootstrap for estimating the variance of the IPSW and stratified estimators.

TABLE 4.1

Summary of Simulation Study Results for Estimators of $\mathfrak{S}^1(t)$ in the Target Population at $t = 3$ for $X = 1$ in 5,000 Simulated Datasets with $m = 4,000$ and $n \approx 1,000$ per Dataset with Independent Censoring. Scenarios are Described in Section 4.4. For Scenarios 1 and 2, $\mathfrak{S}^1(t) = 0.46$, for Scenarios 3 and 4, $\mathfrak{S}^1(t) = 0.47$, for Scenarios 5 and 6, $\mathfrak{S}^1(t) = 0.44$, and for Scenarios 7 and 8, $\mathfrak{S}^1(t) = 0.45$.

	Covariate	(β, e^α)	$\hat{\mathfrak{S}}^1_{KM}(t)$				$\hat{\mathfrak{S}}^1_S(t)$				$\hat{\mathfrak{S}}^1_{IPSW}(t)$			
			Bias	ESE	ASE	ECP	Bias	ESE	ASE	ECP	Bias	ESE	ASE	ECP
1	Binary	(0.4,4)	0.05	3.5	3.5	0.76	2e–4	3.3	3.3	0.95	2e–4	3.5	3.6	0.95
2	Binary	(1,4)	0.13	3.1	3.1	0.03	–1e–4	3.3	3.3	0.95	–2e–4	3.5	3.5	0.95
3	Binary	(0.4,6)	0.05	3.5	3.5	0.75	2e–4	3.3	3.3	0.96	3e–4	3.6	3.5	0.96
4	Binary	(1,6)	0.13	3.0	3.0	0.02	1e–4	3.3	3.3	0.95	–2e–5	3.5	3.5	0.95
5	Continuous	(0.4,4)	0.15	3.1	3.1	<0.01	6e–3	2.4	2.5	0.94	8e–4	3.1	3.1	0.95
6	Continuous	(1,4)	0.34	2.2	2.2	<0.01	0.02	2.5	2.6	0.89	1e–3	3.5	3.8	0.93
7	Continuous	(0.4,6)	0.15	3.0	3.0	<0.01	7e–3	2.3	2.3	0.95	1e–3	3.0	3.0	0.95
8	Continuous	(1,6)	0.34	2.1	2.1	<0.01	0.02	2.3	2.4	0.89	1e–3	3.5	3.7	0.93

Note: ASE = average estimated standard error (×100); ECP = empirical coverage probability; ESE = empirical standard error (×100); IPSW = inverse probability of sampling weighted; KM = within-trial Kaplan Meier; S = stratified.

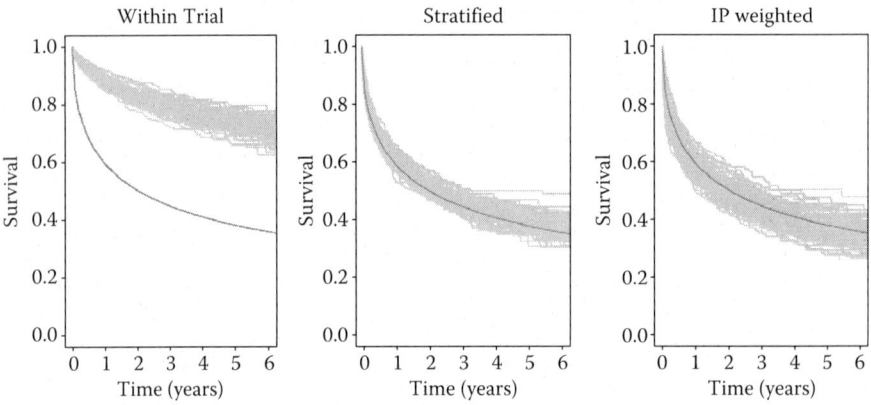

FIGURE 4.1
Comparison of the distributions of within-trial Kaplan–Meier estimator $\hat{\mathfrak{S}}^1_{KM}(t)$, stratified estimator $\hat{\mathfrak{S}}^1_S(t)$, and inverse probability (IP) of sampling weighted estimator $\hat{\mathfrak{S}}^1_{IPSW}(t)$ for $X = 1$ based on 100 simulated datasets where the sampling score model is correctly specified with one continuous covariate, $\beta = (-7, 1)$ and $e^\alpha = 6$ (Scenario 8) (darker line is the true survival curve in the target population).

4.5 Applications

In this section, the methods described in Section 4.3 are applied to generalize results from two different ACTG randomized clinical trials, ACTG 320 and ACTG A5202. Two different target populations are considered, namely all women currently living with HIV in the United States and all people currently living with HIV in the United States.

4.5.1 Cohort and Trial Data

The ACTG 320 trial examined the safety and efficacy of adding a protease inhibitor (PI) to an HIV treatment regimen with two nucleoside analogues. A total of 1,156 participants were enrolled in ACTG 320 between January 1996 and January 1997 and were recruited from 33 AIDS clinical trial units and 7 National Hemophilia Foundation sites in the United States and Puerto Rico (Hammer et al. 1997). These participants were HIV positive, highly active antiretroviral therapy (HAART) naïve, and had CD4 cell counts < 200 cells/mm^3 at screening. Of the 1,156 participants, 200 were women. Participants were followed until AIDS, death, drop-out, or administrative censoring, whichever came first. Among the 1,156 participants, 96 (8%) died or developed AIDS by 1 year, with 33 of those randomized to a regimen with a PI and 63 of those randomized to a regimen without a PI; 203 (18%) dropped out within the first 6 months of the study. The baseline characteristics of the ACTG 320 participants are shown in Table 4.2.

TABLE 4.2

Characteristics of Participants in the WIHS, CNICS, and ACTG 320

Variable	WIHS (m = 493)	ACTG 320 Women (n = 200)	CNICS (m = 6,158)	ACTG 320 Men and Women (n = 1,156)
Male sex—no. (%)	0 (0)	0 (0)	4,909 (80)	956 (83)
Race or ethnic group—no. (%)				
White, non-Hispanic	87 (18)	61 (31)	2,436 (40)	598 (52)
Black, non-Hispanic	272 (55)	95 (48)	2,690 (44)	328 (28)
Hispanic	124 (25)	42 (21)	734 (12)	205 (18)
Asian/other	10 (2)	2 (1)	298 (5)	25 (2)
Median age—yr (Q1–Q3)	40 (35–45)	36 (30–42)	41 (34–47)	38 (33–44)
Age group—no. (%)				
[16, 30) yr	35 (7)	46 (23)	714 (12)	142 (12)
[30, 40) yr	211 (43)	88 (44)	2,108 (34)	536 (47)
[40, 50) yr	196 (40)	53 (27)	2,315 (37)	350 (30)
[50,·) yr	51 (10)	13 (7)	1,021 (17)	128 (11)
Injection drug use—no. (%)	180 (37)	36 (18)	1,241 (20)	184 (16)
Median CD4 count (Q1–Q3)	108 (41–172)	82 (26–139)	89 (27–172)	75 (23–137)
Baseline CD4 count—no. (%)				
(0, 50) cells/mm^3	148 (30)	72 (36)	2,237 (36)	453 (39)
[50, 100) cells/mm^3	83 (17)	43 (22)	1,047 (17)	248 (22)
[100, 200) cells/mm^3	182 (37)	73 (37)	1,818 (30)	372 (32)
[200, ·) cells/mm^3	80 (16)	12 (6)	1,056 (17)	82 (7)

Note: ACTG = AIDS Clinical Trials Group; CNICS = Center for AIDS Research Network of Integrated Clinical Systems; WIHS = the Women's Interagency HIV Study.

The ACTG A5202 trial examined the equivalence of abacavir–lamivudine (ABC-3TC) or tenofovir disoproxil fumarate–emtricitabine (TDF-FTC) plus efavirenz or ritonavir-boosted atazanavir. A total of 1,857 participants were enrolled in ACTG A5202 between September 2005 and November 2007, recruited from 59 ACTG sites in the United States and Puerto Rico (Sax et al. 2009, 2011). These participants were HIV positive, antiretroviral therapy (ART) naïve, and had viral load > 1,000 copies/mL at screening. Of the 1,857 participants, 322 were women. Participants were followed until virologic failure (defined as confirmed HIV-1 RNA level ≥ 1,000 copies/mL at or after 16 weeks and before 24 weeks, or ≥ 200 copies/mL at or after 24 weeks), dropout, or administrative censoring, whichever came first. Among the 1,857 participants, 219 (12%) experienced virologic failure by week 48 with 131 of those randomized to ABC-3TC and 88 of those randomized to TDF-FTC and 431 (23%)

TABLE 4.3

Characteristics of Participants in the WIHS, CNICS, and ACTG A5202

Variable	WIHS (m = 1,012)	ACTG A5202 Women (n = 322)	CNICS (m = 12,302)	ACTG A5202 Men and Women (n = 1,857)
Male sex—no. (%)	0 (0)	0 (0)	10,063 (82)	1,535 (83)
Race or ethnic group[a]—no. (%)				
White, non-Hispanic	171 (17)	57 (18)	5,567 (45)	746 (46)
Black, non-Hispanic	586 (58)	172 (53)	4,682 (38)	615 (33)
Hispanic	222 (22)	82 (26)	1,420 (12)	429 (23)
Asian/other	33 (3)	11 (3)	633 (5)	62 (3)
Median age—yr (Q1–Q3)	39 (33–44)	39 (31–46)	39 (31–46)	38 (31–45)
Age group—no. (%)				
[16, 30) yr	123 (12)	57 (18)	2,454 (20)	404 (22)
[30, 40) yr	435 (43)	110 (34)	4,225 (34)	625 (34)
[40, 50) yr	345 (34)	107 (33)	3,896 (32)	573 (31)
[50, ·) yr	109 (11)	48 (15)	1,727 (14)	255 (14)
Injection drug use—no. (%)	388 (38)	18 (6)	2,042 (17)	162 (9)
Hepatitis B/C—no. (%)	356 (35)	25 (8)	2,245 (18)	165 (9)
AIDS diagnosis—no. (%)	373 (37)	62 (19)	2,834 (23)	312 (17)
CD4 count[b]—no. (%)				
(0, 50) cells/mm^3	102 (10)	61 (18)	2,000 (16)	339 (18)
(50, 100) cells/mm^3	61 (6)	24 (7)	720 (7)	150 (8)
(100, 200) cells/mm^3	164 (16)	55 (17)	1,692 (14)	311 (17)
(200, 350) cells/mm^3	293 (29)	130 (40)	3,262 (27)	656 (35)
(350, ·) cells/mm^3	392 (39)	52 (16)	4,428 (36)	400 (22)
Median CD4 count (Q1–Q3)	290 (162–423)	226 (87–313)	271 (109–427)	230 (90–334)
Viral load—no. (%)				
(0, 50, 000) cp/mL	552 (55)	187 (58)	6,450 (52)	1,000 (54)
(50, 000, 100, 000) cp/mL	144 (14)	62 (19)	1,861 (15)	391 (21)
(100, 000, 300, 000) cp/mL	193 (19)	38 (12)	2,232 (18)	203 (11)
(300, 000, 500, 000) cp/mL	55 (5)	9 (3)	744 (6)	72 (4)
(500, 000, ·) cp/mL	68 (7)	26 (8)	1,015 (8)	191 (10)
Median log$_{10}$ viral load (Q1–Q3)	4.61 (4.04–5.11)	4.58 (4.07–4.93)	4.64 (3.95–5.18)	4.66 (4.33–5.01)

Note: ACTG = AIDS Clinical Trials Group; CNICS = Center for AIDS Research Network of Integrated Clinical Systems; WIHS = the Women's Interagency HIV Study.

[a] Five A5202 participants were missing race.

[b] One A5202 participant was missing CD4 cell count.

dropped out within the first 50 weeks of the study. The baseline characteristics of A5202 participants are shown in Table 4.3.

Participants in the WIHS and Center for AIDS Research (CFAR) Network of Integrated Clinical Systems (CNICS) were considered to be representative samples of the target populations (i.e., all women living with HIV in the United States and all people living with HIV in the United States, respectively). A total of 4,129 women (1,065 HIV uninfected) were enrolled in WIHS between October 1994 and December 2012 at six US sites (Bacon et al. 2005). The CNICS captures comprehensive and standardized clinical data from point-of-care electronic medical record systems for population-based HIV research (Kitahata et al. 2008). The CNICS cohort includes over 27,000 HIV-infected adults (at least 18 years of age) engaged in clinical care since January 1, 1995, at eight CFAR sites in the United States. For generalizing results from ACTG 320, the analysis included cohort participants who were HIV positive, HAART naïve, and had CD4 cell counts $\leq$ 200 cells/mm^3 at the previous visit (m = 493 women and m = 6,158 women and men combined). For generalizing results from A5202, the analysis included cohort participants who were HIV positive, ART naïve, and had viral load > 1,000 copies/mL at the previous visit (m = 1,012 women and m = 12,302 women and men combined). Table 4.2 displays the characteristics of the participants in the WIHS and CNICS samples used to generalize results from ACTG 320. Likewise, the characteristics of the participants in the WIHS sample and the participants in the CNICS sample used to generalize results from ACTG A5202 are shown in Table 4.3.

4.5.2 Analysis

The IPSW and stratified estimators were employed to generalize the causal risk differences (RDs) and causal risk ratios (RRs) observed among women in the trials to all women currently living with HIV in the United States and among all participants in the trials to all people currently living with HIV in the United States. For comparison purposes, the within-trial and stratified estimators were also computed, although based on the empirical results in the previous section these estimators are not in general expected to be consistent for the treatment effects in the target population. Based on Centers for Disease Control and Prevention (2012) estimates, the size of the first target population was assumed to be 280,000 women and the size of the second target population was assumed to be 1.1 million people.

The RDs and RRs in the target population were estimated using the IPSW and stratified estimators described in Section 4.3.2. In the model for the sampling scores, the outcome was trial participation and the possible covariates included sex, race/ethnicity, age, history of injection drug use (IDU), and baseline CD4 for ACTG 320 and sex, race/ethnicity, age, history of IDU, hepatitis B/C, AIDS diagnosis, baseline CD4, and baseline log$_{10}$ viral load for ACTG A5202. Variables associated with trial participation, the outcome, or effect modifiers, as well as all pairwise interactions, were included in the sampling score model. Due to violation of the positivity assumption, sex was excluded from the analysis generalizing the trial results among women.

4.5.3 Results

Estimates of the RDs and RRs based on the within-trial KM estimators among women and all participants are given in Tables 4.4 and 4.5. Among women in ACTG 320, the risk of AIDS or death at 1 year was not

TABLE 4.4

Estimated Risk Differences (RD) and Corresponding 95% Confidence Intervals in Two Target Populations[a]

		Risk Difference (95% CI)		
Cohort	Trial	$\widehat{RD}_{KM}$	$\widehat{RD}_S$	$\widehat{RD}_{IPSW}$
WIHS	320[b]	−0.03 (−0.11, 0.05)	−0.01 (−0.12, 0.09)	−0.02 (−0.08, 0.04)
WIHS	A5202[c]	0.04 (−0.03, 0.11)	0.12 (−0.10, 0.26)	0.08 (−0.12, 0.28)
CNICS	320	−0.06 (−0.10, −0.02)	−0.06 (−0.09, −0.02)	−0.05 (−0.09, −0.01)
CNICS	A5202	0.05 (0.03, 0.08)	0.07 (0.01, 0.10)	0.06 (0.02, 0.10)

Note: IPSW = inverse probability weighted; KM = within-trial Kaplan Meier; S = stratified.

[a] Target populations were all men and women combined and all women living with HIV in the United States. Based on data from the AIDS Clinical Trials Group (ACTG) trials.

[b] For 320, the treatment contrast was protease inhibitor (PI) ($X = 1$) vs. no PI ($X = 0$).

[c] For A5202, the treatment contrast was abacavir-lamivudine (ABC-3TC) ($X = 1$) vs. tenofovir disoproxil fumarate-emtricitabine (TDF-FTC) ($X = 0$) plus efavirenz or ritonavir-boosted atazanavir.

TABLE 4.5

Estimated Risk Ratios (RR) and Corresponding 95% Confidence Intervals in Two Target Populations[a]

		Risk Ratio (95% CI)		
Cohort	Trial	$\widehat{RR}_{KM}$	$\widehat{RR}_S$	$\widehat{RR}_{IPSW}$
WIHS	320[b]	0.70 (0.23, 2.09)	0.85 (0.12, 2.84)	0.58 (0.09, 3.84)
WIHS	A5202[c]	1.43 (0.73, 2.78)	2.32 (0.54, 6.00)	1.80 (0.54, 6.05)
CNICS	320	0.51 (0.34, 0.77)	0.48 (0.32, 0.85)	0.52 (0.31, 0.86)
CNICS	A5202	1.83 (1.33, 2.52)	2.02 (1.16, 2.88)	1.83 (1.23, 2.72)

Note: IPSW = inverse probability weighted; KM = within-trial Kaplan Meier; S = stratified.

[a] Target populations were all men and women combined and all women living with HIV in the United States. Based on data from the AIDS Clinical Trials Group (ACTG) trials.

[b] For 320, the treatment contrast was protease inhibitor (PI) ($X = 1$) vs. no PI ($X = 0$).

[c] For A5202, the treatment contrast was abacavir-lamivudine (ABC-3TC) ($X = 1$) vs. tenofovir disoproxil fumarate-emtricitabine (TDF-FTC) ($X = 0$) plus efavirenz or ritonavir-boosted atazanavir.

significantly different between the two treatment groups. However, among the 1,156 total participants, the risk of AIDS or death at 1 year was lower for those on a regimen with a PI ($\widehat{RD}$ = −0.06) or a 49% risk reduction as compared to those on a regimen without a PI. Among the 322 women in A5202, there was not a statistically significant difference between the treatment groups. However, among all participants in ACTG A5202, the risk of virologic failure at 48 weeks among those on ABC-3TC was higher ($\widehat{RD}$ = 0.05) or 1.8 times the risk compared to those on TDF-FTC. Although we used different estimators, these results are in agreement with the primary analyses from each trial (Hammer et al. 1997; Sax et al. 2009, 2011).

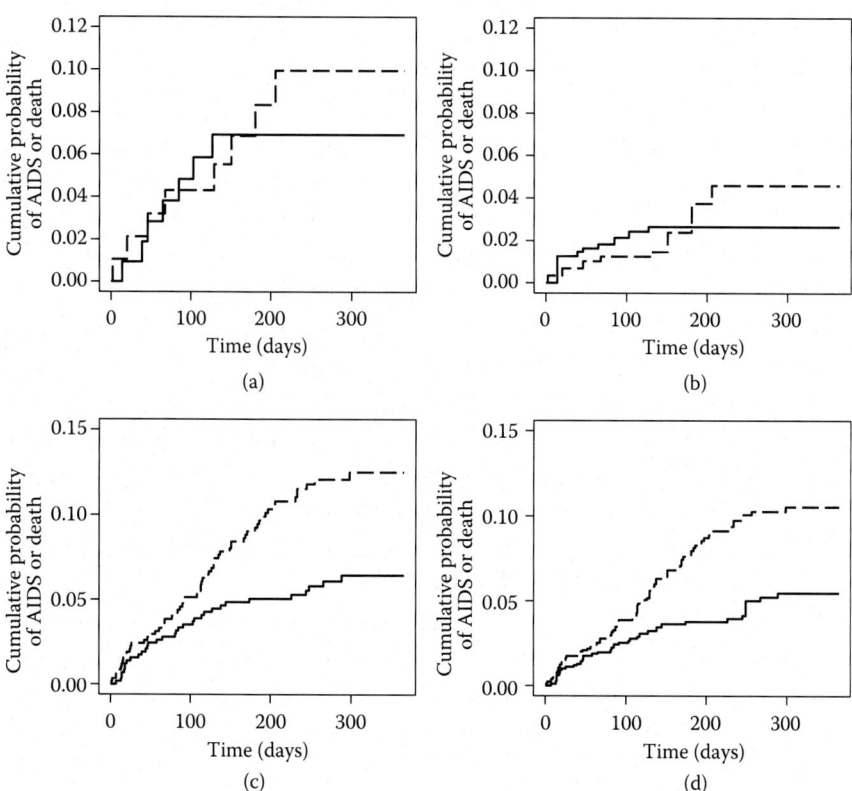

FIGURE 4.2
Estimates of cumulative probability of AIDS or death (i.e., $1 - S^x(t)$ for x = 0, 1) based on data among participants randomized to a regimen with a protease inhibitor (PI) (solid curves) and without a PI (dashed curves). AIDS Clinical Trials Group (ACTG) 320 Study 1996–1997, United States, using the within-trial estimators (a) among women and (c) among both men and women combined and inverse probability of sampling weighted estimators to generalize to (b) all women living with HIV in the United States and (d) all people living with HIV in the United States.

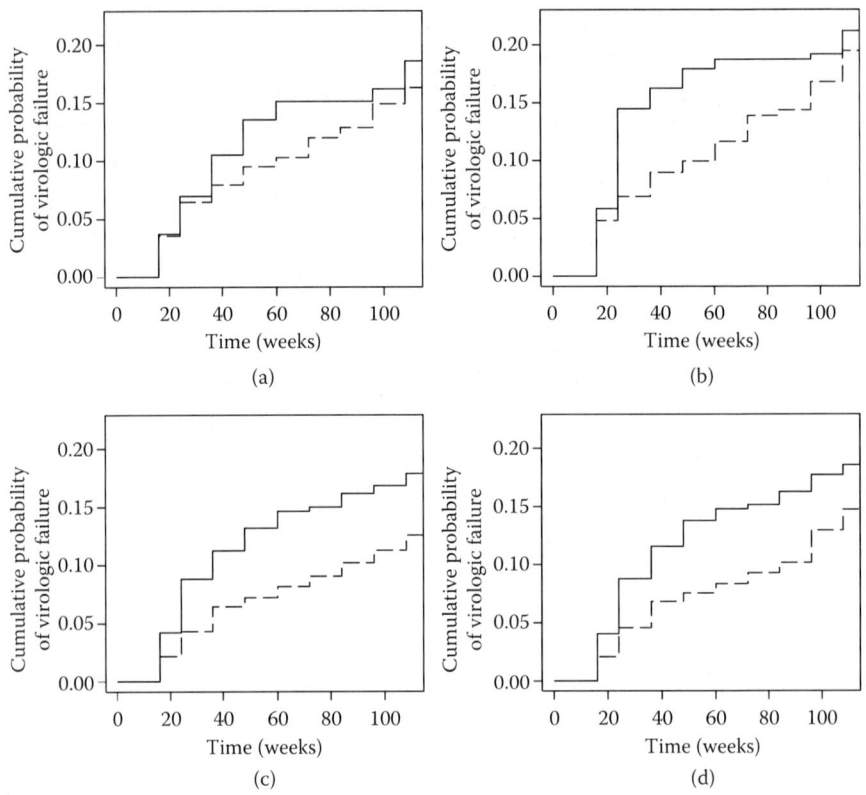

FIGURE 4.3
Estimates of cumulative probability of virologic failure (i.e., $1-\mathfrak{S}^x(t)$ for $x = 0, 1$) among those randomized to abacavir-lamivudine (solid curves) and tenofovir disoproxil fumarate–emtricitabine (dashed curves), AIDS Clinical Trials Group (ACTG) 320 Study, 2005-2007, United States, using the within-trial estimators (a) among women and (c) among both men and women combined, and inverse probability of sampling weighted estimators to generalize to (b) all women living with HIV in the United States and (d) all people living with HIV in the United States.

Tables 4.4 and 4.5 also display the estimated RDs and RRs in the target populations using the IPSW and stratified estimators. Figures 4.2 and 4.3 display $1 - \mathfrak{S}^x(t)$ for $x = 0, 1$ using the within-trial estimators and inverse probability of selection-weighted estimators generalized to both target populations based on data among participants in the two ACTG trials. Based on the ACTG 320 data, the relative difference between the two treatment groups in the target population is comparable to that in the trial; however, the marginal curves for each study arm are attenuated in the target population, as compared to the within-trial estimated survival curves. Based on the ACTG A5202 among women, the difference between the two study arm survival curves is larger in the target population, as compared to the within-trial estimated survival curves.

In the target population of all women living with HIV in the US, the IPSW estimate was comparable to the within-trial estimate observed in ACTG 320 on the difference scale. On the ratio scale, the IPSW estimator indicated a stronger protective effect of (PIs $\widehat{RR}_{IPSW}$ = 0.58 compared to $\widehat{RR}_{KM}$ = 0.70), suggesting that the within-trial result may underestimate the effects of PIs in all HIV-infected women in the US. The IPSW estimate of the effect of ABC-3TC (vs. TDF-FTC) on the difference scale was approximately double the within-trial estimate ($\widehat{RD}_{IPSW}$ = 0.08 compared to $\widehat{RD}_{KM}$ = 0.04) and also indicated a stronger effect on the ratio scale ($\widehat{RD}_{IPSW}$ = 1.80 compared to $\widehat{RD}_{KM}$ = 1.43), providing evidence that this ART combination may be associated with a higher risk of virologic failure than what was observed in the trial. In the target population of all people living with HIV in the US, the IPSW estimates were comparable to the within-trial effect estimates, suggesting that both the effect of PIs and the effect of the ART combination ABC-3TC (vs. TDF-FTC) from the trials may be generalizable to all people living with HIV in the US. In summary, these results suggest the ACTG trial results are more generalizable for US men with HIV than US women with HIV.

4.6 Discussion

In this chapter, we considered generalizing results from a randomized trial to a specific target population. Estimators that employ sampling scores and their corresponding confidence intervals provide inferences about the treatment effect in the target population, that is, a contrast in the survival outcome had (contrary to fact) everyone in the target population received treatment compared to the outcome if everyone in the target population did not receive treatment. In a simulation study, the IPSW outperformed the stratified estimator when the sampling score model was correctly specified. The IPSW was unbiased for all scenarios and the confidence intervals exhibited coverage approximately at the nominal level. With a continuous covariate, the confidence interval of the stratified estimator had coverage below the nominal level.

In the illustrative example, the IPSW estimator was employed to generalize results for right-censored outcomes in the ACTG to all people currently living with HIV in the United States. For both trials, the within-trial effect was comparable to the effect estimated with the IPSW. Thus, the ACTG 320 and A5202 results appear to be generalizable to all people living with HIV in the United States. However, the results among women were markedly different in the target population, as compared to the trial.

Among women in A5202, the RD doubled when estimated with the IPSW estimator, as compared to the within-trial KM estimator ($\widehat{RD}$ = 0.08 vs.

$\widehat{RD} = 0.04$, respectively). The marginal event rates typically had a larger change in magnitude than the relative measures (i.e., risk difference and risk ratio). Results were not sensitive to the specification of the size of the target population.

When applying this method, the analysis is subject to the following considerations. For the right-censored outcome, the nonparametric bootstrap standard error was used to estimate the variance. Additional research to demonstrate the large sample properties of this estimator for right-censored data could allow for a closed-form expression of the variance. The absence of unmeasured covariates associated with the trial participation mechanism and treatment effect modifiers is an untestable assumption. In trials with non-negligible rates of noncompliance, effect estimates based on IPSW or stratification should be interpreted as estimates of treatment assignment rather than treatment receipt. Future research could entail extending these estimators to account for noncompliance. The sampling score model was assumed to be correct (e.g., correct covariate functional forms); however, this is not guaranteed in practice. Because some degree of model misspecification is inevitable, sensitivity analysis of inferences about the treatment effect in the population to the sample score model specification is recommended. The stratified estimator (O'Muircheartaigh and Hedges 2013; Tipton et al. 2014) requires that individuals sharing the same stratum of the distribution of sampling scores can be identified, which may be difficult in practice. This estimator may be biased when there is residual confounding within strata, and it is therefore not a consistent estimator of the PATE in some cases (e.g., a continuous covariate in the sampling score model) (Lunceford and Davidian 2004). Weighted logistic regression was used to estimate the sampling scores. Future research could entail instead using machine learning methods as in Westreich et al. (2010) to estimate the sampling scores. Additional research to develop an augmented estimator could improve efficiency (Zhang et al. 2008).

In the application, the cohort study was assumed to be a random sample (i.e., representative) of the target population. Although considered to be representative of women living with HIV and at risk for HIV in the US, the WIHS is an epidemiological study with prospective data collection and participants were required to have enrolled and continued to engage with the study. Because the study includes visits and assessments beyond recommended treatment and care, these patients may not be representative of those engaged with HIV care nor those living with HIV. Because CNICS captures electronic medical health record data from geographically and ethnically diverse HIV care and treatment centers, the data collected better reflects health outcomes of HIV-infected patients engaged with care in the HAART era; however, these patients may not be representative of the typical person living with HIV, specifically those not actively engaged with care. If the cohort is not representative, one possibility is weighting the cohort data to the distribution of covariates in a census (e.g., Centers for Disease Control and Prevention [CDC] estimates). A limitation of this approach is that the census may not have covariate information as rich as the cohort data. The CDC estimates used to quantify the size of the target population in the example were for all people living with HIV. Use of surveillance studies that report on the number of ART and HAART naïve HIV patients in the US could further sharpen the information about the target population.

In conclusion, we considered estimators that employ sampling scores to estimate marginal survival curves, risk differences, and risk ratios in a target population. Quantitative methods for generalizability is a growing field of statistical research and methods for right-censored data are essential to address questions in HIV/AIDS research (Keiding and Louis 2016). We hope that this chapter will be useful for implementation of these methods and increasing interest in quantitative methods for generalizability of trial results.

Acknowledgments

These findings are presented on behalf of the Women's Interagency HIV Study (WIHS), the Center for AIDS Research (CFAR) Network of Integrated Clinical Trials (CNICS), and the AIDS Clinical Trials Group (ACTG). We would like to thank all of the WIHS, CNICS, and ACTG investigators, data management teams, and participants who contributed to this project. Funding for this study was provided by National Institutes of Health (NIH) grants R01AI100654, R01AI085073, U01AI042590, U01AI069918, R56AI102622, 5 K24HD059358-04, 5 U01AI103390-02 (WIHS), R24AI067039 (CNICS), and P30AI50410 (The University of North Carolina at Chapel Hill (UNC) CFAR). The views and opinions of the authors expressed in this manuscript do not necessarily state or reflect those of the NIH.

Data in this manuscript were collected by the WIHS. WIHS (principal investigators): UAB-MS WIHS (Michael Saag, Mirjam-Colette Kempf, and Deborah Konkle-Parker), U01-AI-103401; Atlanta WIHS (Ighovwerha Ofotokun and Gina Wingood), U01-AI-103408; Bronx WIHS (Kathryn Anastos), U01-AI-035004; Brooklyn WIHS (Howard Minkoff and Deborah Gustafson), U01-AI-031834; Chicago WIHS (Mardge Cohen and Audrey French), U01-AI-034993; Metropolitan Washington WIHS (Mary Young), U01-AI-034994; Miami WIHS (Margaret Fischl and Lisa Metsch), U01-AI-103397; UNC WIHS (Adaora Adimora), U01-AI-103390; Connie Wofsy Women's HIV Study, Northern California (Ruth Greenblatt, Bradley Aouizerat, and Phyllis Tien), U01-AI-034989; WIHS Data Management and Analysis Center (Stephen Gange and Elizabeth Golub), U01-AI-042590; Southern California WIHS (Joel Milam), U01-HD-032632 (WIHS I WIHS IV). The WIHS is funded primarily by the National Institute of Allergy and Infectious Diseases (NIAID), with additional co-funding from the Eunice Kennedy Shriver National Institute of Child Health and Human Development (NICHD), the National Cancer Institute (NCI), the National Institute on Drug Abuse (NIDA), and the National

Institute on Mental Health (NIMH). Targeted supplemental funding for specific projects is also provided by the National Institute of Dental and Craniofacial Research (NIDCR), the National Institute on Alcohol Abuse and Alcoholism (NIAAA), the National Institute on Deafness and Other Communication Disorders (NIDCD), and the NIH Office of Research on Women's Health. WIHS data collection is also supported by UL1-TR000004 (UCSF CTSA) and UL1-TR000454 (Atlanta CTSA).

References

Bacon, M. C., von Wyl, V., Alden, C., Sharp, G., Robison, E., and Hessol, N. (2005). The Women's Interagency HIV Study: An observational cohort brings clinical sciences to the bench. *Clinical and Diagnostic Laboratory Immunology*, 12, 1013–1019.

Bareinboim, E. and Pearl, J. (2013). A general algorithm for deciding transportability of experimental results. *Journal of Causal Inference*, 1, 107–134.

Buchanan, A. L., Hudgens, M. G., Cole, S. R., Mollan, K., Sax, P. E., Daar, E., Adimora, A. A., Eron, J., and Mugavero, M. (2015). Generalizing evidence from randomized trials using inverse probability of sampling weights. *The University of North Carolina at Chapel Hill Department of Biostatistics Technical Report Series*, Working Paper 45.

Centers for Disease Control and Prevention (2012). *Diagnoses of HIV infection and AIDS in the United States and dependent areas*. HIV Surveillance Report, 17.

Cole, S. R. and Hernan, M. A. (2004). Adjusted survival curves with inverse probability weights. *Computer Methods and Programs in Biomedicine*, 75, 45–49.

Cole, S. R. and Stuart, E. A. (2010). Generalizing evidence from randomized clinical trials to target populations: The ACTG 320 trial. *American Journal of Epidemiology*, 172, 107–115.

Efron, B. and Tibshriani, R. (1994). *An Introduction to the Bootstrap*. London: Chapman Hall.

Gandhi, M., Ameli, N., Bacchetti, P., Sharp, G. B., French, A. L., and Young, M. (2005). Eligibility criteria for HIV clinical trials and generalizability of results: The gap between published reports and study protocols. *AIDS*, 19, 1885–1896.

Greenblatt, R. M. (2011). Priority issues concerning HIV infection among women. *Women's Health Issues*, 21, S266–S271.

Greenhouse, J. B., Kaizar, E. E., Kelleher, K., Seltman, H., and Gardner, W. (2008). Generalizing from clinical trial data: A case study. The risk of suicidality among pediatric antidepressant users. *Statistics in Medicine*, 27, 1801–1813.

Grodstein, F., Manson, J. E., Colditz, G. A., Willett, W. C., Speizer, F. E., and Stampfer, M. J. (2000). A prospective, observational study of postmenopausal hormone therapy and primary prevention of cardiovascular disease. *Annals of Internal Medicine*, 133, 933–941.

Grodstein, F., Stampfer, M. J., Manson, J. E., Colditz, G. A., Willett, W. C., Rosner, B., Speizer, F. E., and Hennekens, C. H. (1996). Postmenopausal estrogen and progestin use and the risk of cardiovascular disease. *New England Journal of Medicine*, 335, 453–461.

Hammad, T. A., Laughren, T., and Racoosin, J. (2006). Suicidality in pediatric patients treated with antidepressant drugs. *Archives of General Psychiatry*, 63, 332–339.

Hammer, S. M., Squires, K. E., Hughes, M. D., Grimes, J. M., Demeter, L. M., and Currier, J. S. (1997). A controlled trial of two nucleoside analogues plus indinavir in persons with HIV infection and CD4 cell counts of 200 per cubic millimeter or less. *New England Journal of Medicine*, 337, 725–733.

Hernan, M. A. (2010). The hazards of hazard ratios. *Epidemiology*, 21, 13–15.

Hernán, M. A., Alonso, A., Logan, R., Grodstein, F., Michels, K. B., Stampfer, M. J., Willett, W. C., Manson, J. E., and Robins, J. M. (2008). Observational studies analyzed like randomized experiments: An application to postmenopausal hormone therapy and coronary heart disease. *Epidemiology*, 19, 766.

Hernán, M. A. and Robins, J. M. (2006). Estimating causal effects from epidemiological data. *Journal of Epidemiology and Community Health*, 60, 578–586.

Hernan, M. A. and VanderWeele, T. J. (2011). Compound treatments and transportability of causal inference. *Epidemiology*, 22, 368–377.

Kalbfleisch, J. D. and Prentice, R. L. (2002). *The Statistical Analysis of Failure Time Data*. Hoboken, NJ: Wiley-Interscience.

Kaufman, J. S. (2010). Marginalia: Comparing adjusted effect measures. *Epidemiology*, 21, 490–493.

Keiding, N. and Louis, T. A. (2016). Perils and potentials of self-selected entry to epidemiological studies and surveys. *Journal of the Royal Statistical Society: Series A (Statistics in Society)*, 179, 319–376.

Kitahata, M. M., Rodriguez, B., Haubrich, R., Boswell, S., Mathews, W. C., and Lederman, M. M. (2008). Cohort profile: The Centers for AIDS Research Network of Integrated Clinical Systems. *International Journal of Epidemiology*, 37, 948–955.

Lunceford, J. K. and Davidian, M. (2004). Stratification and weighting via the propensity score in estimation of causal treatment effects: A comparative study. *Statistics in Medicine*, 23, 2937–2960.

Manson, J. E., Hsia, J., Johnson, K. C., Rossouw, J. E., Assaf, A. R., Lasser, N. L., Trevisan, M., et al. (2003). Estrogen plus progestin and the risk of coronary heart disease. *New England Journal of Medicine*, 349, 523–534.

Neyman, J. (1923). On the application of probability theory to agricultural experiments: Essay on principles, Section 9. *Statistical Science*, 5, 463–480, 1990.

O'Muircheartaigh, C. and Hedges, L. V. (2013). Generalizing from unrepresentative experiments: A stratified propensity score approach. *Journal of the Royal Statistical Society: Series C (Applied Statistics)*, 63, 195–210.

Robins, J. M. and Finkelstein, D. M. (2000). Correcting for noncompliance and dependent censoring in an AIDS clinical trial with inverse probability of censoring weighted log rank tests. *Biometrics*, 56, 779–788.

Rothman, K. J., Gallacher, J. E., and Hatch, E. E. (2013). Why representativeness should be avoided. *International Journal of Epidemiology*, 42, 1012–1014.

Rothman, K. J., Greenland, S., and Lash, T. L. (2008). *Modern Epidemiology*. Philadelphia, PA: Lippincott Williams & Wilkins.

Rubin, D. B. (1978). Bayesian inference for causal effects: The role of randomization. *The Annals of Statistics*, 7, 34–58.

Rubin, D. B. (1980). Comment on "Randomization analysis of experimental data in the Fisher randomization test" by Basu. *J. American Statistical Association*, 75, 591–593.

Sax, P. E., Tierney, C., Collier, A. C., Daar, E. S., Mollan, K., Budhathoki, C., Godfrey, C., et al. (2011). Abacavir/lamivudine versus tenofovir DF/emtricitabine as part of combination regimens for initial treatment of HIV: Final results. *Journal of Infectious Diseases*, 204, 1191–1201.

Sax, P. E., Tierney, C., Collier, A. C., Fischl, M. A., Mollan, K., Peeples, L., Godfrey, C., et al. (2009). Abacavir–lamivudine versus tenofovir–emtricitabine for initial HIV-1 therapy. *New England Journal of Medicine*, 361, 2230–2240.

Scott, A. J. and Wild, C. (1986). Fitting logistic models under case control or choice based sampling. *Journal of the Royal Statistical Society: Series B (Methodological)*, 48, 170–182.

Simon, G. E., Savarino, J., Operskalski, B., and Wang, P. S. (2006). Suicide risk during antidepressant treatment. *American Journal of Psychiatry*, 163, 41–47.

Stuart, E. A., Bradshaw, C. P., and Leaf, P. J. (2015). Assessing the generalizability of randomized trial results to target populations. *Prevention Science*, 16, 475–485.

Stuart, E. A., Cole, S. R., Bradshaw, C. P., and Leaf, P. J. (2011). The use of propensity scores to assess the generalizability of results from randomized trials. *Journal of the Royal Statistical Society: Series A (Statistics in Society)*, 174, 369–386.

Tipton, E. (2013). Improving generalizations from experiments using propensity score subclassification assumptions, properties, and contexts. *Journal of Educational and Behavioral Statistics*, 38, 239–266.

Tipton, E., Hedges, L., Vaden-Kiernan, M., Borman, G., Sullivan, K., and Caverly, S. (2014). Sample selection in randomized experiments: A new method using propensity score stratified sampling. *Journal of Research on Educational Effectiveness*, 7, 114–135.

Valuck, R.J., Libby, A. M., Sills, M. R., Giese, A. A., and Allen, R. R. (2004). Antidepressant treatment and risk of suicide attempt by adolescents with major depressive disorder. *CNS Drugs*, 18, 1119–1132.

Westreich, D. and Cole, S. R. (2010). Invited commentary: Positivity in practice. *American Journal of Epidemiology*, 171, 674–677.

Westreich, D., Lessler, J., and Funk, M. J. (2010). Propensity score estimation: Neural networks, support vector machines, decision trees (cart), and meta-classifiers as alternatives to logistic regression. *Journal of Clinical Epidemiology*, 63, 826–833.

Xie, J. and Liu, C. (2005). Adjusted Kaplan–Meier estimator and log rank test with inverse probability of treatment weighting for survival data. *Statistics in Medicine*, 24, 3089–3110.

Zhang, M., Tsiatis, A. A., and Davidian, M. (2008). Improving efficiency of inferences in randomized clinical trials using auxiliary covariates. *Biometrics*, 64, 707–715.

5

Statistical Tests of Regularity among Groups with HIV Self-Test Data

John Rice
University of Rochester, Rochester, NY

Robert L. Strawderman
University of Rochester, Rochester, NY

Brent A. Johnson
University of Rochester, Rochester, NY

CONTENTS

5.1 Introduction

The HIV epidemic continues to disproportionately affect men who have sex with men (MSM). Recent studies suggest MSM have a 44-fold increase in the rate of infection relative to other men and account for 61% of new HIV diagnoses (Purcell et al. 2012). Many newly diagnosed MSM report not having been tested for HIV for at least 12 months and being unaware of their serostatus. The U.S. Centers for Disease Control and Prevention (CDC) has responded by calling for annual HIV testing among sexually active MSM and even more frequent testing among high-risk MSM (CDC 2010). The government has sponsored interventions and strategies to increase regular HIV testing among MSM but, as we explain below, those charged with quantitatively evaluating the degree of regularity in HIV testing face several challenges.

First, there are challenges in nomenclature. HIV testing performed once every month or once every year can both be considered regular testing, but the frequency of the former is 12 times the latter. Both *regular* and *routine* testing are common phrases often used interchangeably in everyday vernacular and in the scientific literature, but this is not always the case. Recently, Gilead Sciences, Inc., launched the FOCUS program that aims to promote routine HIV and Hepatitis C (HCV) testing in clinics, hospitals, and other health care institutions. In this context, the intended interpretation of routine testing is that clinic staff screen for HIV/HCV in most patients who come to the emergency department (ED). Statisticians might rephrase this use of routine testing as complete or totality testing.

A related point is that the same individual may be no risk for a period of time, then high risk, before returning to a period of low or no risk. If the regularity of HIV testing changes with sexual risk-taking, it may not be sensible to follow exactly the guidelines specified for high risk versus low risk. The reason is because once a person becomes infected, it may take months or years for viremia to rise to detectable levels. In order to increase the probability of detecting a new case as early as possible, one may suggest more frequent HIV testing even if the individual has already returned to a lifestyle of no sexual risk-taking.

In addition to HIV testing, assessing the regularity of a sequence of events over time is relevant to other public health problems. Cancer screening such as mammograms or lower endoscopies is recommended to be performed at certain regular intervals (Centers for Disease Control and Prevention 2003; Davis et al. 2010). However, there is no commonly accepted definition of "regular," and therefore no way of objectively assessing whether or not patients are following these recommendations. In this chapter, we propose an approach based on counting processes for objectively assessing regularity of a population's behavior when we have very "coarse" data, in a sense that will be defined below. This work is important because there is a need for a unified, theoretically grounded statistical method for determining whether or not populations are adhering to recommended screening regimens. Our motivating study is a CDC-sponsored study designed to evaluate the use of text messaging to increase retention in a cohort study of a population of HIV-negative MSM, where data was also collected on whether each subject had performed an HIV self-test during each 2-month period over the course of 1 year (Khosropour et al. 2013). The study randomized eligible men to either receive text message (SMS) or online follow-up and collected data at

2-month intervals for a period of 12 months. The CDC currently recommends yearly testing for HIV in MSM (Centers for Disease Control and Prevention 2010) and more frequent testing for those at increased risk (Mitchell and Horvath 2015). We are interested in two questions:

1. Does either treatment group self-test in a regular manner?
2. Do the two groups differ from one another in their patterns of self-testing?

5.2 Statistical Background

We define a *regular* process to be a Poisson process with constant rate, that is, a homogeneous Poisson process. Mathematically, the key concept in this definition is the hazard or rate function, familiar from survival analysis (Kalbfleisch and Prentice 2002), which quantifies the frequency with which events occur. Assessment of regularity of a stochastic process is therefore straightforward when the precise timing of the events is known (e.g., Moran 1951) and is essentially a test of constant hazard rate over time. The situation is complicated if one does not have access to the exact event times. For example, data for which we may only observe the count of events in each of a set of time intervals is known as panel count data. Many methods have been proposed for the estimation and testing of the hazard function in this setting. Lawless and Zhan (1998) assume a mixed Poisson process, which is essentially a nonhomogeneous Poisson process with a multiplicative random effect; they restrict the rate function to be piecewise constant, but the number of segments in this function is allowed to vary as a trade-off between parametric and nonparametric methods. Sun and Fang (2003) develop a test for equality of hazard functions between several samples that amounts to a score test of the regression parameter for the group indicators being equal to 0 when the processes are Poisson. Zhang (2002) focuses on the estimation of the rate function, developing an estimation procedure under the assumption that the counting process driving the recurrent events is nonhomogeneous Poisson, but goes on to show that the method is consistent for any counting process.

In our motivating problem, however, we only observe the presence or absence of any events in each interval, that is, a binary time series for each subject. Our approach is to treat this observed data as a coarsening of a stochastic process in continuous time. By "coarsening," we specifically mean two distinct operations: discretization and clipping (Foufoula-Georgiou and Lettenmaier 1986). The former is due to the grouping of data within disjoint time intervals, and the latter to grouping events within intervals into the categories *zero* or *at least one* (rather than observing the count of events in each, which would place us in the setting of panel count data; see Sun and Fang (2003) for a test of equality of hazards for this sort of data). An early reference is Davison and Hemphill (1987), who model the probability of at least one ozone exceedance event in a day assuming that these events occur according to a Poisson process.

Guttorp (1986) introduces the zero probability function in this context, which is defined as the probability that no events will occur in some interval. This may be used as a basis for a generalized linear model (GLM) (McCullagh and Nelder 1989) for the observed data. Foufoula-Georgiou and Lettenmaier (1986) compare approaches for continuous-time and discrete-time analysis of point process data, concluding that analyzing discretized time series data using continuous-time methods can result in misleading inferences. Building on such work, Davison and Ramesh (1996) propose a doubly stochastic Poisson process for modeling binary time series data. Cheuvart (1988) proposes such a model, using the logistic link, for recurrent events (such as the presence of one or more tumors following treatment for bladder cancer) when subjects are given follow-up exams according to a predefined schedule. Similarly, Valim et al. (2008) model vaccine efficacy for preventing recurrent infection events: if susceptibility to infection increases with some measure of exposure and if these exposures are distributed as Poisson in each time interval, then the authors show that the model is a binomial GLM with the complementary log–log link.

The connection between the proportional hazards model for survival data and the binomial model with complementary log–log link is also made by Lindsey (1995) and Collett (2003, Sections 9.2 and 9.3), among others, although the earliest such discussion seems to be by Prentice and Gloeckler (1978). This is the basis for our approach as well.

Instead of modeling the probability of compliance with a recommended screening regimen, with "compliance" defined arbitrarily, we propose to directly model the probability of being screened in each time interval; a chi-square likelihood ratio (LR) test is then used to determine if time, included as a categorical covariate, has a significant effect on this probability. This approach is conceptually simple and easily implemented in standard statistical software. In addition, unlike (say) a naïve test for equal proportions, it also allows for nonparametric estimation of the distribution of screening times.

The intuition behind this approach is that, for a population attending screenings regularly, approximately the same proportion of the population should be attending screenings in each of the time intervals composing the study period. In principle, any binary response model for longitudinal data could be used to evaluate regularity in this context, with approximately the same results as what our method will give. Our aim in this chapter, then, is to show that this approach is justified by certain assumptions about the underlying event process in continuous time. Additionally, the use of this approach allows for a much more detailed understanding of the nature of this latent process, specifically in the form of a one-to-one transformation of model parameters into the unspecified baseline hazard of the process, evaluated at fixed points defined by the observation times of the study.

5.3 Model

Suppose that events occur for each of the m subjects under study according to a Poisson process $\{N_i(t),\ t \geq 0\}$ conditional on a p-dimensional covariate vector $\mathbf{z}_i$ with intensity

$$\lambda_i(t) = \tilde{g}_0(t)\exp\{\mathbf{z}_i'\beta\}. \qquad (5.1)$$

where $\tilde{g}_0(t) > 0$ for $t \geq 0$ is otherwise unspecified. This is the multiplicative intensity model widely used in survival analysis (Kalbfleisch and Prentice 2002) with corresponding baseline intensity $\tilde{g}_0(t)$. Without loss of generality, we take the study period to be the interval $[0, 1]$.

Alternatively and equivalently, we can take

$$\lambda_i(t) = g_0(t)\exp\{\beta_0 + \mathbf{z}_i'\beta\}, \qquad (5.2)$$

where $\beta_0 = \log\int_0^1 \tilde{g}_0(t)dt \in (-\infty, \infty)$ and $\int_0^1 g_0(t)dt = 1$. The latter formulation is convenient because it simplifies the interpretation of the model. In particular, for any Poisson process, given that exactly one event has occurred during $[0, 1]$ (i.e., the study period), the conditional distribution of this event time T is easily shown to be

$$P[T \leq t | N_i(1) = 1] = \frac{\int_0^t \lambda_i(s)ds}{\int_0^1 \lambda_i(s)ds} = \frac{\int_0^t g_0(s)\exp\{\beta_0 + \mathbf{z}_i'\beta\}ds}{\int_0^1 g_0(s)\exp\{\beta_0 + \mathbf{z}_i'\beta\}ds} = \frac{\int_0^t g_0(s)ds}{\int_0^1 g_0(s)ds} = \int_0^t g_0(s)ds.$$

Therefore, $g_0(\cdot)$ represents the conditional density of an event time in $[0, 1]$ given the occurrence of exactly one event in $[0, 1]$.

More generally, given that n events occur on this same interval, the sequence of event times has the same distribution as the set of n order statistics from an independent and identically distributed sample from g_0. In the case where the Poisson process is homogeneous, the indicated normalization implies that e^{β_0} is the relevant baseline rate and that $g_0(t) = 1$ for $t \in [0, 1]$.

In our setting, the process $N_i(t)$ is unobserved. Instead, the study period $[0, 1]$ is divided into k intervals, with endpoints $0 \equiv t_0 < t_1 < \ldots < t_k \equiv 1$. The observed data consist of a series of binary indicators of the event $N_{ij} \equiv N_i(t_j) - N_i(t_j - 1) > 0$ for $j = 1, \ldots, k$. Specifically, we observe

$$Y_{ij} = \begin{cases} 1, & N_i(t_j) - N_i(t_{j-1}) > 0, \\ 0, & N_i(t_j) - N_i(t_{j-1}) = 0. \end{cases}$$

Although we develop these ideas for equally spaced intervals (i.e., we assume that $t_j - t_{j-1} = 1/k$ for all j), this is not essential. We do require that the intervals be the same for all subjects, however. This considerably simplifies matters from a statistical perspective, although it only allows us to estimate the hazard function's value nonparametrically at specific points (in contrast to, e.g., Zhang 2002; Sun and Fang 2003, in the panel count setting). Lindsey (1995) allows for different units of observation across subjects but is primarily concerned with Poisson (count) rather than binomial (indicator) models and so is able to incorporate the appropriate offset terms into the estimation procedure.

5.3.1 Hypothesis Testing for Regularity

We are interested in testing the null hypothesis that subjects are behaving in a regular manner. In this chapter, we will interpret regularity as attending screenings according to a homogeneous Poisson process. The reasoning behind this definition is that for such a process, given the number of events in an interval, the distribution of the times of those events will be uniform on that interval (Ross 1996, p. 67). For a sample of size $n = N_i(1)$ from a uniform distribution on the unit interval (i.e., n is the number of events experienced by the ith subject in the totality of the study period), the jth order statistic has expectation $j/(n + 1)$, implying on average equal spacing of tests over the study period (see, e.g., Casella and Berger 2001, theorem 5.4.4).

Assuming that intervals are of equal length, define

$$G_j = \int_{(j-1)/k}^{j/k} g_0(t)dt, \quad j = 1, \ldots, k; \tag{5.3}$$

under our assumptions on $g_0(\cdot)$, it follows that $G_j > 0$ for each j and $\sum_{j=1}^{k} G_j = 1$. Therefore, the expected number of events in the jth interval is $\mathbb{E}[N_i(t_j) - N_i(t_{j-1})] = \int_{(j-1)/k}^{j/k} \lambda_i(t)dt = G_j \exp\{\beta_0 + z_i'\beta\}$. The probability that any tests have occurred for the ith subject in the jth interval is then

$$P(Y_{ij} = 1|z_i) = \mathbb{E}(Y_{ij}|z_i) = 1 - e^{-G_j \exp\{\beta_0 + z_i'\beta\}}, \tag{5.4}$$

which corresponds to a binomial GLM with a complementary log–log link function [see Prentice and Gloeckler (1978), who originally suggested a similar model in the context of grouped survival data without recurrent events in an attempt to deal more rigorously with data with many tied failure times]. In this formulation, there are $k + p$ free parameters, namely β_0, G_2, ..., G_k, and the p-dimensional regression parameter β.

We propose to use an LR test for the effect of time on the probability of experiencing at least one event in a given interval. This is similar to the approach of Brown (1975), although we use the complementary log–log link rather than the logistic because of the proportional hazards structure of our model. As in Brown (1975), we introduce a set of $k - 1$ dummy variables for the k observation intervals, with associated coefficients $\boldsymbol{\gamma} = (\gamma_2, \ldots, \gamma_k)'$, so that

$$\mathbb{E}(Y_{ij}|\mathbf{z}_i) = \begin{cases} 1 - e^{-\exp\{\beta_0^* + \mathbf{z}_i'\boldsymbol{\beta}\}}, & j = 1 \\ 1 - e^{-\exp\{\beta_0^* + \mathbf{z}_i'\boldsymbol{\beta} + \gamma_j\}}, & 2 \leq j \leq k, \end{cases}$$

where $\beta_0^* = \beta_0 + \log G_1$. In this formulation, $e^{\gamma_j} = G_j/G_1, j = 2, \ldots, k$. It is shown in Section 5.3.2 why one can estimate $\beta_0^*, \gamma_2, \ldots, \gamma_k$ in place of $\beta_0, G_2, \ldots, G_k$; we also relate these parameterizations to estimation under (5.1) with the same time-grouped structure.

Under the assumption that testing for subject i follows a homogeneous Poisson process, we recall that $g_0(t) = 1$ for $t \in [0, 1]$ and hence that $G_1 = G_2 = \ldots = G_k = 1/k$. Consequently, in the LR test of interest, our null hypothesis corresponds to $H_0 : \gamma_2 = \gamma_3 = \ldots = \gamma_k = 0$. This means that the ratios of the probability mass falling in each of the intervals $j = 2, \ldots, k$ to the mass in the first interval are all equal to 1. As a result, conditional on the occurrence of one event during the study period, that event is equally likely to occur in any interval.

Note that although this test may exclude the possibility of the underlying event process being homogeneous Poisson, failure to reject does not necessarily imply the converse. This is because with a fixed set of k observation times, we are unable to make any statements whatsoever about the behavior of the process within observation intervals.

Our approach, paralleling the suggestion of Brown (1975), is similar to one of the models discussed by Lindsey (1995) with the restriction that the only time-dependent covariate that may be included in the model is time itself (or, as we will see in the two-sample case, the interaction between time and the group indicator). This is an important distinction, as inclusion of any other time-dependent covariates would mean that Equation 5.2 would no longer factor into a common hazard function and a subject-specific multiplier.

5.3.2 Identifiability of Model Parameters

Considering the model (5.1), define

$$\tilde{G}_j = \int_{(j-1)/k}^{j/k} \tilde{g}_0(t)\,dt, \quad j = 1, \ldots, k, \tag{5.5}$$

and observe that $\tilde{G}_j = e^{\beta_0} G_j$ for $j = 1, \ldots, k$. Starting with the unconstrained model parameterization involving the $k + p$ free parameters $(\tilde{G}_1, \ldots, \tilde{G}_k$ and the p-dimensional regression parameter $\boldsymbol{\beta}$, excluding β_0), observe that

$$
\log[-\log P(Y_{ij} = 0|\mathbf{z}_i)] = \log\tilde{G}_j + \mathbf{z}_i'\boldsymbol{\beta} =
\begin{cases}
\log \tilde{G}_1 + \mathbf{z}_i'\boldsymbol{\beta}, & j = 1 \\[2mm]
\log \tilde{G}_1 + \log \dfrac{\tilde{G}_j}{\tilde{G}_1} + \mathbf{z}_i'\boldsymbol{\beta}, & 2 \le j \le k
\end{cases}
$$

(5.6)

Using the facts that $\tilde{G}_j = e^{\beta_0} G_j$ for $j = 1, \ldots, k$ and $\Sigma_{j=1}^k G_j = 1$, we may now rewrite Equation 5.6 as

$$
\log[-\log P(Y_{ij} = 0|\mathbf{z}_i)] =
\begin{cases}
\beta_0 + \log(1 - \Sigma_{v=2}^k G_v) + \mathbf{z}_i'\boldsymbol{\beta}, & j = 1 \\[2mm]
\beta_0 + \log(1 - \Sigma_{v=2}^k G_v) + \log \dfrac{G_j}{1 - \Sigma_{v=2}^k G_v} + \mathbf{z}_i'\boldsymbol{\beta}, & 2 \le j \le k
\end{cases}
$$

$$
=
\begin{cases}
\beta_0^* + \mathbf{z}_i'\boldsymbol{\beta}, & j = 1 \\
\beta_0^* + \gamma_j + \mathbf{z}_i'\boldsymbol{\beta}, & 2 \le j \le k,
\end{cases}
$$

(5.7)

where $\beta_0^* = \beta_0 + \log G_1$ and $e_j^\gamma = G_j/G_1$, $j = 2, \ldots, k$. We see that (5.7) is just a reparameterization of (5.6) with the $k + p$ free parameters $\beta_0^*, \gamma_2, \ldots, \gamma_k$ and the p-dimensional regression parameter $\boldsymbol{\beta}$.

The reparameterization of the linear predictor in (5.6) and (5.7) shows why it is sufficient to estimate $\beta_0^*, \gamma_2, \ldots, \gamma_k$ in place of either $\beta_0^*, G_2, \ldots, G_k$ or β_0, $G_2, \ldots, G_k$; calculation of the maximum likelihood estimators (MLEs) in one parameterization allows one to recover the MLEs in another. To see this, we only need to be able to recover
$(G_1, G_2, \ldots, G_k)$ from $(\gamma_2, \ldots, \gamma_k)$. Recall that $\Sigma_{j=1}^k G_j = 1$; therefore,

$$
\sum_{j=2}^k e^{\gamma_j} = \frac{1}{G_1} \sum_{j=2}^k G_j = \frac{1 - G_1}{G_1}.
$$

Solving for G_1, we get

$$
G_1 = \frac{1}{1 + \Sigma_{j=2}^k e^{\gamma_j}},
$$

implying that

$$
G_j = \frac{e^{\gamma_j}}{1 + \Sigma_{v=2}^k e^{\gamma_v}}, \quad j = 2, \ldots, k.
$$

(5.8)

It follows from these calculations that estimation of $\gamma_2, \ldots, \gamma_k$ is equivalent to $G_1, \ldots, G_k$ under the constraint $\Sigma_{j=1}^k G_j = 1$. The result (5.8) also shows directly why $G_j = 1/k$ for all j under $H_0: \gamma_2 = \ldots = \gamma_k$.

5.4 LR Tests for Uniformity

5.4.1 One-Sample Problem

Let

$$\eta_{ij}(\beta_0^*, \boldsymbol{\beta}, \boldsymbol{\gamma}) = \begin{cases} \beta_0^* + z_i'\boldsymbol{\beta}, & j = 1 \\ \beta_0^* + z_i'\boldsymbol{\beta} + \gamma_j, & 2 \leq j \leq k, \end{cases} \tag{5.9}$$

The full log-likelihood contribution for the ith subject is $\sum_{j=1}^{k} \ell_{ij}(\beta_0^*, \boldsymbol{\beta}, \boldsymbol{\gamma})$, where

$$\ell_{ij}(\beta_0^*, \boldsymbol{\beta}, \boldsymbol{\gamma}) = Y_{ij} \log\left(1 - e^{-\exp\{\eta_{ij}(\beta_0^*, \boldsymbol{\beta}, \boldsymbol{\gamma})\}}\right) - (1 - Y_{ij}) \exp\{\eta_{ij}(\beta_0^*, \boldsymbol{\beta}, \boldsymbol{\gamma})\}. \tag{5.10}$$

Because we are assuming a Poisson process for testing events, independent increments imply that we may treat observations within a subject as independent from one another.

Now, letting $\log L(\beta_0^*, \boldsymbol{\beta}, \boldsymbol{\gamma}) = \sum_{i=1}^{m} \sum_{j=1}^{k} \ell_{ij}(\beta_0^*, \boldsymbol{\beta}, \boldsymbol{\gamma})$,

$$-2 \log \frac{\sup_{\beta_0^* \in \mathbb{R}, \boldsymbol{\beta} \in \mathbb{R}^p} L(\beta_0^*, \boldsymbol{\beta}, \mathbf{0})}{\sup_{\beta_0^* \in \mathbb{R}, \boldsymbol{\beta} \in \mathbb{R}^p, \boldsymbol{\gamma} \in \mathbb{R}^{k-1}} L(\beta_0^*, \boldsymbol{\beta}, \boldsymbol{\gamma})} \sim \chi_{k-1}^2 \tag{5.11}$$

asymptotically under H_0 (McCullagh and Nelder 1989). To accommodate intervals of differing widths, this statistic may be modified to

$$-2\log \frac{\sup_{\beta_0^* \in \mathbb{R}, \boldsymbol{\beta} \in \mathbb{R}^p} L(\beta_0^*, \boldsymbol{\beta}, \boldsymbol{\gamma}^0)}{\sup_{\beta_0^* \in \mathbb{R}, \boldsymbol{\beta} \in \mathbb{R}^p, \boldsymbol{\gamma} \in \mathbb{R}^{k-1}} L(\beta_0^*, \boldsymbol{\beta}, \boldsymbol{\gamma})} \sim \chi_{k-1}^2,$$

where $\boldsymbol{\gamma}^0 = (\gamma_2^0, ..., \gamma_k^0)'$ and $\gamma_j^0 = \log(t_j - t_{j-1}) - \log(t_1)$, $j = 2, ..., k$.

5.4.2 Two-Sample Problem

Now suppose we would like to compare the regularity of testing between two groups. There are two possible questions of interest now:

1. Do the two groups differ from one another in their regularity of testing?
2. Does either group differ from uniformity in its testing patterns?

The first question does not make reference to any baseline definition of uniformity, and will fail to reject the null hypothesis even if both groups are substantially different from uniform in their testing patterns as long as they deviate from uniformity in roughly the same way. The second question is more restrictive, but is perhaps more important from a practical standpoint, as it will reject the null hypothesis if there is any deviation from uniformity in either or both of the groups with respect to testing patterns.

To formulate this in terms of model parameters, let $\gamma_2, \ldots, \gamma_k$ be, as before, the parameters corresponding to the dummy variables for interval in the first group, with sample size m_1; and let $\delta_2, \ldots, \delta_k$ be the same parameters for the second group, with sample size m_2. To address our first question, the null hypothesis is

$$H_0 : \gamma_2 = \delta_2, \ldots, \gamma_k = \delta_k, \tag{5.12}$$

while for the second question, the null hypothesis is

$$H_0 : \gamma_2 = \cdots = \gamma_k = \delta_2 = \cdots = \delta_k = 0. \tag{5.13}$$

Now let x_i be the treatment indicator, that is, the covariate taking value 1 if the subject is in the treated group and 0 if control. Let

$$\eta_{ij}(\beta_0^*, \boldsymbol{\beta}, \boldsymbol{\gamma}, \boldsymbol{\delta}) = \begin{cases} \beta_0^* + x_i(\alpha_0^* - \beta_0^*) + \mathbf{z}_i'\boldsymbol{\beta}, & j = 1 \\ \beta_0^* + x_i(\alpha_0^* - \beta_0^*) + \mathbf{z}_i'\boldsymbol{\beta} + \gamma_j + x_i(\delta_j - \gamma_j), & 2 \leq j \leq k, \end{cases}$$

and let $\mathbf{z}_i$ now include all covariates as well as all treatment-by-covariate interactions, with $\boldsymbol{\beta}$ likewise appropriately augmented; this means that $\boldsymbol{\beta}$ now has dimension 2_p. The parameter $\alpha_0^* - \beta_0^*$ is the main effect of treatment, so that for a subject in the treatment group, $\alpha_0^* = \alpha_0 + \log F_1$, where α_0 is analogous to β_0 in (5.2), and F_j is analogous to G_j in Equation 5.3.

To test the null hypothesis (5.12), we have

$$-2\log \frac{\sup_{\beta_0^* \in \mathbb{R}, \alpha_0^* \in \mathbb{R}, \boldsymbol{\beta} \in \mathbb{R}^{2p}, \boldsymbol{\gamma} \in \mathbb{R}^{k-1}} L(\beta_0^*, \alpha_0^*, \boldsymbol{\beta}, \boldsymbol{\gamma}, \boldsymbol{\gamma})}{\sup_{\beta_0^* \in \mathbb{R}, \alpha_0^* \in \mathbb{R}, \boldsymbol{\beta} \in \mathbb{R}^{2p}, \boldsymbol{\gamma} \in \mathbb{R}^{k-1}, \boldsymbol{\delta} \in \mathbb{R}^{k-1}} L(\beta_0^*, \alpha_0^*, \boldsymbol{\beta}, \boldsymbol{\gamma}, \boldsymbol{\delta})} \sim \chi_{k-1}^2. \tag{5.14}$$

Likewise, to test (5.13), we have

$$-2\log \frac{\sup_{\beta_0^* \in \mathbb{R}, \alpha_0^* \in \mathbb{R}, \boldsymbol{\beta} \in \mathbb{R}^{2p}} L(\beta_0^*, \alpha_0^*, \boldsymbol{\beta}, 0, 0)}{\sup_{\beta_0^* \in \mathbb{R}, \alpha_0^* \in \mathbb{R}, \boldsymbol{\beta} \in \mathbb{R}^{2p}, \boldsymbol{\gamma} \in \mathbb{R}^{k-1}, \boldsymbol{\delta} \in \mathbb{R}^{k-1}} L(\beta_0^*, \alpha_0^*, \boldsymbol{\beta}, \boldsymbol{\gamma}, \boldsymbol{\delta})} \sim \chi_{2(k-1)}^2, \tag{5.15}$$

The test in (5.14) is equivalent to a test of the time-by-treatment interaction in a longitudinal analysis (Fitzmaurice et al. 2004). The test in (5.15), by contrast, is a joint test of the hypothesis of no time effect in either treatment group. Note that in neither test are we concerned with the main effect for treatment. We thereby allow for the baseline rate of the process to differ between the two treatment groups, as we are only interested in the pattern of testing over time. The fact that the probability mass falling into first interval does not appear separately in the set of parameters (i.e., $\gamma_2, \ldots, \gamma_k$,

$\delta_2, \ldots, \delta_k$) used for the test is not relevant, because both null hypotheses imply their equivalence between the two treatment groups: if, as in null hypothesis (5.12), $\gamma_j = \delta_j$ for all $j \geq 2$, then $\log \frac{G_j}{G_1} = \log \frac{F_j}{F_1}$, which implies that $\log \frac{G_j}{F_j} = \log \frac{G_1}{F_1}$ for all $j \geq 2$ as well. Therefore, if $\gamma_j = \delta_j$ for all $j \geq 2$, $G_1 = F_1$ also. The same argument applies for null hypothesis (5.13), since this is a special case of (5.12) with $\gamma_j = \delta_j = 0$ for all $j \geq 2$, so $G_1 = F_1 = 1/k$.

5.5 Application to a Study of Self-Testing for HIV

We applied the proposed method to the data set originally analyzed by Khosropour et al. (2013). There were a total of 329 subjects in the online treatment group and 317 in the SMS treatment group. Variables on which data were collected included baseline demographic variables such as age, education level, and race, as well as whether a subject had self-tested for HIV during each of the 2-month intervals for which that subject was followed. In our notation, Y_{ij} is the variable indicating that the ith subject has self-tested for HIV during the jth interval, $j = 1, \ldots, k = 6$.

Table 5.1 presents interval-specific summaries of the data. Specifically, the table shows the proportion of subjects in each interval for whom any data was recorded (reflecting response or participation rate for that interval), as well as the proportion of subjects who reported testing in that interval. It is clear from this table that the response rate declined over time for both treatment groups. We are also able to see the difference in testing patterns between the two treatment groups, at least in one respect: the online group had a large spike in tests in the first interval, which thereafter declined to roughly the same level as for the SMS group. The SMS group, by contrast, seems to have tested less in the first interval than in subsequent intervals. A slightly different perspective is obtained by examining the distribution of number of testing intervals by subject: this reveals that a much larger proportion of the SMS group never tested compared with the online group (50% vs. 16%).

The results of the LR chi-square tests for regularity described in Section 5.4 are displayed in Table 5.2; the models are adjusted for baseline covariates (race, education, and age). It is not surprising that we have highly significant evidence against the null hypothesis of uniformity for both groups, due primarily to the testing behavior of subjects in the first interval. As noted above, the online subjects seem to have tested at a much greater rate in this interval than in subsequent intervals, while those in the SMS group tested at a somewhat lower rate in the first interval compared with later intervals.

For a more direct perspective on this, see Table 5.3, which gives the estimated $\hat{G}_j$ for each group, along with their standard errors. This table mirrors

TABLE 5.1

Summary Statistics Pertaining to Intervals

	Interval					
	1	2	3	4	5	6
Online response rate	0.991	0.936	0.903	0.875	0.860	0.830
SMS response rate	0.987	0.946	0.921	0.880	0.852	0.590
Online testing rate (conditional)	0.715	0.227	0.178	0.181	0.201	0.198
SMS testing rate (conditional)	0.109	0.210	0.144	0.204	0.181	0.246
Online testing rate (marginal)	0.708	0.213	0.161	0.158	0.173	0.164
SMS testing rate (marginal)	0.107	0.199	0.132	0.180	0.155	0.145

Note: The response rate is the proportion of unique subjects in the data set with data on the interval in question; the testing rates labeled "conditional" are the proportion of subjects who reported testing in that interval, given that data were recorded on that subject for the interval; and the testing rates labeled "marginal" are the testing rates obtained by filling in missing values with 0, that is, assuming that subjects not reporting in an interval did not test in that interval.

the information shown in the conditional testing rate rows of Table 5.1, at least in terms of the relative magnitudes of the estimated probabilities in each interval.

Table 5.3 shows that the conditional distribution of the time of any test given its occurrence during the study period is heavily skewed in the case of the online group, with half the mass concentrated in the first interval. The density for the SMS group is somewhat flatter, although there is relatively more mass in the second through sixth intervals in this group compared with the first interval. Note that for this table, the null hypothesis would assign mass of $1/k \approx 0.167$ to each interval.

To examine the impact of the first interval on our results, Table 5.2 also shows the results of the LR tests for this data set with the analysis restricted to Intervals 2–6. All significance disappears, with only the SMS group coming at all close to being significantly different from uniform. Therefore, we conclude that it is indeed the subjects' behavior during the first interval which is causing the observed deviation from uniformity seen with the full data set.

Since, as we see in Table 5.1, there is substantial dropout for this data set (especially in the SMS group in the final interval), we also conducted the analysis assuming that any intervals for which a subject was missing data were intervals for which that subject had not self-tested. The LR test results for this analysis are given in Table 5.2, but our conclusions do not differ substantially. It seems as though this assumption results in the online group appearing to deviate slightly more from uniformity and the SMS group slightly less, but overall it appears that the method is robust to our treatment of missing data, at least for this data set.

TABLE 5.2

Likelihood Ratio Chi-Square Tests for Uniformity in Testing Patterns

	LR Statistic	DF	*P*-value
All Intervals, Ignoring Missing Data			
Online: deviation from uniformity	323.6	5	0.0000
SMS: deviation from uniformity	23.0	5	0.0003
Deviation in testing patterns between online and SMS	187.8	5	0.0000
Either online or SMS: deviation from uniformity	346.6	10	0.0000
Excluding First Interval, Ignoring Missing Data			
Online: deviation from uniformity	2.9	4	0.5689
SMS: deviation from uniformity	9.1	4	0.0585
Deviation in testing patterns between online and SMS	3.8	4	0.4329
Either online or SMS: deviation from uniformity	12.0	8	0.1494
All Intervals, Assuming Missing Data Indicates No Self-Testing			
Online: deviation from uniformity	367.1	5	0.0000
SMS: deviation from uniformity	13.3	5	0.0204
Deviation in testing patterns between online and SMS	175.6	5	0.0000
Either online or SMS: deviation from uniformity	380.4	10	0.0000

Note: LR, likelihood ratio; DF, degrees of freedom.

TABLE 5.3

Estimates of G_j for Each Group (Standard Errors Are Given Below the Value for $\hat{G}_j$)

Group		1		2	3	3	5	6
Online	Estimate	0.540	Missing	0.108	0.082	0.083	0.094	0.093
	Std. err.	0.023		0.013	0.011	0.011	0.012	0.012
	Estimate	0.569	Filled	0.108	0.079	0.078	0.086	0.080
	Std. err.	0.023		0.013	0.011	0.011	0.011	0.011
SMS	Estimate	0.094	Missing	0.194	0.127	0.188	0.165	0.232
	Std. err.	0.016		0.022	0.019	0.023	0.022	0.029
	Estimate	0.113	Filled	0.221	0.142	0.198	0.168	0.158
	Std. err.	0.018		0.025	0.020	0.024	0.022	0.021

Note: Recall that this provides an estimate of the probability mass between the points t_{j-1} and t_j in the conditional distribution of an event time given its occurrence; because in this study we have $k = 6$ equally spaced intervals, this is the probability mass between $(j - 1)/k$ and j/k. Estimates are provided for each of the two ways of addressing the issue of missing data: "missing" indicates the estimates obtained by treating missing data as ignorable, while "filled" indicates estimates obtained after filling in 0 as the outcome for all subjects with missing data (i.e., assuming that not reporting implied not self-testing).

Although it seems from Table 5.2 that there is less evidence of deviation from uniformity for the SMS group than for the online group, this is only one aspect of the problem from a public health perspective. While it is desirable for individuals to self-test regularly, it is also important that they be testing frequently; this is the concept of "routine" versus "regular" as we have defined it. The statistics $\hat{G}_1, ..., \hat{G}_k$ only provide information on regularity of testing; we need to examine the full regression model for information on frequency of testing.

From the form of the model in Equation 5.4 and with $\hat{\eta}_{ij} \equiv \eta_{ij}(\widehat{\beta_0^*}, \widehat{\beta}, \hat{\gamma})$ defined as in Equation 5.9, we may predict the number of tests for a given subject over the course of the study by $\mathbb{E}\, N_i(1) = \Sigma_{j=1}^k\, e^{\widehat{\eta_{ij}}}$. Boxplots of these fitted values are shown in Figure 5.1. This figure shows the expected number of self-testing events for each subject over the course of the study as if each subject had been followed for the entire 12-month period. Clearly, the SMS group self-tests at a much lower rate than the online group, regardless of which assumption regarding missing data is made. The main effect of assuming that missing data indicate that no tests were performed seems to be a modest shift to the left in the distribution of self-testing rates, with subjects predicted to have the highest rates in the incomplete data analysis exhibiting the greatest changes.

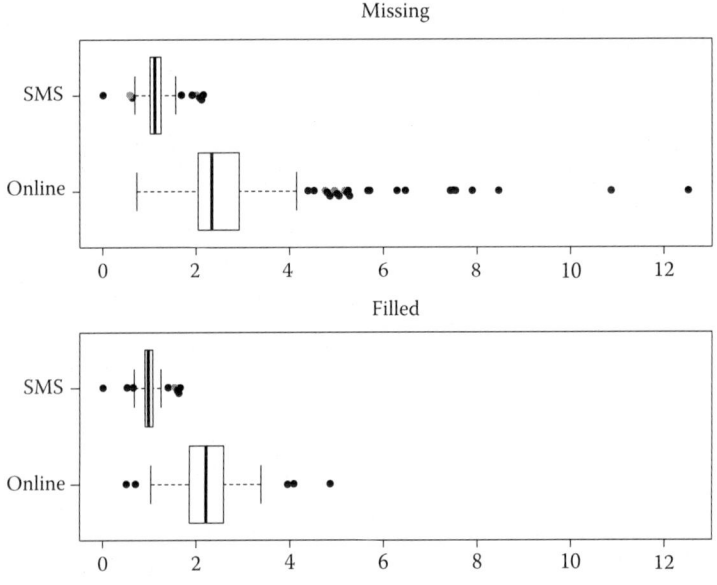

FIGURE 5.1
Expected number of tests by treatment group. "Missing" indicates analysis of the data set as it is, with ignorable missingness, while "filled" indicates analysis following the replacement of missing outcomes with 0.

These predicted numbers of tests allow us to assess whether subjects are testing frequently enough. Although we reject the null hypothesis of regularity for both the online and SMS groups, in the online group more than 99% of subjects are predicted to have tested at least once, which is the current CDC recommendation for MSM (Centers for Disease Control and Prevention 2010), regardless of how missing data are dealt with. In the SMS group, however, analyzing the data as-is leads to a conclusion that roughly 76% of men are testing at least once per year, while filling in the missing outcomes with 0 results in a decrease of that figure to 48%.

5.6 Simulation Studies

Standard asymptotic arguments for MLE in GLMs apply to our model, so that simulation results comparing estimated parameter values to the truth and estimated to observed standard errors are omitted. However, we wish to evaluate the performance of the proposed method with respect to power in detecting departures from regularity. We therefore performed simulations to examine the rejection rate of the null hypothesis that each of two groups was experiencing events according to a homogeneous Poisson process, as well as the two-sample null hypotheses (5.12) and (5.13). We compare results for four values of k (3, 4, 6, and 12) to determine what effect the granularity of the data has on power and five simulation settings corresponding to the true data-generating mechanism.

All $m = 100$ subjects in each of the two groups had a number of events $N_i(1)$ over the course of the study generated according to a Poisson distribution with mean $e^{z_i'1}$ where z_i was composed of two independent Bernoulli variables with mean 1/2 for the first group and two independent standard normal variables for the second group. Then the times of the events were generated independently from a beta distribution with parameters a_1, b_1 for the first group and a_2, b_2 for the second group. (The beta density here corresponds to g_0 above.) We used the following combinations of beta parameters:

1. $a_1 = b_1 = a_2 = b_2 = 1$: both groups are uniform, so all four null hypotheses are true.

2. $a_1 = b_1 = 1$, $a_2 = b_2 = 0.8$: the first group is uniform, but the second group is more inclined to experience events at the beginning and end of the study period.

3. $a_1 = b_1 = 1$, $a_2 = 0.8$, $b_2 = 1$: the first group is uniform, but the second group is more likely to experience events at the beginning of the study period.

4. $a_1 = b_1 = a_2 = b_2 = 0.8$: both groups are more inclined to experience events at the beginning and end of the study period.

5. $a_1 = 0.8, b_1 = a_2 = 1, b_2 = 0.8$: the first group is more likely to experience events at the beginning of the study period, while the second group is more likely to experience events at the end of the study period.

See Figure 5.2 for a graphical presentation of the testing patterns of each group under each of these scenarios. Results of the simulation studies are presented in Table 5.4. We see that under Scenario 1, when all null hypotheses are true (since both groups have the same pattern of events, and that pattern is uniform), rejection rates are close to the nominal significance level. The slight deviations from 5% are most likely the result of the relatively small sample size considered here.

We are also able to detect a clear trend of increasing power with increasing k, so that the number of intervals per subject seems to add considerably to our ability to detect deviations from regularity. This is also what intuition would lead us to expect, as with more intervals, we are able to resolve the process to a finer level of detail.

Power in the one-sample test of uniformity appears to be considerably greater when detecting asymmetric patterns of events (compare Scenarios 2 and 3). The generally greater power seen in the one-sample tests for Group 1

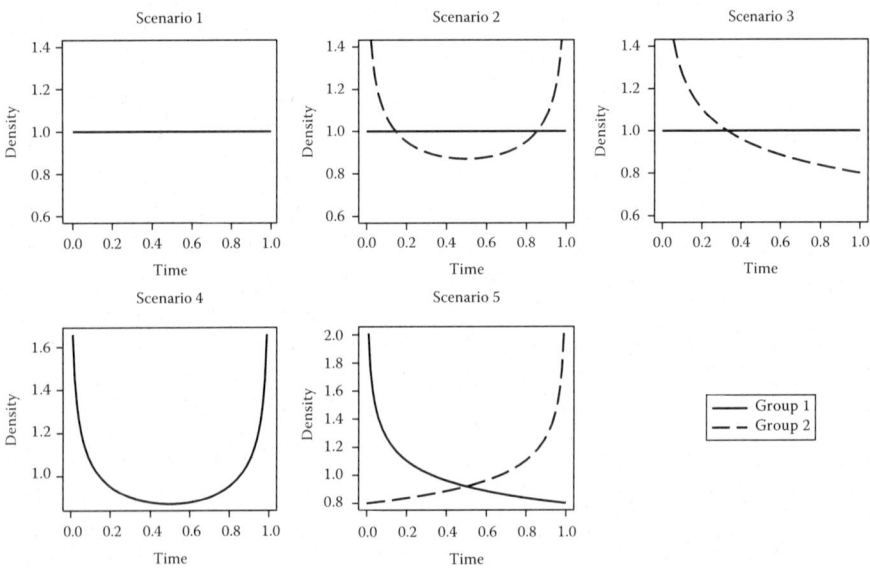

FIGURE 5.2
Densities g_0 corresponding to each of the five simulation scenarios. These are proportional to the hazard rate λ_0 and so are reflective of when subjects are relatively more or less likely to experience an event.

TABLE 5.4

Simulation Results

Null Hypothesis	k	Scenario 1	2	3	4	5
Group 1 is uniform	3	0.050	0.056	0.059	0.161	0.459
	4	0.072	0.040	0.057	0.233	0.541
	6	0.046	0.051	0.058	0.312	0.568
	12	0.042	0.052	0.055	0.384	0.616
Group 2 is uniform	3	0.066	0.126	0.274	0.111	0.293
	4	0.057	0.123	0.305	0.171	0.309
	6	0.061	0.176	0.356	0.213	0.347
	12	0.055	0.233	0.404	0.216	0.404
Groups are the same	3	0.057	0.100	0.193	0.055	0.565
	4	0.060	0.086	0.223	0.057	0.651
	6	0.066	0.139	0.240	0.073	0.683
	12	0.044	0.145	0.265	0.051	0.743
Both groups are uniform	3	0.062	0.101	0.215	0.190	0.528
	4	0.076	0.083	0.236	0.278	0.623
	6	0.056	0.144	0.273	0.388	0.672
	12	0.055	0.178	0.289	0.460	0.738

Note: This table shows the rejection rate of the likelihood ratio test under each of the null hypotheses described above at a nominal significance level of 5%.

under Scenarios 4 and 5 (where this group deviates from the null hypothesis) is due to the fact that it experiences a slightly higher rate of events due to its covariate distribution (Bernoulli vs. standard normal).

The power for the two-sample test for both groups having the same pattern of events is higher when neither group is uniform (compare Scenarios 2 and 3 with Scenario 5), which is also what intuition would suggest. The test for both groups jointly being uniform also has greater power when neither is uniform (as in Scenario 5), but power is reduced when the two groups both deviate from uniformity in the same way (Scenario 4).

5.7 Discussion

In this chapter, we have proposed a method for evaluation of regularity of an event process using binary outcome data corresponding to serial observations of whether or not some event of interest has occurred. We assume that the data come from a (possibly nonhomogeneous) Poisson process, and propose the use of an LR test of the effect of time on the probability of experiencing at least one event in order to assess the regularity of the underlying event process. The use of this particular model also allows us to obtain nonparametric estimates of the conditional distribution of the event times, as seen in Table 5.3 for the HIV self-testing data set.

Our test is comparable to a test for a constant hazard rate (in the one-sample case), which for binary data becomes a test of equality of proportions (Cheuvart 1988). In the two-sample case, it is comparable to a test of equal hazards [as in Sun and Fang (2003), for panel count data]. The distinction is that, with fixed observation intervals, we are unable to determine the behavior of the underlying process within these intervals, so that while rejecting our null hypothesis implies a rejection of the null hypothesis that a homogeneous Poisson process has generated the data, failing to reject does not imply the converse.

We see this work as providing a firm theoretical justification for the analysis of binary serial data on screening when the aim is to assess adherence to a recommended regular regimen. The literature on regular screening exams as a whole does not seem to have addressed the problem from the perspective of recurrent events, but rather categorizes subjects on the basis of some more or less subjective definition of regularity. Often only two categories are used (e.g., Davis et al. 2010), which is convenient from an analyst's perspective since it allows for the use of logistic regression, but greatly reduces the available information about regularity by dichotomizing the outcome. Even when more categories are used (e.g., Zapka et al. 1991; Johnson et al. 1996), they must be somehow ranked in order of "degree of compliance" or the like, which introduces another level of subjectivity into the analysis.

What we have proposed instead is a means of unifying the study of regularity into an objective framework based on a Poisson process model for the event times. It is not necessary to restrict the testing to one- or two-sample tests as we have discussed here; it can in principle be generalized to test the association of any covariate with regularity. A limiting factor here would be the number of parameters we would need to estimate, which could be quite large in the case of categorical covariates. However, in many of the studies on regularity available in the literature, the analysis can be distilled into a very small number of intervals, so that $k = 2$ or $k = 3$ is common.

As much of the literature on regularity in screening is based on responses to survey questions which are often formulated in terms of the time of the most recent exam, it would be interesting to extend this work to be able to deal with cases in which the first interval did not have a definite left endpoint. For example, although the analysis in Davis et al. (2010) used a binary measure of regularity, the surveys from which their data were derived collected more detail, corresponding to $k = 5$, with the first interval not having a defined length, the second interval of length 2 years, and the third through fifth intervals of 1 year each.

A potential shortcoming of the method is that it provides no way to detect departures from regularity on the subject level, as it assumes a common rate of testing within each interval across all subjects within each treatment group. It is not obvious how to evaluate a single subject's binary time series from the perspective of regularity, making this a potentially interesting area for future research.

We have used one particular definition of regularity, motivated by a uniformity property of the homogeneous Poisson process based on equal expected spacing of events. However, other definitions are possible, and perhaps preferable. Use of such definitions as equal *observed* (as opposed to expected) spacing of events with binary data would not be straightforward, providing another fruitful direction for further study.

Acknowledgments

The authors acknowledge and thank Dr. Patrick Sullivan for providing the HIV self-test data from the *Checking In!* study in Section 5.5. The project described in this publication was supported by the University of Rochester CTSA award (UL1 TR000042) from the National Center for Advancing Translational Sciences of the National Institutes of Health.

References

Brown, C. C. (1975). On the use of indicator variables for studying the time-dependence of parameters in a response-time model. *Biometrics* 31, 863–872.

Casella, G. and Berger, R. L. (2001). *Statistical Inference*. Pacific Grove, CA: Duxbury, second edition.

Centers for Disease Control and Prevention. (2003). Colorectal cancer test use among persons aged ≥ 50 years—United States, 2001. *Morbidity and Mortality Weekly Report* 52, 193–196.

Centers for Disease Control and Prevention. (2010). Sexually transmitted diseases treatment guidelines, 2010. *Morbidity and Mortality Weekly Report: Recommendations and Reports* 59, 1–109.

Cheuvart, B. (1988). A nonparametric model for multiple recurrences. *Journal of the Royal Statistical Society, Series C (Applied Statistics)* 37, 157–168.

Collett, D. (2003). *Modelling Survival Data in Medical Research*. London, UK: Chapman & Hall/CRC, second edition.

Davis, W. W., Parsons, V. L., Xie, D., Schenker, N., Town, M., Raghunathan, T. E., and Feuer, E. J. (2010). State-based estimates of mammography screening rates based on information from two health surveys. *Public Health Reports* 125, 567–578.

Davison, A. C. and Hemphill, M. W. (1987). On the statistical analysis of ambient ozone data when measurements are missing. *Atmospheric Environment* 21, 629–639.

Davison, A. C. and Ramesh, N. I. (1996). Some models for discretized series of events. *Journal of the American Statistical Association* 91, 601–609.

Fitzmaurice, G. M., Laird, N. M., and Ware, J. H. (2004). *Applied Longitudinal Analysis*. Hoboken, NJ: John Wiley & Sons.

Foufoula-Georgiou, E. and Lettenmaier, D. P. (1986). Continuous-time versus discrete-time point process models for rainfall occurrence series. *Water Resources Research* 22, 531–542.

Guttorp, P. (1986). On binary time series obtained from continuous time point processes describing rainfall. *Water Resources Research* 22, 897–904.

Johnson, M. M., Hislop, T. G., Kan, L., Coldman, A. J., and Lai, A. (1996). Compliance with the screening mammography program of British Columbia: Will she return? *Canadian Journal of Public Health/Revue Canadienne de Santé Publique* 87, 176–180.

Kalbfleisch, J. D. and Prentice, R. L. (2002). *The Statistical Analysis of Failure Time Data*. Hoboken, NJ: John Wiley & Sons, second edition.

Khosropour, C. M., Johnson, B. A., Ricca, A. V., and Sullivan, P. S. (2013). Enhancing retention of an Internet-based cohort study of men who have sex with men (MSM) via text messaging: Randomized controlled trial. *Journal of Medical Internet Research* 15, e194.

Lawless, J. F. and Zhan, M. (1998). Analysis of interval-grouped recurrent-event data using piecewise constant rate functions. *The Canadian Journal of Statistics* 26, 549–565.

Lindsey, J. K. (1995). Fitting parametric counting processes by using log-linear models. *Journal of the Royal Statistical Society, Series C (Applied Statistics)* 44, 201–212.

McCullagh, P. and Nelder, J. A. (1989). *Generalized Linear Models*. London:UK, Chapman & Hall, second edition.

Mitchell, J. W. and Horvath, K. J. (2015). Factors associated with regular HIV testing among a sample of US MSM with HIV-negative main partners. *Journal of Acquired Immune Deficiency Syndromes* 64, 417–423.

Moran, P. (1951). The random division of an interval—Part II. *Journal of the Royal Statistical Society, Series B (Methodological)* 13, 147–150.

Prentice, R. L. and Gloeckler, L. A. (1978). Regression analysis of grouped survival data with application to breast cancer data. *Biometrics* 34, 57–67.

Purcell, D. W., Johnson, C. H., Lansky, A., Prejean, J., Stein, R., Prejean, J, Denning, P, Gau, Z., Weinstock, H., Su, J., and Crepaz, N. (2012). Estimating the population size of men who have sex with men in the United States to obtain HIV and syphilis rates. *Open AIDS J* 6, 98–107.

Ross, S. M. (1996). *Stochastic Processes*. Hoboken, NJ: John Wiley & Sons, second edition.

Sun, J. and Fang, H.-B. (2003). A nonparametric test for panel count data. *Biometrika* 90, 199–208.

Valim, C., Mezzetti, M., Maguire, J., Urdaneta, M., and Wypij, D. (2008). Estimation of vaccine efficacy in a repeated measures study under heterogeneity of exposure or susceptibility to infection. *Philosophical Transactions of the Royal Society A* 366, 2347–2360.

Zapka, J. G., Stoddard, A., Maul, L., and Costanza, M. E. (1991). Interval adherence to mammography screening guidelines. *Medical Care* 29, 697–707.

Zhang, Y. (2002). A semiparametric pseudolikelihood estimation method for panel count data. *Biometrika* 89, 39–48.

Section II

Quantitative Methods for Analysis of Laboratory Assays

6

Estimating Partial Correlations between Logged HIV RNA Measurements Subject to Detection Limits

Robert H. Lyles

The Rollins School of Public Health of Emory University, Atlanta, GA

CONTENTS

6.1 Introduction

Human immunodeficiency virus (HIV) studies frequently emphasize the quantification of HIV ribonucleic acid (HIV RNA) copy numbers per unit volume of biospecimens (e.g., plasma, semen). Viral load assay sensitivity has improved substantially with time, and reaching a nondetectable level is often used as a surrogate endpoint in clinical studies of HIV infection. However, the issue of left censoring due to values below detection limits continues to pose challenges to the analysis of continuous HIV RNA data despite improved assays. This is due in part to the effectiveness of modern therapeutic regimens, which can successfully suppress the virus below detectable levels for a reasonable proportion of patients in cohort or clinical studies of patients with access to them.

Laboratory assay nondetectables are pervasive enough in multiple areas of science to have spawned statistical research encompassing books and book chapters (e.g., Helsel 2005; Looney and Hagan 2015), dissertations in biostatistics or statistics (e.g., McCracken 2013; Moore 2006; Zheng 2002), and a myriad of journal articles. Although we do not undertake an exhaustive review here, many of these articles can be categorized in terms of the underlying statistical estimation and inferential focus. For example, early work concentrated on the estimation of univariate means and variances, often motivated by problems in environmental science or occupational health (e.g., Cohen 1959, 1961; Hornung and Reed 1990).

To deal with bivariate problems such as those arising in HIV or environmental epidemiology, considerable subsequent attention was paid to parametric approaches for estimating crude correlation coefficients in addition to means and variances when one or both variables are subject to nondetectables (e.g., Li et al. 2005; Lyles et al. 2001a, 2001b; Lynn 2001). The need to extend these considerations over a broader range of problems arising in practice also engendered efforts to deal with nondetectables when calculating nonparametric measures of correlation (e.g., Nie et al. 2008; Williamson et al. 2010), to account for a preponderance of nondetectables via mixture models (e.g., Chu et al. 2005; Moulton and Halsey 1995; Taylor et al. 2001), and to deal with nondetectables when estimating biomarker discriminatory properties and receiver operating curves (ROCs) (Perkins et al. 2009, 2011; Vexler et al. 2008).

Beginning with forward-thinking work by Pettit (1986), many recent efforts have focused upon dealing with left censoring in longitudinal or otherwise repeated measures studies of exposure. The goals of these analyses include the traditional estimation of mixed model regression parameters and variance components, prediction of random effects, estimating correlation matrices for multivariate data, joint modeling of longitudinal exposure data and health outcomes, and Bayesian inference (e.g., Albert 2008; Chu et al. 2010; Hughes 1999; Jacqmin-Gadda et al. 2000; Lee et al. 2012; Lee et al. 2014; Lyles et al. 2000; Moore et al. 2010; Nie et al. 2009; Sun et al. 2015; Thiebaut et al. 2004; Wannemuehler and Lyles 2005; Xie et al. 2012).

In what follows, we focus on an extension of likelihood-based methods for estimating the crude correlation between two biomarkers (Y and X), both of which may be subject to assay nondetectables. We examine a motivating example involving longitudinal HIV RNA data collected as part of the HIV Epidemiology Research Study (HERS), in which it is of interest to obtain a measure of association between viral load measurements across consecutive visits among subjects who were consistently on highly active antiviral treatment. Other examples relevant to HIV epidemiology come easily to mind, such as studies focused on associating viral load measurements taken from different reservoirs within the same patient. The methodological extension considered here is to incorporate covariates so as to focus on the corresponding partial (rather than crude) correlation and/or regression coefficient. The approach might be viewed as a special case of mixed linear model analysis for left-censored repeated measures data, again with particular emphasis on estimation and inference about the adjusted association parameters relating Y and X.

6.2 Methods

6.2.1 Basic Modeling Framework for Estimating the Partial Correlation

In the absence of nondetectables, we begin with a simple paradigm based on the following two multiple linear regression (MLR) models:

$$Y = \mu_{y|xc} + \varepsilon_{y|xc} = \beta_0 + \sum_{t=1}^{T} \beta_t C_t + \beta_{T+1} X + \varepsilon_{y|xc} \qquad (6.1)$$

and

$$X = \mu_{x|c} + \varepsilon_{x|c} = \psi_0 + \sum_{t=1}^{T} \psi_t C_t + \varepsilon_{x|c}, \qquad (6.2)$$

where the error terms $\varepsilon_{y|xc}$ and $\varepsilon_{x|c}$ are each assumed i.i.d. with mean 0 and homogeneous variances $\sigma^2_{y|xc}$ and $\sigma^2_{x|c}$, respectively. The vector $\mathbf{C}$ is a T-dimensional set of covariates (e.g., possible confounders), so that models (6.1) and (6.2) characterize the conditional distributions of $Y|X,\mathbf{C}$ and $X|\mathbf{C}$. Given that $E(Y|\mathbf{C}) = E_{X|\mathbf{C}}[E(Y|X, \mathbf{C})]$ and $\text{Var}(Y|\mathbf{C}) = E_{X|\mathbf{C}}[\text{Var}(Y|X,\mathbf{C})] + \text{Var}_{X|\mathbf{C}}[E(Y|X, \mathbf{C})]$, the above specifications also imply the following MLR model characterizing the distribution of $Y|\mathbf{C}$:

$$Y = \mu_{y|c} + \varepsilon_{y|c} = \gamma_0 + \sum_{t=1}^{T} \gamma_t C_t + \varepsilon_{y|c} \tag{6.3}$$

with i.i.d. homogeneous errors $\varepsilon_{y|c}$ of mean 0 and variance $\sigma^2_{y|c}$. These specifications (without yet positing further distributional assumptions on the errors in the three models) are sufficient to characterize the partial correlation ($\rho_{yx|c}$) between Y and X conditional on $\mathbf{C}$ as follows:

$$\rho^2_{yx|c} = \frac{\sigma^2_{y|c} - \sigma^2_{y|xc}}{\sigma^2_{y|c}} \tag{6.4}$$

where $\sigma^2_{y|c} = \text{Var}(Y|\mathbf{C}) = \beta^2_{T+1}\sigma^2_{x|c} + \sigma^2_{y|xc}$. Equivalently, we can write

$$\rho_{yx|c} = \frac{\beta_{T+1}\sigma_{x|c}}{\sqrt{\beta^2_{T+1}\sigma^2_{x|c} + \sigma^2_{y|xc}}}. \tag{6.5}$$

Standard practice (e.g., Kleinbaum et al. 2008; Kutner et al. 2005) dictates estimation of the squared partial correlation in Equation 6.4 based on the error sums of squares from models (6.1) and (6.3), that is,

$$\hat{\rho}^2_{yx|c} = \frac{\text{SSE}_{y|c} - \text{SSE}_{y|xc}}{\text{SSE}_{y|c}}, \tag{6.6}$$

with the estimator $\hat{\rho}_{yx|c}$ taken as the positive or negative square root of Equation 6.6 to correspond with the sign of the ordinary least squares estimate of β_{T+1} from the fit of model (6.1).

6.2.2 Likelihood-Based Methods for Bivariate Data Incorporating Covariates and Nondetectables

Our goal is to consider estimation of $\rho_{yx|c}$ and/or β_{T+1} when either Y or X or both are subject to left censoring due to assay detection limits, and we explore two basic strategies. The first is based upon a fully specified conditional bivariate normal (BVN) model, whereas the second relies on univariate normal models with exclusion of records with nondetectables on X.

6.2.2.1 Maximum Likelihood Method 1: A Conditional BVN Model

As a primary framework for handling nondetectables in this setting, we extend the maximum likelihood (ML) approach outlined by Lyles et al. (2001b) for estimating the crude correlation ρ_{yx} based on a BVN model. The extension to incorporate the covariates in $\mathbf{C}$ assumes models (6.2) and (6.3) for the conditional means of X and Y, respectively, with a further BVN assumption as follows:

$$(Y, X | \mathbf{C}) \sim N_2 \left[\begin{pmatrix} \mu_{y|c} \\ \mu_{x|c} \end{pmatrix}, \begin{pmatrix} \sigma^2_{y|c} & \sigma_{yx|c} \\ \sigma_{yx|c} & \sigma^2_{x|c} \end{pmatrix} \right], \tag{6.7}$$

where the conditional covariance $\sigma_{yx|c} = \rho_{yx|c}\sigma_{y|c}\sigma_{x|c}$.

Aside from the incorporation of covariates, the approach relies on the same four types of observations (records) described in Lyles et al. (2001b). Denoting the respective lower limits of detection as LD_x and LD_y, we refer to these records as Type 1 (both Y and X observed), Type 2 (Y observed and $X < LD_x$), Type 3 (X observed and $Y < LD_y$), and Type 4 ($X < LD_x$ and $Y < LD_y$). Individual likelihood contributions attributable to experimental unit i are based on the following for records of Types 1–4, respectively: $f(y_i, x_i | c_i)$, $\Pr(Y < LD_y | x_i, c_i) \times f(x_i | c_i)$, $\Pr(X < LD_x | y_i, c_i) \times f(y_i | c_i)$, and $\Pr(Y < LD_y \cap X < LD_x | c_i)$.

Letting n_j represent the number of observations of type j ($j = 1, 2, 3, 4$), we present the log-likelihood contributions attributed to the sets of records of each type as follows:

$$\text{Type 1}: -n_1\ln(2\pi\sigma_{x|c}\sigma_{y|xc}) - (2\sigma^2_{y|xc})^{-1}\sum_{i=1}^{n_1}(y_i - \mu_{y|x_i,c_i})^2 - (2\sigma^2_{x|c})^{-1}\sum_{i=1}^{n_1}(x_i - \mu_{x|c_i})^2$$

$$\text{Type 2}: -0.5n_2\ln(2\pi\sigma^2_{x|c}) - (2\sigma^2_{x|c})^{-1}\sum_{i=n_1+1}^{n_{2\bullet}}(x_i - \mu_{x_i|c_i})^2 + \sum_{i=n_1+1}^{n_{2\bullet}}\ln\left\{\Phi\left(\frac{LD_y - \mu_{y|x_i,c_i}}{\sigma_{y|xc}}\right)\right\}$$

$$\text{Type 3}: -0.5n_3\ln(2\pi\sigma^2_{y|c}) - (2\sigma^2_{y|c})^{-1}\sum_{i=n_{2\bullet}+1}^{n_{3\bullet}}(y_i - \mu_{y_i|c_i})^2 + \sum_{i=n_{2\bullet}+1}^{n_{3\bullet}}\ln\left\{\Phi\left(\frac{LD_x - \mu_{x|y_i,c_i}}{\sigma_{x|yc}}\right)\right\}$$

$$\text{Type 4}: -0.5n_4\ln(2\pi\sigma^2_{y|c}) + \sum_{i=n_{3\bullet}+1}^{n_{4\bullet}}\ln\left\{\int_{-\infty}^{LD_y}\left[\Phi\left(\frac{LD_x - \mu_{x|y,c_i}}{\sigma_{x|yc}}\right) \times e^{-(y-\mu_{y|c_i})^2/2\sigma^2_{y|c}}\right]dy\right\}.$$

Here, we let $n_{k\bullet} = \sum_{j=1}^{k} n_j$ ($k = 2,3,4$) and assume observations are ordered and indexed by i such that records of Type 1 come first, followed by those of

Types 2, 3, and 4. The 2T + 5 parameters to be estimated include the regression coefficients ψ and γ in models (6.2) and (6.3), the residual variances $\sigma^2_{y|c}$ and $\sigma^2_{x|c}$, and the partial correlation coefficient $\rho_{yx|c}$. These primary parameters make up the following terms involved in the above expressions:

$$\mu_{y|x_i,c_i} = \mu_{y|c_i} + \left(\frac{\rho_{yx|c}\sigma_{y|c}}{\sigma_{x|c}}\right)(x_i - \mu_{x|c_i}), \quad \sigma^2_{y|xc} = \sigma^2_{y|c}(1 - \rho^2_{yx|c})$$

$$\mu_{x|y_i,c_i} = \mu_{x|c_i} + \left(\frac{\rho_{yx|c}\sigma_{x|c}}{\sigma_{y|c}}\right)(y_i - \mu_{y|c_i}), \text{ and } \sigma^2_{x|yc} = \sigma^2_{x|c}(1 - \rho^2_{yx|c})$$

Aside from the additional 2T regression parameters, this modeling framework is similar to that discussed by Lyles et al. (2001b) for estimating the unadjusted correlation between Y and X. One noteworthy difference, however, is that in principle the integrals reflected in the Type 4 log-likelihood contributions must now be calculated separately for each subject each time the likelihood is evaluated. Exceptions would occur, for example, if all covariates in C are binary, in which case the integral needs to be calculated once for each unique covariate combination in order to evaluate the likelihood.

As in prior implementations of ML for the BVN setting without covariates (e.g., Li et al. 2005; Lyles et al. 2001b), we apply functions available in the SAS IML software (SAS Institute, Inc., 2008) for optimization. Specifically, we applied the QUAD function for numerical integration of Type 4 contributions at each iteration, the NLPQN routine for quasi-Newton optimization, and the NLPFDD function for close approximation of second derivatives to evaluate the observed information matrix in order to estimate standard errors (SEs).

6.2.2.2 Confidence Intervals for the Partial Correlation Coefficient under ML Method 1

In large samples, we can apply a typical normal theory-based confidence interval (CI) for $\rho_{yx|c}$:

$$\hat{\rho}_{yx|c} \pm z_{1-\alpha/2}\widehat{SE}(\hat{\rho}_{yx|c}) \qquad (6.8)$$

Given the small-sample limitations of Wald-type CIs and the inherent lack of variance stabilization, Lyles et al. (2001b) suggested profile-likelihood–based intervals for the crude correlation ρ_{yx} and gave empirical evidence suggesting improvements in overall coverage and coverage balance relative to the CIs in Equation 6.8. However, a computationally faster and simpler approach would be to apply Fisher's z-transformation here, despite the fact that left censoring in Y and X precludes the argument that it fully stabilizes the variance.

This leads to the following alternative CI, based on back-transforming the limits of a standard Wald interval for the parameter $\rho^*_{yx|c} = 0.5 \ln\left(\frac{1 + \rho_{yx|c}}{1 - \rho_{yx|c}}\right)$:

$$\left(\frac{\exp(2LL_{\rho*}) - 1}{\exp(2LL_{\rho*}) + 1}, \frac{\exp(2UL_{\rho*}) - 1}{\exp(2UL_{\rho*}) + 1}\right), \qquad (6.9)$$

where

$$(LL_{\rho*}, UL_{\rho*}) = \widehat{\rho}^*_{yx|c} \pm z_{1-\alpha/2} \widehat{SE}(\widehat{\rho}^*_{yx|c}). \qquad (6.10)$$

Although $\widehat{SE}(\widehat{\rho}^*_{yx|c})$ could be obtained by reparameterizing the likelihood based on the Type 1–4 contributions directly in terms of $\rho^*_{yx|c}$, a virtually identical approach is to base it on a familiar delta method–based approximation:

$$\widehat{Var}(\widehat{\rho}^*_{yx|c}) = \frac{\widehat{Var}(\widehat{\rho}_{yx|c})}{(1 - \widehat{\rho}^2_{yx|c})^2}$$

In an effort to further improve upon the CI based on Equations 6.9 and 6.10 in the crude correlation case, Li et al. (2005) proposed an alternate pivotal quantity by further refining a Taylor series expansion for $\widehat{\rho}_{yx} - \rho_{yx}$. Applying this refinement in the partial correlation case considered here, one would use Equation 6.9 to back-transform the limits of the following alternative CI for $\rho^*_{yx|c}$:

$$(LL_{\rho*}, UL_{\rho*}) = (\widehat{\rho}^*_{yx|c} - \widehat{A} - z_{1-\alpha/2}\widehat{B}, \ \widehat{\rho}^*_{yx|c} - \widehat{A} + z_{1-\alpha/2}\widehat{B}) \qquad (6.11)$$

where

$$\widehat{A} = (1 - \widehat{\rho}^2_{yx|c})^{-2} \widehat{\rho}_{yx|c} \widehat{Var}(\widehat{\rho}_{yx|c})$$

$$\widehat{B} = (1 - \widehat{\rho}^2_{yx|c})^{-2} \widehat{SE}(\widehat{\rho}_{yx|c}) \sqrt{2\widehat{\rho}^2_{yx|c} \widehat{Var}(\widehat{\rho}_{yx|c}) + (1 - \widehat{\rho}^2_{yx|c})^2}.$$

In Section 6.4, we explore the coverage and coverage balance properties of CIs based on Equations 6.8 through 6.11 empirically using simulated data.

6.2.2.3 *ML Method 2: Univariate Normal Models Ignoring Records with Nondetectables on X*

An alternative to the full conditional BVN specification is to base estimation of $\rho_{yx|c}$ directly upon Equation 6.4 using the model for $Y \mid X,C$ in Equation 6.1 and the model for $Y \mid C$ in Equation 6.3. Specifically, assuming normal errors in models (6.1) and (6.3), we can obtain maximum likelihood estimates (MLEs) for the residual variances $\sigma^2_{y|xc}$ and $\sigma^2_{y|c}$ by appropriately accounting for nondetectables when fitting those models. Applying ML to model (6.3) is straightforward. Observations with Y detected make the usual likelihood contribution based on the normal density $f(y_i|c_i)$, whereas those with Y unobserved contribute $\Phi\left(\frac{LD_y - \mu_{y|c_i}}{\sigma_{y|c}}\right)$, where $\Phi(.)$ denotes the standard normal *cdf*.

For ML Method 2, we avoid dealing with nondetectables in X by dropping those observations prior to fitting model (6.1), accounting for left censoring in Y. This strategy is valid for estimating $\sigma^2_{y|xc}$ (as well as the regression coefficients comprising $\mu_{y|xc}$), because it induces missing records by a mechanism that depends only on a variable (X) that is conditioned upon in model (6.1) (e.g., Little and Rubin 2002; Nie et al. 2010). However, it naturally sacrifices some precision in the estimate of $\sigma^2_{y|xc}$; the loss may be small or substantial, depending upon the percentage of records with X nondetected. The analysis of the remaining records under model (6.1) proceeds straightforwardly in the same manner as ML under model (6.3). Here, observations with Y detected make the standard likelihood contribution based on the normal density $f(y_i|x_i, c_i)$, whereas those with Y unobserved contribute $\Phi\left(\frac{LD_y - \mu_{y|x_ic_i}}{\sigma_{y|xc}}\right)$.

To complete estimation of $\rho_{yx|c}$ via ML Method 2, we insert the MLEs into Equation 6.4 and take the positive or negative square root as dictated by the sign of the MLE for the partial regression coefficient β_{T+1} based on our fit of model (6.1) as described above. Clearly, Method 2 should be valid whenever Method 1 is valid, with an advantage being a simpler implementation of ML methods without the need for numerical integration. One operational disadvantage of ML Method 2, however, is that standard error estimation is not immediate; for this, we suggest standard bootstrap-based percentile CIs (Efron and Tibshirani 1993). We could also speculate as to whether Method 2 could potentially offer some robustness advantage, given that it does not rely explicitly on a full BVN assumption. In Section 6.4, we provide some limited empirical results to explore this question as well as the precision loss relative to Method 1 when the BVN model holds.

6.2.2.4 *Partial Regression Coefficient Estimation*

If the parameter of interest is the partial regression coefficient β_{T+1}, one approach is to reparameterize the BVN model in terms of models (6.1) and (6.3) based on the factorization $f(Y,X|C) = f(Y|X,C)f(X|C)$. The total number of parameters characterizing the likelihood contributions of Types 1–4 remains the same in this equivalent parameterization, with β_{T+1} appearing as a primary parameter instead of the partial correlation coefficient $\rho_{yx|c}$ and $\sigma^2_{y|xc}$ in place of $\sigma^2_{y|c}$. To specify the four types of BVN log-likelihood contributions from Section 6.2.2.1, we need only replace $\rho_{yx|c}$ with $\beta_{T+1}\sigma_{x|c}/\sigma_{y|c}$ and then make the following other changes to the expressions:

$$\mu_{y|x_i c_i} = \beta_0 + \sum_{t=1}^{T} \beta_t c_{it} + \beta_{T+1} x_i, \quad \mu_{y|c_i} = \mu_{y|x_i,c_i} - \beta_{T+1}(x_i - \mu_{x|c_i}),$$

$$\mu_{x|y_i,c_i} = \mu_{x|c_i} + \beta_{T+1}\sigma_{x|c}^2 (y_i - \mu_{y|c_i})/\sigma_{y|c}^2, \quad \text{and} \quad \sigma_{y|c}^2 = \beta_{T+1}^2\sigma_{x|c}^2 + \sigma_{y|xc}^2.$$

Nevertheless, it is virtually equivalent numerically to estimate β_{T+1} as the following function of the MLEs based on the original parameterization in Section 6.2.2.1:

$$\widehat{\beta}_{T+1} = g(\widehat{\rho}_{y|xc}, \widehat{\sigma}_{y|c}^2, \widehat{\sigma}_{x|c}^2) = \frac{\widehat{\rho}_{y|xc}\widehat{\sigma}_{y|c}}{\widehat{\sigma}_{x|c}}. \tag{6.12}$$

We then estimate the standard error using the following multivariate delta method approximation:

$$\widehat{\mathrm{Var}}(\widehat{\beta}_{T+1}) = \widehat{\mathbf{D}}\widehat{\mathbf{\Sigma}}\widehat{\mathbf{D}}'$$

where

$$\widehat{\mathbf{D}} = (\widehat{dg}/d\sigma_{x|c}^2 \;\; \widehat{dg}/d\sigma_{y|c}^2 \;\; \widehat{dg}/d\rho_{y|xc}) \quad \text{and} \quad \widehat{\mathbf{\Sigma}} = \widehat{\mathrm{Var}}\begin{pmatrix} \widehat{\sigma}_{x|c}^2 \\ \widehat{\sigma}_{y|c}^2 \\ \widehat{\rho}_{y|xc} \end{pmatrix}.$$

We obtain the 3×3 variance–covariance matrix $\widehat{\Sigma}$ via the numerically derived Hessian for the full BVN likelihood, and the estimated first derivatives are as follows:

$$\widehat{dg}/d\sigma_{x|c}^2 = -0.5\widehat{\rho}_{y|xc}\widehat{\sigma}_{y|c}\widehat{\sigma}_{x|c}^{-3}, \quad \widehat{dg}/d\sigma_{y|c}^2 = 0.5\widehat{\rho}_{y|xc}\widehat{\sigma}_{x|c}^{-1}\widehat{\sigma}_{y|c}^{-1}, \quad \widehat{dg}/d\rho_{y|xc} = \widehat{\sigma}_{y|c}\widehat{\sigma}_{x|c}^{-1}$$

Although the above provides the analogue to ML Method 1 for estimating the partial regression coefficient, an obvious approach somewhat akin to ML Method 2 is immediately available. Namely, one can estimate β_{T+1} validly based on the left-censored likelihood for model (6.1) after dropping records with X nondetected, as described in Section 6.2.2.3. We expect the precision loss in this estimate of β_{T+1} when there is substantial left censoring on X to be relatively more extreme here than the corresponding loss in the estimation of $\rho_{yx|c}$ based on ML Method 2. Again, however, one may speculate as to the possible robustness advantage of this computationally simple approach relative to the BVN model, and one may favor this approach when there is little censoring on X. We compare the two proposed estimators for β_{T+1} empirically in Section 6.4.

6.2.3 Alternative Univariate Models Adjusting for Covariates

One way to judge the appropriateness of a univariate normal model for left-censored data is via a Q–Q plot (e.g., Chu et al. 2005; Lyles et al. 2001b). We recommend comparing observed quantiles versus those expected based on a truncated normal model for the observed data (truncated at the normal-scale limit of detection [LOD]) and using the estimated truncated normal parameters to compute a predicted number of nondetectables to compare against the number observed (Lyles et al. 2001b). As it is fairly common for the number of nondetectables to exceed what would be expected under the normal model, it can also be informative to compare Q–Q plots in which the expected quantiles are estimated using MLEs for the mean and variance based on a truncated versus a left-censored normal model (see Section 6.3). Alternatives to the left-censored model to account for a preponderance of nondetectables include mixture models assuming a point mass at zero or some other value below the LOD on the raw scale (e.g., Chu et al. 2005; Chu and Nie 2005; Moulton and Halsey 1995; Taylor et al. 2001) and models assuming a mixture of two normal distributions (e.g., Chu et al. 2005). In this section, we briefly outline "extended mixture models" of this type for univariate left-censored data, with the extension being the straightforward incorporation of covariates.

6.2.3.1 *Mixture of Two Normal Models*

Consider a normal mixture model for the variable X conditional on covariates **C**, where X is subject to nondetectables. We assume model (6.2) for the two separate components of the mixture, where in general each ψ coefficient as well as the residual variance $\sigma^2_{x|c}$ could differ in the lower and upper components. However, given numerical challenges to optimizing a mixture of normal likelihood for small to moderate sample sizes, here we account for the excessive number of nondetectables by allowing the intercept alone to vary. That is, we assume the two components f_L and f_U, where $f_L(X|\mathbf{C}) \sim N(\psi_{CL}, \sigma^2_{x|c})$ and $f_U(X|\mathbf{C}) \sim N(\psi_{CU}, \sigma^2_{x|c})$, with

$$\psi_{CL} = \psi_{0L} + \sum_{t=1}^{T} \psi_t C_t \quad \text{and} \quad \psi_{CU} = \psi_{0U} + \sum_{t=1}^{T} \psi_t C_t$$

Then, letting ω represent the mixing proportion, observations with X observed $(X > LD_x)$ make the likelihood contribution $\omega f_L(X|\mathbf{C}) + (1-\omega)f_U(X|\mathbf{C})$. Nondetectables $(X < LD_x)$, by contrast, make the contribution

$$\omega\Phi\left(\frac{LD_x - \psi_{CL}}{\sigma_{x|c}}\right) + (1-\omega)\Phi\left(\frac{LD_x - \psi_{CU}}{\sigma_{x|c}}\right)$$

Chu et al. (2005) considered a bivariate version of the above mixture model, without covariates, which also incorporated simplifying assumptions in order to facilitate numerical optimization. Although we do not pursue it here, we note that the expectation–maximization (EM) algorithm (Dempster et al. 1977) could provide a computational alternative to overcome numerical challenges to the reliable fit of more general versions of univariate and/or bivariate normal mixture models under left censoring.

6.2.3.2   *Mixture Model Assuming a Point Mass below the LOD*

With an excessive number of nondetectables under a lognormal assumption for a raw-scale variable e^X, a "lower" mixture component is sometimes taken to be a point mass at 0 (e.g., Taylor et al. 2001). For the variable X, we will assume the point mass occurs at some unspecified value below the log-scale LOD. For incorporating covariates, we continue to assume an "upper" component $f_U(X|\mathbf{C}) \sim \mathrm{N}(\psi_{\mathrm{CU}}, \sigma^2_{x|c})$. In general we can incorporate covariates into the mixture probability as well, for example, through a logistic model for the mixture proportion:

$$\mathrm{logit}(\omega) = \eta_0 + \sum_{t=1}^{T} \eta_t C_t$$

where ω is the probability that X resides in the lower component. In this case, observations with $X > LD_x$ contribute $(1-\omega)f_U(X|\mathbf{C})$ to the likelihood, whereas those with $X < LD_x$ contribute

$$\omega + (1-\omega)\Phi\left(\frac{LD_x - \psi_{\mathrm{CU}}}{\sigma_{x|c}}\right)$$

6.2.3.3   *Partial Correlation and Regression Coefficient Estimation under Alternative Models*

In this section, we briefly consider the scenario in which a left-censored normal model is deemed reasonable for the $Y|X,\mathbf{C}$ distribution (i.e., model (6.1) holds) but one of the aforementioned mixture models is more appropriate for the $X|\mathbf{C}$ distribution. If the normal mixture model specified in Section 6.2.3.1 is assumed for $X|\mathbf{C}$, we recommend ML based on the factorization $f(Y,X|\mathbf{C}) = f(Y|X,\mathbf{C})f(X|\mathbf{C})$ as in Section 6.2.2.4. In that case, both the partial correlation coefficient ($\rho_{yx|c}$) and the partial regression coefficient (β_{T+1}) should be unique and validly estimable via ML because of the assumption that $\sigma^2_{x|c}$ is identical for the lower and upper components. One would obtain MLEs of β_{T+1}, $\sigma^2_{y|xc}$ and $\sigma^2_{x|c}$ directly based on the ML factorization and then compute the MLE of the partial correlation coefficient via the relation $\rho_{yx|c} = \beta_{T+1}\sigma_{x|c}/\sigma_{y|c}$, where $\sigma^2_{y|c} = \beta_{T+1}\sigma^2_{x|c} + \sigma^2_{y|xc}$.

By contrast, if the mixture model with a point mass below the LOD as described in Section 6.2.3.2 is assumed to hold for $X|\mathbf{C}$, we recommend the use of the partial regression coefficient β_{T+1} based on model (6.1) as the measure of covariate-adjusted association between Y and X. This is because $\sigma^2_{x|c}$ will no longer be homogeneous with respect to the covariates **C**, making it problematic to define a single unique partial correlation coefficient $\rho_{yx|c}$. Estimation of β_{T+1} could proceed according to ML Method 2 as described in Section 6.2.2.4, where records with X nondetected are dropped. In Section 6.4, we consider a simulation study to evaluate this approach in comparison to ML Method 1 in this mixture model scenario, where the robustness of the latter could be called into question given the incorrect assumption of a left-censored normal model for X | **C**.

In Section 6.3, we use Akaike's information criterion (AIC; Akaike 1974) as a gauge of relative fit for candidate models to real HIV RNA data at two visits from a longitudinal study of HIV infection among women. In addition to the covariate-adjusted mixture models described above, we evaluate the fit of single left-censored normal models with and without covariate adjustment, mixture models with a point mass below the LOD without covariates, and mixture models with a point mass below the LOD with covariates used only to model the normal component mean.

6.3 Example

6.3.1 HERS Data

Data for the motivating example come from the HERS, a longitudinal study that enrolled over 1,300 women in four US cities (Baltimore, Providence, New York, and Detroit) during the early to mid-1990s (Smith et al. 1997). Specifically, we use HIV RNA data from two consecutive visits (HERS Visits 8 and 9), which were obtained between September 1996 and December 1999. The analysis includes a total of 63 HIV-positive women who were all on highly active antiretroviral therapy and who had complete data on HIV RNA and CD4 cell counts at both visits. HIV RNA was quantified using a branched-chain DNA signal amplification assay (Chiron Corporation), with a detection limit of 50 copies/mL. The primary focus is upon estimating the partial correlation between the two consecutive $\log_{10}$(HIV RNA) measurements, adjusting for three covariates: HIV risk group (1 = injection drug use [IDU], 0 = sexual activity), age in years at Visit 8, and CD4 count/100 at Visit 8.

Of the 63 women, 27 (43%) were in the IDU risk group. At Visit 8, the average age was 40.2 years and the average CD4 count/100 was 3.5. Letting X and Y represent $\log_{10}$(HIV RNA) at Visits 8 and 9, respectively, assay nondetectables were obtained on X for 14 of 63 women (22%) and on Y for 16 of 63 women (25%). Forty-three subjects had detectable viral loads at both visits (Type 1), whereas 6 had nondetectables only at Visit 9 (Type 2), 4 had nondetectables only at Visit 8 (Type 3), and 10 had nondetectables at both visits (Type 4).

6.3.2 HERS Example: Crude and Partial Correlation Estimates

Table 6.1 displays crude and partial correlation estimates based on the $\log_{10}$(HIV RNA) data at HERS Visits 8 and 9. *Ad hoc* Method 1 refers to simply dropping all subjects who had nondetectables at either visit and computing a standard Pearson's or MLR-based partial correlation coefficient using data from the 43 Type 1 subjects. For *ad hoc* Method 2, we replaced all nondetectables with the base 10 log-scale limit of detection (i.e., $\log_{10}(50) = 1.699$, which is also the value of LD_x and LD_y in the notation of Section 6.2).

TABLE 6.1

Crude and Partial Correlation Estimates for HERS Example[a]

| Method[b] | Crude Correlation between Y and X | | |
	Estimate	Standard Error	95% CI
Ad hoc 1	0.663	–	–
Ad hoc 2	0.664	–	–
ML[c]	0.698	0.072	(0.557, 0.838)
			(0.529, 0.813)
			(0.517, 0.810)[d]

| Method[e] | Partial Correlation between Y and X, Adjusting for (C_1, C_2, C_3) | | |
	Estimate	Standard Error	95% CI
Ad hoc 1	0.628	–	–
Ad hoc 2	0.615	–	–
ML 1	0.651	0.080	(0.494, 0.807)
			(0.466, 0.781)
			(0.454, 0.777)[d]
ML 2	0.648	0.106[f]	(0.433, 0.824)[f]

Note: BVN, bivariate normal; CI, confidence interval; HERS, HIV Epidemiology Research Study; LOD, limit of detection; ML, maximum likelihood; MLE, maximum likelihood estimate.

[a] Total sample size = 63, with 43, 6, 4, and 10 observations of Types 1–4, respectively; C_1 = risk cohort (1 = IDU, 0 = sex); C_2 = age (years) at Visit 8; C_3 = CD4 count/100 at Visit 8.

[b] *Ad hoc* 1: Dropping all records with X or Y nondetected; *ad hoc* 2: replacing nondetectables by LOD.

[c] Using ML based on BVN likelihood described in Lyles et al. (2001b).

[d] The first interval is standard Wald CI; the second is based on Fisher's z-transformation (Equation 6.10); the third uses the approach of Li et al. (2005) (see Equation 6.11).

[e] ML Methods 1 and 2 as detailed in Sections 6.2.2.2 and 6.2.2.3; Method 1 MLEs for $(\psi_0, \psi_1, \psi_2, \psi_3, \gamma_0, \gamma_1, \gamma_2, \gamma_3, \sigma^2_{x|c}, \sigma^2_{y|c})$ = (5.20, −0.25, −0.04, −0.23, 5.27, −0.03, −0.05, −0.19, 1.15, 1.64).

[f] Bootstrap standard error and percentile-based CI.

ML refers to the BVN-based approach in Lyles et al. (2001b) for estimating the crude correlation accounting for nondetectables, whereas ML 1 and ML 2 are the partial correlation estimators described in Sections 6.2.2.1 and 6.2.2.3, respectively. Table 6.1 omits SEs and CIs in conjunction with the biased *ad hoc* methods. For the ML and ML 1 methods, CIs are calculated in three ways for comparison (standard Wald CI, delta method based on Fisher's z-transformation, and the refinement of the latter based on the pivotal quantity in Li et al. [2005]; see Section 6.2.2.2). A standard nonparametric bootstrap based on 1,000 resamples with replacement was applied to obtain the estimated standard error for the ML 2 estimate, with a corresponding bootstrap percentile-based CI.

As seen in the top half of Table 6.1, the two *ad hoc* approaches produce nearly identical point estimates of the crude correlation in this case, whereas the MLE is larger in magnitude by approximately 5%. In the bottom half of the table, we see that the *ad hoc* partial correlation estimates are somewhat smaller than their crude *ad hoc* counterparts. The ML estimates of the partial correlation are also smaller than the crude MLE but larger than the *ad hoc* partial estimates. The ML 1 and ML 2 point estimates are very similar, whereas the former is more precise (as expected). In comparing the three CIs accompanying the ML and ML 1 estimates, we note that the standard delta method-based interval using Fisher's z-transformation is shifted to the left relative to the typical Wald interval (but of very similar width). The CI based on the Li et al. (2005) approach is further shifted to the left and is somewhat wider.

6.3.3 HERS Example: Partial Regression Coefficient Estimates

Table 6.2 presents MLEs for the partial regression coefficient that captures association between base 10 log viral load measurements at Visits 8 and 9, adjusting for the three covariates. In this table, the ML 1 method corresponds to the estimate in Equation 6.12, based on the generalized BVN likelihood, with the standard error obtained via the delta method. Both the estimated

TABLE 6.2

Partial Regression Coefficient Estimates for HERS Example[a]

Method[b]	Estimate	Standard Error	95% CI
ML 1	0.775	0.136	(0.510, 1.041)
ML 2	0.710	0.186	(0.345, 1.075)

Note: CI, confidence interval; ML, maximum likelihood; HERS, HIV Epidemiology Research Study.

[a] Total sample size = 63, with 43, 6, 4, and 10 observations of Types 1–4, respectively. C_1 = risk cohort (1 = IDU, 0 = sex); C_2 = age (years) at Visit 8; C_3 = CD4 count/100 at Visit 8.

[b] ML Methods 1 and 2 as discussed in Section 6.2.2.4.

coefficient and its standard error were virtually identical to those obtained by the reparameterization of the likelihood discussed in Section 6.2.2.4. As also described in that section, the ML 2 method is based on the fit of a left-censored MLR model for the distribution of $Y|X,C$ after dropping the 14 women who had nondetected log viral loads (X) at Visit 8. Although this is a valid estimate assuming model (6.1) with normal errors, its sacrifice of efficiency relative to ML 1 is apparent when comparing the estimated standard errors and corresponding CI widths.

6.3.4 HERS Example: Relative Fit of Candidate Univariate Models

Figures 6.1 and 6.2 show Q–Q plots with observed quantiles based on the detected $\log_{10}$(HIV RNA) data at Visits 8 and 9, where expected quantiles are calculated based on a truncated normal model with a single mean and variance (e.g., Lyles et al. 2001b). In Figure 6.1, MLEs for the mean and variance from fitting the truncated normal model to the data are utilized in computing the expected quantiles. These MLEs are as follows: $\hat{\mu} = 3.16$, $\hat{\sigma}^2 = 0.81$ (Visit 8); $\hat{\mu} = 2.95$, $\hat{\sigma}^2 = 1.44$ (Visit 9). Note that both plots seem to suggest a

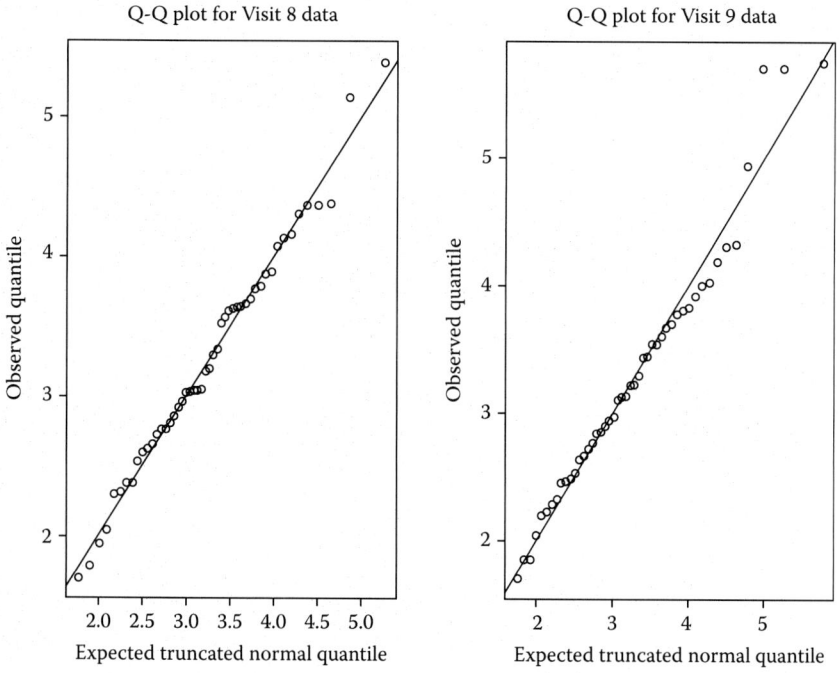

FIGURE 6.1
Q–Q plots for HERS Visit 8 and Visit 9 $\log_{10}$(HIV RNA) data, using truncated normal expected quantiles with MLEs for mean and variance calculated via truncated normal likelihood.

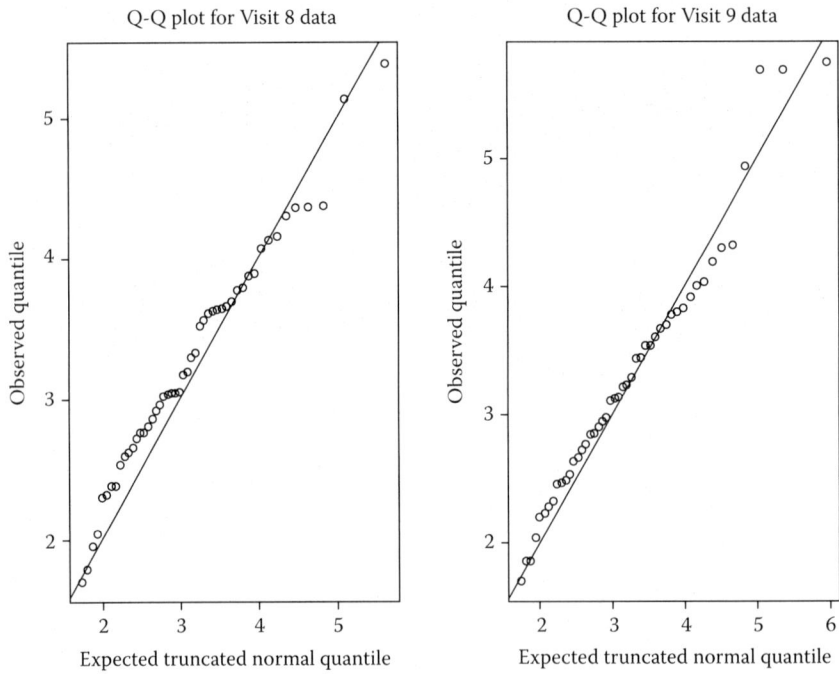

FIGURE 6.2
Q–Q plots for HERS Visit 8 and Visit 9 $\log_{10}$(HIV RNA) data, using truncated normal expected quantiles with MLEs for mean and variance calculated via left-censored normal likelihood.

reasonable fit, with points roughly following a 45-degree line. Using these truncated normal MLEs to estimate the proportion of subjects expected to have nondetectable measurements, we obtain predictions of 5.2% and 9.4% at Visits 8 and 9, respectively.

In Figure 6.2, the only change is that MLEs used to compute the expected truncated normal quantiles are now based on the fit of left-censored normal models to the data. These MLEs are as follows: $\hat{\mu} = 2.77$, $\hat{\sigma}^2 = 1.42$ (Visit 8); $\hat{\mu} = 2.67$, $\hat{\sigma}^2 = 1.88$ (Visit 9). Although it is not necessarily surprising to see lower estimated means and higher estimated variances in each case compared with those based on the truncated normal model, the two sets of estimates would be expected to be similar in large samples (though more precise under the left-censored normal model), if the left-censored model truly generated the data. The discrepancy is more extreme at Visit 8 (particularly with regard to the variance). Perhaps correspondingly, the discrepancy between the expected and observed proportions of subjects with nondetectables is somewhat more marked at Visit 8 (5.2% vs. 22%) than at Visit 9 (9.4% vs. 25%), and the Q–Q plot for Visit 8 in Figure 6.2 now suggests lack of fit while the plot for Visit 9 remains more similar to the version in Figure 6.1.

TABLE 6.3

Univariate Model AIC Comparisons for HERS Example[a,b]

Model Number	Model	Number of Parameters	AIC (Visit 8)	AIC (Visit 9)
1	Left-censored normal (no covariates)	2	189.36	198.07
2	Mixture with point mass (no covariates)	3	187.26	199.44
3	Mixture with point mass (covariates for both normal mean and mixture probability)	9	184.11	202.80
4	Normal mixture (with covariates)	7	183.32	199.27
5	Left-censored normal (with covariates)	5	181.47	196.31
6	Mixture with point mass (covariates for normal mean only)	6	180.94	197.27

Note: AIC, Akaike's information criterion; HERS, HIV Epidemiology Research Study.
[a] Covariates are as follows: C_1 = risk cohort (1 = IDU, 0 = sex); C_2 = age (years) at Visit 8; C_3 = CD4 count/100 at Visit 8.
[b] Model 3 as described in Section 6.2.3.2; Model 4 as described in Section 6.2.3.1.

Table 6.3 presents the results of univariate model fit comparisons based separately on the Visits 8 and 9 data, as judged by AIC. Models 1 and 2 in Table 6.3 utilize no covariates; note that a mixture model with a point mass below the LOD appears to be favored at Visit 8, whereas a standard left-censored normal model is favored at Visit 9. This is qualitatively consistent with the impressions suggested by the Q–Q plots in Figures 6.1 and 6.2. However, at both visits, multiple models that account for covariates appear to provide a better fit.

Note in particular that Model 5 (Table 6.3) is the univariate model most consistent with the assumptions of the BVN modeling strategy underlying the ML 1 approach in Tables 6.1 and 6.2. This model is favored overall at Visit 9 and produces the second lowest AIC value at Visit 8; this suggests that the proposed BVN model may not be unreasonable for these data. The model favored overall at Visit 8 on the basis of AIC is a simplified version of the covariate-adjusted mixture model described in Section 6.2.3.2, in which the covariates are used to model the normal component mean but no covariates model the mixing probability. This is likely consistent with the notion that the number of nondetectables obtained at Visit 8 is somewhat higher than would be expected based on the best fitting left-censored normal model for the data.

6.4 Simulation Study

6.4.1 Evaluating Partial Correlation Estimators

Table 6.4 presents the results of simulations designed to examine relative performance of several estimators of the partial correlation coefficient $\rho_{yx|c}$,

TABLE 6.4

Results of Simulations to Evaluate Partial Correlation Estimators in Settings Mimicking HERS Example[a]

Sample Size = 63, $LD_x = LD_y = \log_{10}(50)$ Average Number of Type 1–4 Observations: 42.7, 8.1, 4.5, 7.7		
Method[b,c]	Mean Estimate (SD)	95% CI Coverage[d,e]
Complete data	0.645 (0.076)	95.9%
Ad hoc 1	0.503 (0.128)	74.6%
Ad hoc 2	0.620 (0.087)	92.6%
ML 1	0.648 (0.083)	92.8% (1.2%, 5.9%)
		94.5% (2.6%, 3.0%)
		95.0% (2.9%, 2.1%)
ML 2	0.654 (0.086)	–

Sample Size = 63, $LD_x = LD_y = \log_{10}(200)$ Average Number of Type 1–4 Observations: 30.3, 9.5, 6.6, 16.5		
Method	Mean Estimate (SD)	95% CI Coverage
Ad hoc 1	0.452 (0.165)	71.7%
Ad hoc 2	0.600 (0.101)	86.6%
ML 1	0.655 (0.092)	89.1% (1.7%, 9.2%)
		92.1% (3.2%, 4.7%)
		92.9% (3.6%, 3.4%)
ML 2	0.667 (0.104)	–

Note: CI, confidence interval; HERS, HIV Epidemiology Research Study; LD, limit of detection; ML, maximum likelihood; SD, empirical standard deviation; SE, standard error.

[a] 2,500 simulation replicates in each case; Covariates C_1, C_2, C_3 generated as described in Section 6.4; true $\rho = 0.65$; other parameters set equal to ML 1 method estimates (see footnote to Table 6.1).

[b] *Ad hoc* 1: Dropping all records with X or Y nondetected; *ad hoc* 2: replacing nondetectables by LOD.

[c] ML Methods 1 and 2 as detailed in Sections 6.2.2.2 and 6.2.2.3.

[d] CIs for complete data and *ad hoc* methods based on standard Fisher's z-transformation; numbers in parentheses represent percentages of times CIs "missed" on the low and high side, respectively.

[e] The first ML 1 interval is standard Wald CI; the second is based on Fisher's z-transformation (Equation 6.10); the third uses the approach of Li et al. (2005) (see Equation 6.11).

under conditions closely mimicking the HERS example. Although generated as independent for convenience, the marginal distributions of the three covariates included in the simulations were based on the HERS data (C_1, "risk group" ~ Bernoulli [0.43]; C_2, "age" ~ N[40.2, 6.6^2]; C_3, "CD4/100" ~ N [3.5, 2.1^2]). A total of 2,500 datasets, each with a sample size of 63 records, were generated according to the BVN model specifications in Equation 6.7. As in the HERS example, limits of detection (LD_x and LD_y) of $\log_{10}(50)$ were assumed in the first set of simulations. A second set was then performed in which the LODs were increased to $\log_{10}(200)$. The true value of $\rho_{yx|c}$ was 0.65 in each case, and the true values of all other model parameters were set equal to the MLEs listed in the footnotes to Table 6.1. The estimation approaches considered include the *ad hoc* 1 and 2 and the ML 1 and 2 methods (see Section 6.3.4). CI approaches considered in Table 6.1 were evaluated with respect to overall coverage, as well as coverage balance (i.e., proportions of times the intervals missed the true parameter on the low and high side). Due to computing time, the bootstrap procedure used to analyze the example data under the ML 2 method was not evaluated in the simulations.

The top half of Table 6.4 shows that, under conditions very similar to the example, the ML 1 and ML 2 methods perform the best overall. In particular, both show little bias in the estimate of $\rho_{yx|c}$; the ML 1 method also loses rather little precision (measured by the empirical standard deviation, SD) relative to the complete data. The *ad hoc* methods suffer as expected in terms of bias and overall CI coverage, although these deficiencies are relatively minor for the *ad hoc* 2 approach with the LOD at $\log_{10}(50)$. Overall CI coverage and coverage balance for ML 1 are clearly better based on the two approaches founded on Fisher's z-transformation, as compared to the standard Wald CI. These impressions largely carry over to the lower half of Table 6.4, summarizing a repeat of the simulation study with the LODs raised to $\log_{10}(200)$. In this case, the bias issues associated with the *ad hoc* 2 method are somewhat more apparent, as are the potential small-sample CI coverage benefits associated with the approach of Li et al. (2005).

Table 6.5 repeats the simulation conditions of Table 6.4, except with a larger sample size (200) at each replication. We conducted 1,500 replications in these scenarios, due to computing time associated with the need for numerical integration to calculate the contribution for every observation at each evaluation of the log-likelihood. Estimates are predictably more precise given the increase in sample size, which accentuates the poor CI coverage properties associated with the *ad hoc* approaches. In this case the ML 1 and ML 2 estimators are both virtually unbiased, while overall coverage and CI balance in conjunction with ML 1 is relatively similar for the two intervals based on Fisher's z-transformation. The standard Wald CI for $\rho_{yx|c}$ continues to exhibit poor coverage balance, with a large proportion of intervals missing on the high side.

6.4.2 Evaluating Partial Regression Coefficient Estimators

Table 6.6 evaluates the ML 1 and 2 estimators of the partial regression coefficient (Section 6.2.2.4) associating Y with X, based on the same four sets of simulated data summarized in Tables 6.1 and 6.2.

Both display minimal bias, but the ML 1 estimator is markedly more precise. Wald CIs associated with ML 1 also displayed better overall coverage in each case compared to those based on ML 2.

TABLE 6.5

Results of Simulations to Evaluate Partial Correlation Estimators in Settings Mimicking HERS Example[a]

Sample Size = 200, $LD_x = LD_y = \log_{10}(50)$ Average Number of Type 1–4 Observations: 135.6, 25.5, 14.4, 24.5		
Method[b,c]	Mean Estimate (SD)	95% CI Coverage[d,e]
Complete data	0.649 (0.041)	95.8%
Ad hoc 1	0.509 (0.067)	33.6%
Ad hoc 2	0.623 (0.046)	89.7%
ML 1	0.650 (0.044)	94.2% (1.1%, 4.7%)
		95.3% (1.9%, 2.8%)
		95.6% (2.1%, 2.3%)
ML 2	0.651 (0.047)	–

Sample Size = 200, $LD_x = LD_y = \log_{10}(200)$ Average Number of Type 1–4 Observations: 95.6, 30.7, 21.5, 52.2		
Method	Mean Estimate (SD)	95% CI Coverage
Ad hoc 1	0.451 (0.092)	25.9%
Ad hoc 2	0.600 (0.055)	74.9%
ML 1	0.649 (0.049)	94.6% (1.3%, 4.1%)
		95.0% (2.3%, 2.7%)
		95.1% (2.6%, 2.3%)
ML 2	0.653 (0.056)	–

Note: CI, confidence interval; HERS, HIV Epidemiology Research Study; ML, maximum likelihood; LD, limit of detection; SD, empirical standard deviation; SE, standard error.

[a] 1,500 simulation replicates in each case; covariates C_1, C_2, C_3 generated as described in Section 6.4; true $\rho = 0.65$; other parameters set equal to ML 1 method estimates (see footnote to Table 6.1).

[b] *Ad hoc* 1: Dropping all records with X or Y nondetected; *ad hoc* 2: replacing nondetectables by LOD.

[c] ML Methods 1 and 2 as detailed in Sections 6.2.2.2 and 6.2.2.3.

[d] CIs for complete data and *ad hoc* methods based on standard Fisher's z-transformation; numbers in parentheses represent percentages of times CIs "missed" on the low and high side, respectively.

[e] The first ML 1 interval is standard Wald CI; the second is based on Fisher's z-transformation (Equation 6.10); the third uses the approach of Li et al. (2005) (see Equation 6.11).

6.4.3 Evaluating Partial Regression Coefficient Estimators under Mixture Model for X | C

As seen in Table 6.3, AIC slightly favored a mixture model with a point mass below the LOD over the left-censored normal model with covariates in the HERS example for the X | C distribution (i.e., log viral load at Visit 8). This mixture model utilized the covariates to model the mean of the normal

TABLE 6.6

Results of Simulations to Evaluate Partial Regression Coefficient Estimators in Settings Mimicking HERS Example[a,b]

Method	Mean Estimate (SD)	Mean Estimated SE	95% CI Coverage
	2,500 Simulations; Sample Size = 63, LD_x = LD_y = $\log_{10}(50)$		
ML 1	0.780 (0.138)	0.134	94.4%
ML 2	0.774 (0.178)	0.168	93.4%
	2,500 Simulations; Sample Size = 63, LD_x = LD_y = $\log_{10}(200)$		
ML 1	0.794 (0.166)	0.155	93.3%
ML 2	0.787 (0.244)	0.221	92.0%
	1,500 Simulations; Sample Size = 200, LD_x = LD_y = $\log_{10}(50)$		
ML 1	0.776 (0.077)	0.075	93.9%
ML 2	0.772 (0.096)	0.094	93.5%
	1,500 Simulations; Sample Size = 200, LD_x = LD_y = $\log_{10}(200)$		
ML 1	0.780 (0.088)	0.087	95.4%
ML 2	0.783 (0.126)	0.123	93.5%

Note: CI, confidence interval; HERS, HIV Epidemiology Research Study; LD, limit of detection; ML, maximum likelihood; SD, empirical standard deviation; SE, standard error.
[a] Results based on simulation datasets summarized in Tables 6.4 and 6.5; true β = 0.776.
[b] ML Methods 1 and 2 as detailed in Section 6.2.2.4.

component, while using a single parameter (ω) to capture the mixing proportion. In Section 6.2.3.3, we recommend a focus upon the partial regression coefficient (β_{T+1}) if this mixture model is assumed for $X \mid C$, given the lack of a unique partial correlation coefficient. The two proposed ML methods (1 and 2; Sections 6.2.2.4 and 6.2.3.3) for this circumstance were fit to the HERS data and summarized in Table 6.2. Although less efficient, ML Method 2 might arguably be preferable on the grounds of robustness in this scenario given that it does not rely upon a particular (e.g., left-censored normal) $X \mid C$ distributional assumption.

In Table 6.7, we evaluate this robustness question through simulations designed to roughly mimic the conditions of the HERS example with respect to the parameterization $f(Y,X \mid C) = f(Y \mid X,C)f(X \mid C)$, with parameters chosen to be similar to MLEs obtained via the real data. Specifically, the true value of the partial regression coefficient was taken to be 0.8. Although Table 6.7 considers only one scenario that is similar to the motivating example, the suggestion is that under those conditions there is little or no concern with regard to the robustness of the ML 1 method despite the fact that the $X \mid C$ data were generated according to the mixture model. The ML 1 method is also markedly more precise than ML 2 in this case. We note that mean estimated SEs for both methods appear slightly small relative to the corresponding empirical SDs, likely leading to the CI coverage rates observed to be below the nominal level. This might suggest an alternative approach (e.g., the bootstrap) for SE and CI estimation in this context. Nevertheless, CI coverage was

TABLE 6.7

Results of Simulations to Evaluate Partial Regression Coefficient (β_4) Estimators under Mixture Model for $X \mid C$ Distribution[a,b]

Method[c]	Mean Estimate (SD)	Mean Estimated SE	95% CI Coverage
	2,500 Simulations; Sample Size = 63, $LD_x = LD_y = \log_{10}(50)$		
ML 1	0.795 (0.189)	0.175	92.3%
ML 2	0.798 (0.374)	0.324	91.1%
	1,500 Simulations; Sample Size = 200, $LD_x = LD_y = \log_{10}(50)$		
ML 1	0.787 (0.097)	0.096	93.9%
ML 2	0.805 (0.185)	0.175	94.1%

Note: CI, confidence interval; ML, maximum likelihood; HERS, HIV Epidemiology Research Study; LD, limit of detection; SD, empirical standard deviation; SE, standard error.
[a] Covariates C_1, C_2, C_3 generated as described in Section 6.4; $X \mid C$ generated via mixture model with point mass below LOD (Section 6.2.3.2) with covariates modeling only the normal mean, then $Y \mid X, C$ generated via model (6.1).
[b] True parameters as follows: $(\psi_0, \psi_1, \psi_2, \psi_3, \beta_0, \beta_1, \beta_2, \beta_3, \beta_4, \sigma_{x|c}^2, \sigma_{y|xc}^2, \omega)$ = (5, −0.2, −0.05, −0.25, 1.3, 0.2, −0.02, −0.02, 0.8, 0.8, 1, 0.3).
[c] ML Methods 1 and 2 as detailed in Section 6.2.2.4.

better for ML 1 than ML 2 under smaller sample size conditions ($n = 63$), and coverage improved for both methods with a larger sample size ($n = 200$).

Overall, the analyses summarized in Table 6.3 appear relatively supportive of the BVN-based ML 1 estimates of $\rho_{yx|c}$ and β_{T+1} reported in Tables 6.1 and 6.2, respectively. If taking a cautious view in light of some suggestion of a preponderance of nondetectables at Visit 8, one might prefer to rely on the partial regression coefficient as the measure of association between Y and X for the HERS data.

6.5 Discussion

Laboratory nondetectables are a common occurrence in epidemiologic and clinical health-related research, notably in HIV/AIDS studies that monitor HIV viral load. As such, there continues to be considerable interest in statistical methods that account for left censoring in a defensible manner. This chapter offers an overview (though far from exhaustive) of relevant literature on the analytic handling of assay nondetectables and extends an accessible ML approach for estimating the correlation between two left-censored variables by incorporating covariates as motivated by an example based on viral loads at consecutive visits in the HERS.

With a focus upon estimating the partial correlation and/or partial regression coefficient associating two left-censored variables, we have considered two main approaches (labeled *ML 1* and *ML 2*). The ML 1 method is a natural generalization of the BVN modeling approach taken in Lyles et al. (2001b), whereas ML 2 works with separate univariate models for the $Y|C$ and $Y|X,C$ distributions. The ML 2 approach is predictably less efficient when the BVN assumptions hold, given that it involves ignoring records with X nondetected. However, it is simpler computationally and there is some motivation to explore its potential to be more robust. Our simulation studies are by no means fully conclusive in this regard, but we have seen no empirical evidence to suggest a robustness advantage to ML 2 sufficient to recommend it over ML 1. Both methods appear relatively robust, at least to mild departures from the BVN model assumptions as dictated by univariate modeling exercises undertaken using the HERS data (Table 6.3). Nevertheless, certain alternative models (e.g., a mixture model for $X|C$ with a point mass below the LOD) can preclude defining a unique partial correlation coefficient and may dictate a focus on the partial regression coefficient in its stead (e.g., Table 6.7). In the current study, we did not examine robustness with respect to inappropriateness of a left-censored normal model for the $Y|X,C$ distribution.

We hope that this investigation will be of use to HIV researchers seeking to associate bivariate HIV RNA measurements taken over time or in different reservoirs, when there is a need to take covariates into account in a natural way. Further research into alternative models and robust approaches, building upon the growing literature on the handling of laboratory assay nondetectables would seem valuable and welcome.

Acknowledgments

Drs. Caroline King and Li Tang provided access to the HERS data, along with valuable insight and advice pertaining to the motivating example. The author also thanks the HERS participants and the HERS Research Group, which consists of Robert S. Klein, MD, Ellie Schoenbaum, MD, Julia Arnsten, MD, MPH, Robert D. Burk, MD, Chee Jen Chang, PhD, Penelope Demas, PhD, and Andrea Howard, MD, MSc, from Montefiore Medical Center and the Albert Einstein College of Medicine; Paula Schuman, MD, and Jack Sobel, MD, from the Wayne State University School of Medicine; Anne Rompalo, MD, David Vlahov, PhD, and David Celentano, PhD, from the Johns Hopkins University School of Medicine; Charles Carpenter, MD, and Kenneth Mayer, MD, from the Brown University School of Medicine; Ann Duerr, MD, Caroline C. King, PhD, Lytt I. Gardner, PhD, Charles M. Heilig, PhD, Scott Holmberg, MD, Denise Jamieson, MD, Jan Moore, PhD, Ruby Phelps, BS, Dawn Smith, MD, and Dora Warren, PhD, from the CDC; and Katherine Davenny, PhD from the National Institute of Drug Abuse. This research was supported in part by the National Center for Advancing Translational Sciences (UL1TR000454), and by the Emory Center for AIDS Research (P30AI050469).

References

Akaike H. A new look at the statistical model identification. *IEEE Transactions on Automatic Control* 1974; **19**:716–723.

Albert PS. Modeling longitudinal biomarker data from multiple assays that have different known detection limits. *Biometrics* 2008; **64**:527–537.

Chu HT, Gange SJ, Li X, et al. The effect of HAART on HIV RNA trajectory among treatment-naïve men and women: A segmental Bernoulli/lognormal random effects model with left censoring. *Epidemiology* 2010; **21**:S25–S34.

Chu HT, Moulton LH, Mack WJ, et al. Correlating two continuous variables subject to detection limits in the context of mixture distributions. *Applied Statistics* 2005; **54**:831–845.

Chu H, Nie L. A note on comparing exposure data to a regulatory limit in the presence of unexposed and a limit of detection. *Biometrical Journal* 2005; **47**:880–887.

Cohen AC. Simplified estimators for the normal distribution when samples are singly censored or truncated. *Technometrics* 1959; **1**:217–237.

Cohen AC. Tables for maximum likelihood estimates: Singly truncated and singly censored samples. *Technometrics* 1961; **3**:535–541.

Dempster AP, Laird NM, and Rubin DB. Maximum likelihood from incomplete data via the EM algorithm (with discussion). *Journal of the Royal Statistical Society B* 1977; **39**:1–38.

Efron B and Tibshirani RJ. *An Introduction to the Bootstrap*. Chapman and Hall: New York, 1993.

Helsel DR. *Nondetects and Data Analysis*. Wiley: Hoboken, NJ, 2005.

Hornung RW and Reed LD. Estimation of average concentration in the presence of nondetectable values. *Applied Occupational and Environmental Hygiene* 1990; **5**:46–51.

Hughes JP. Mixed effects models with censored data with application to HIV RNA levels. *Biometrics* 1999; **55**:625–629.

Jacqmin-Gadda H, Thiebaut R, Chene G and Commenges D. Analysis of left-censored longitudinal data with application to viral load in HIV infection. *Biostatistics* 2000; **1**:355–368.

Kleinbaum DG, Kupper LL, Nizam A and Muller KE. *Applied Regression Analysis and Other Multivariable Methods* (4th Edition), Thomspon Brooks/Cole: Belmont, CA, 2008.

Kutner MH, Nachtsheim CJ, Neter J and Li W. *Applied Linear Statistical Models*. (5th edition), McGraw—Hill/Irwin: New York, NY, 2005.

Lee M-J and Kong L. Quantile regression analysis of censored longitudinal biomarker data subject to left censoring and dropouts. *Communications in Statistics—Theory and Methods* 2014; **43**:4628–4641.

Lee M-J, Kong L and Weissfeld L. Multiple imputation for left-censored biomarker data based on Gibbs sampling method. *Statistics in Medicine* 2012; **31**:1838–1848.

Li L, Wang WWB and Chan ISF. Correlation coefficient inference on censored bioassay data. *Journal of Biopharmaceutical Statistics* 2005; **3**:501–512.

Little RJA and Rubin DB. *Statistical Analysis with Missing Data*. New York, NY; Wiley & Sons, 2002.

Looney SW and Hagan JL. *Analysis of Biomarker Data: A Practical Guide*. Wiley: Hoboken, NJ, 2015.

Lyles RH, Fan D and Chuachoowong R. Correlation coefficient estimation involving a left-censored laboratory assay variable. *Statistics in Medicine* 2001a; **20**:2931–2933.

Lyles RH, Lyles CM and Taylor DJ. Random regression models for human immunodeficiency virus ribonucleic acid data subject to left censoring and informative drop-outs. *Applied Statistics* 2000; **49**:485–497.

Lyles RH, Williams JK and Chuachoowong R. Correlating two viral load assays with known detection limits. *Biometrics* 2001b; **57**:1238–1244.

Lynn HS. Maximum likelihood inference for left-censored HIV RNA data. *Statistics in Medicine* 2001; **20**:33–45.

McCracken CE. *Correlation Coefficient Inference for Left-Censored Biomarker Data with Known Detection Limits.* Unpublished Ph.D. dissertation, Department of Biostatistics, Georgia Regents University, 2013.

Moore RH. *Prediction of Random Effects when Data are Subject to a Detection Limit.* Unpublished Ph.D. dissertation, Department of Biostatistics and Bioinformatics, Emory University, 2006.

Moore RH, Lyles RH and Manatunga AK. Empirical constrained Bayes predictors accounting for non-detects among repeated measures. *Statistics in Medicine* 2010; **29**:2656–2668.

Moulton LH and Halsey NA. A mixture model with detection limits for regression analyses of antibody response to vaccine. *Biometrics* 1995; **51**:1570–1578.

Nie L, Chu H, Cheng Y, et al. Marginal and conditional approaches to multivariate variables subject to limit of detection. *Journal of Biopharmaceutical Statistics* 2009; **19**:1151–1161.

Nie L, Chu H and Korostyshevskiy VR. Bias reduction for nonparametric correlation coefficients under the bivariate normal copula assumption with known detection limits. *Canadian Journal of Statistics* 2008; **3**:427–442.

Nie L, Chu H, Liu C, Cole SR, Vexler A, and Schisterman EF. Linear Regression with an independent variable subject to a detection limit. *Epidemiology* 2010; **21**: S17–S24.

Perkins NJ, Schisterman EF and Vexler A. Generalized ROC curve inference for a biomarker subject to a limit of detection and measurement error. *Statistics in Medicine* 2009; **28**:1841–1860.

Perkins NJ, Schisterman EF and Vexler A. ROC curve inference for best linear combination of two biomarkers subject to limits of detection. *Biometrical Journal* 2011; **53**:464–476.

Pettit AN. Censored observations, repeated measures and mixed effects models: An approach using the EM algorithm and normal errors. *Biometrika* 1986; **73**:635–643.

SAS Institute, Inc. *SAS/IML User's Guide 9.2*, Cary, NC, 2008.

Smith DK, Warren DL, Vlahov D, et al. Design and baseline participant characteristics of the Human Immuondeficiency Virus Epidemiology Research (HER) study: A prospective cohort study of human immunodeficiency virus infection in US women. *American Journal of Epidemiology* 1997; **146**:459–469.

Sun X, Peng L, Manatunga A, et al. Quantile regression analysis of censored longitudinal data with irregular outcome-dependent follow-up. *Biometrics* 2015; **72**:64–73. (DOI: 10.1111/biom12367).

Taylor DJ, Kupper LL, Rappaport SM, et al. A mixture model for occupational exposure mean testing with a limit of detection. *Biometrics* 2001; **57**:681–688.

Thiebaut R and Jacqmin-Gadda H. Mixed models for longitudinal left-censored repeated measures. *Computer Methods and Programs in Biomedicine* 2004; **3**:255–260.

Vexler A, Liu A, Eliseeva E, et al. Maximum likelihood ratio tests for comparing the discriminatory ability of biomarkers subject to limit of detection. *Biometrics* 2008; **64**:895–903.

Wannemuehler KA and Lyles RH. A unified model for covariate measurement error adjustment in an occupational health study while accounting for non-detectable exposures. *Applied Statistics* 2005; **54**:259–271.

Williamson JM, Crawford SB and Lin H-M. A multiple imputation approach for estimating rank correlation with left-censored data. *Statistics in Biopharmaceutical Research* 2010; **2**:540–548.

Xie X, Xue X, Gange SJ, et al. Estimation and inference on correlations between biomarkers with repeated measures and left-censoring due to minimum detection levels. *Statistics in Medicine* 2012; **31**:2275–2289.

Zheng S. *Random regression for longitudinal data subject to left censoring and informative drop-outs using generalized multivariate theory.* Unpublished Ph.D. dissertation, University of Alabama-Birmingham, School of Joint Health Sciences, 2002.

7

Quantitative Methods and Bayesian Models for Flow Cytometry Analysis in HIV/AIDS Research

Lin Lin

Pennsylvania State University, State College, PA

Cliburn Chan

Duke University, Durham, NC

CONTENTS

7.1 Flow Cytometry in HIV/AIDS Research

Flow cytometry is a multiparameter single-cell assay ubiquitous in HIV/AIDS clinical and research settings for evaluating the immune response to the virus, therapy, and vaccination. In clinical practice, flow cytometry is used to monitor the CD4 and CD8 T cell counts of HIV-infected subjects. In research settings, flow cytometry is used to evaluate innate and antigen-specific responses to the HIV virus, so as to better understand pathogenesis, the mechanisms responsible for long-term nonprogression, and to develop effective immune-based interventions. In vaccine development, there is significant interest in the potential of flow-based biomarkers that can serve as surrogate measures of efficacy.

After sample collection and processing, cells in solution labeled by fluorescent dyes are streamed in a cytometer for excitation by multiple lasers, and light scattered from cells and emitted from the relaxation of fluorescent molecules into their resting state is collected via optical detectors and recorded electronically. Fundamentally, the information collected consists of a $n \times p$ matrix, where each of the n rows represents an "event" (typically a cell but also possibly cell aggregates, debris, microparticles, or photon noise) and each of the p columns represents a measure of event characteristics (time, forward and side light scatter, fluorescence intensity in a specific wavelength band). The fluorescence intensity values are of most interest, because these correspond to fluorochromes associated with the cell, often as labels on antibodies targeting cell surface (e.g. CD4) or intracellular (e.g., Tumor Necrosis Factor-α [TNF-α]) proteins. Fluorochromes not attached to antibodies are also used to report cell division (e.g., carboxyfluorescein succinimidyl ester) or viability (e.g., amine dyes).

Because different fluorochromes can emit light with overlapping wavelengths, preprocessing using single-stained samples is necessary to subtract the "spillover" and recover the "true" signal from each fluorochrome. Subtraction of spillover is performed using matrix multiplication and is known as *compensation*. This is generally performed automatically, but sometimes manual fine-tuning is also performed for optimal visual resolution of cell subsets. The distribution of fluorescence intensities is right-skewed, and a log-like transformation is usually applied to correct for this. The most commonly applied data transformations, such as biexponential, preserve linearity at lower intensities but log transform at high intensities.

After preprocessing by compensation and transformation, the data are typically summarized by partitioning events into cell subsets and reporting the count or relative frequency, as well as the mean/median fluorescence intensity (MFI) of each parameter for every cell subset of interest. Overall, the process reduces the $n \times p$ raw data matrix into k counts or percentages and k p-vectors representing the MFIs, where $k \ll n$. Traditionally, the process of event partitioning into cell subsets is done using software for *gating* (e.g., FlowJo, TreeStar, Ashland, OR), a sequential process that visually demarcates events in bounded regions on 1D or 2D projections. For example, a CD4+ T cell can be identified via projection on forward and side scatter to gate for lymphocytes, then on CD3/viability, and finally on a CD4/CD8 projection. The sequence of projections to use is determined by expert knowledge. The exact shape and location of the gates may be chosen according to prior experience or by comparison with reference samples, for example, negative controls such as fluorescence minus one stained samples. Once a gating strategy has been set, it is typically applied in common to all flow cytometry samples in the batch being analyzed. Sometimes, the gates may be adjusted to accommodate individual variability for individual samples. In general, the manual gating approach is subjective, difficult to reproduce, and biased towards the identification of known cell subsets rather than novel ones. Cell subsets can also be defined by combining gates in "Boolean" gating, for example, when enumerating all the 2^m low/high combinations of m markers—this is often done when defining all functional cell subsets in intracellular assays, which use labeled antibodies to intracellular effector proteins such as cytokines as markers. A review of traditional flow cytometry analysis can be found in Herzenberg et al. (2006).

To improve the reproducibility of flow cytometry assays, large-scale proficiency testing programs have been initiated to standardize the complex process, for example, the NIH-sponsored External Quality Assurance Program Oversight Laboratory (EQAPOL) initiative for NIAID-sponsored national and international laboratories conducting HIV/AIDS clinical research (Staats et al. 2014). These programs provide standard protocols for sample processing and analysis, standard lyophilized antibody panels, and provide feedback on the quality of compensation and gating. In the absence of any objective gold standard for flow cytometry analysis, the objective is for laboratories participating in the EQAPOL program to converge to similar results with minimum deviation across laboratories. Flow laboratories are encouraged to participate in this free program to compare their performance relative to other NIH-sponsored laboratories (see https://eqapol.dhvi.duke.edu for participation details).

Although proficiency programs such as EQAPOL are essential, as the number of parameters measured increases, it becomes increasingly difficult to apply the traditional gating techniques as the number of gating sequence permutations possible grows as the factorial of the number of dimensions. Major contributions from the quantitative community have been made to address the challenge of increasing dimensionality, especially for automated cell subset identification, dimension reduction and visualization, and comparative analysis of cell counts. Because there are a number of excellent recent reviews of these areas (Aghaeepour et al. 2013; Bashashati and Brinkman 2009), we will only describe them briefly; rather, we emphasize Bayesian and multilevel approaches that are less well known and a major focus of the authors' own research.

7.2 Brief Review of Automated Analysis

In automated analysis, the goal is usually to develop a computational pipeline from raw data to cell counts or relative frequencies. Quality control and sanity checks are important aspects of any automated pipeline, but usually the focus is on the partitioning of event subsets into distinct groups (clustering) in such a way that the clusters can be identified across different samples (registration). Mapping of clusters to biologically meaningful cell subsets (annotation) is often not part of the pipeline, although the pipeline could potentially be extended with supervised leaning or rule-based approaches to also automate cell subset labeling.

The core interest is to automatically identify groups of similar cells (cell subsets) for further study. This is essentially a clustering procedure and summaries of several clustering methods applied to flow cytometry data can be found in recent publications (Aghaeepour et al. 2013; O'Neill et al. 2013; Verschoor et al. 2015). One of the most popular approaches is the use of mixture models for clustering (Boedigheimer and Ferbas 2008). One appeal of the mixture model strategy is that the goodness of fit to any observed data sample can be evaluated by calculating the likelihood and improved by increasing the number of mixture components. Typically, the mixture components are multivariate distributions, and projection to lower dimensions is not necessary for fitting. Symmetric Gaussian mixture models are often used as the base component, but skewed and heavy-tailed distributions, such as the t distribution, can also be useful (Lo et al. 2008; Pyne et al. 2009). Heavy-tailed distributions are robust to the presence of outliers and can result in more parsimonious models, whereas skew distributions can be applied directly to the flow cytometry data without the need for transformation. Finally, model selection strategies, such as the Akaike information criterion (AIC) and Bayesian information criterion (BIC), are used to determine the number of mixture components and avoid under- or overfitting.

After fitting mixture models, the simplest approach is to assign each mixture component to an individual cell subset. However, the shapes of some cell subsets can be asymmetric and nonconvex, and the use of simple parametric distributions typically provides a poor fit to such populations. Instead, we can use various strategies to merge multiple mixture components to represent an individual cell subset, and this gives a better and more flexible representation of cell subsets with arbitrary shapes (Aghaeepour et al. 2011; Chan et al. 2010; Finak et al. 2009; Lin et al. 2016; Pyne et al. 2009). The count of merged clusters also provides a reasonable estimate of the number of well-separated cell subsets in the data.

Once cell subsets are identified, the next essential step is to align cell subsets across multiple data samples for comparative analysis. These samples may come from different batches, different individuals, and different laboratories in multicenter studies. One intuitive approach is to perform normalization on a set of samples to remove technical between-sample variation before performing any clustering procedures. This facilitates the correct matching of cell subsets across samples (Finak et al. 2014a; Hahne et al. 2010). Another strategy is to perform meta-clustering, a second clustering procedure that uses the identified cell subset features to identify clusters across samples with similar properties (Azad et al. 2012, 2013; Sörensen et al. 2015). The third strategy is through the use of hierarchical mixture models, a Bayesian approach that will be discussed later in this chapter.

The development of various useful visualization tools greatly facilitates the interpretation of automated analysis results (Amir et al. 2013; Lin et al. 2015b;

Qiu et al. 2011; Sarkar et al. 2008). As flow cytometry can generate many, very large datasets, the ability to fit mixture models to increasingly large datasets becomes a key challenge for efficient analysis. Various algorithms have been developed for fast computations (Hyrkas et al. 2015; Naim et al. 2014; Suchard et al. 2010). In addition, the software for most of the automated analysis strategies have open source licenses and are freely available (Kvistborg et al. 2015).

7.3 Introduction to Bayesian Modeling

The essential idea of the Bayesian modeling approach is that every parameter θ in the probabilistic model that we fit to data x is a random variable with a prior distribution $P(\theta)$, either informed by historical data ("informative prior") or left diffuse ("uninformative prior"). Given the data, we can then compute the posterior distribution $P(\theta \mid x)$ from the prior distribution and a likelihood function $P(x \mid \theta)$ using Bayes' theorem:

$$P(\theta|x) = \frac{P(x|\theta)P(\theta)}{P(x)}$$

For high dimensional data, the posterior distribution is nearly always computed numerically using Markov Chain Monte Carlo (MCMC) or variational algorithms that generalize Laplace's approximation. The numerical procedure is designed to eventually generate samples from the posterior distribution. Given these samples from the posterior distribution, we can estimate any statistic of interest for inference about the model by simple averaging. For example, we can estimate a function f such as the posterior mean using $f(\theta) \approx \frac{1}{N} \sum_{i=1}^{N} f(\theta_i)$, where θ_i represents samples from the posterior distribution.

Practically, there are two main advantages of the Bayesian approach. First, we can define a prior distribution based on historical data. This is particularly useful when sample sizes are small, because there is shrinkage towards the prior. It is prudent to evaluate the influence of the prior with a sensitivity analysis in this case. Second, and more importantly, multilevel or hierarchical models are simpler to evaluate with a Bayesian approach. Multiple levels are often the most natural way to model flow cytometry data, allowing us to capture commonalities across groups of cell subsets, samples, and subjects for more robust inference. The use of multilevel Bayesian models can also address the issue of multiple testing naturally, in providing automatic shrinkage and conservative comparisons (Gelman et al. 2012).

The flexibility of Bayesian multilevel models comes at the cost of increased complexity in setting up the model and the computational demands of estimating the posterior distribution. However, both these issues are mitigated by modern software packages such as Stan (Carpenter et al. 2015) and PyMC3 (Wiecki 2013) that provide domain-specific languages for model specification and automatic compilation to multicore or graphical processing unit native code for efficiency.

7.4 Bayesian Models for Cell Subset Identification

We consider each flow cytometry data set as a sample from a complex multimodal multivariate distribution, modeled using a mixture of simple multivariate distributions. Each event is assumed to belong to a group of events (i.e., a component distribution) sharing the same location and scale parameters, and hence this is a simple example of a multilevel (event and group) model. In some contexts, use of fat-tailed distributions such as mixtures of Student t distributions is parsimonious in that fewer mixture components are required to fit the data. In other contexts where it is useful to fit rare event subsets to discrete components, mixtures of multivariate Gaussians are appropriate. In either case, fitting mixtures of multivariate distributions with a fixed number of components is one of the first applications of Bayesian multivariate models to flow cytometry data (Chan et al. 2008). Useful inferences can be derived from the fitted posterior distribution—for example, inferring the quantitative contribution of particular antibody labels towards discrimination of a target cell subset, information useful for optimal development of antibody panels (Chan et al. 2010).

7.4.1 Finite Gaussian Mixture Models

Here, we provide a detailed example to illustrate the concept of Bayesian modeling and posterior computation. We start with a finite Gaussian mixture model. Begin by representing data in a general form, with the following notations and definitions: Let x denote the set of flow cytometry measurements from one sample, where x is a matrix of size $n \times p$, n is the total number of cells measured in one sample, and p is the number of markers measured in the assay. Then $x_i = (x_{i1}, \ldots, x_{ip})$ is the p-dimensional vector representing the measured markers on the ith cell. We typically compensate, transform, and standardize the flow cytometry measurements before performing any statistical analysis; hence, x usually represents the preprocessed flow cytometry data.

The finite Gaussian mixture model with k components may be written as follows:

$$x_i \sim \sum_{j=1}^{k} \pi_j N(x_i | \mu_j, \Sigma_j),$$

where k is the number of mixture components, $\pi_1, \ldots, \pi_k$ are the mixture probabilities that sum to 1, N is the multivariate normal distribution, μ_j is the p-dimensional mean vector of mixture components j, and Σ_j is the corresponding $p \times p$ covariance matrix. The mixture model can be interpreted as arising from a clustering procedure depending on an underlying latent indicator z_i for x_i. That is, $z_i = s$ indicates that x_i was generated from mixture component s, or $x_i | z_i = s \sim N(\mu_s, \Sigma_s)$, and with $P(z_i = s) = \pi_s$. Typically, a number of models with different k are run and the number of mixture components is determined by model selection criterion such as AIC, BIC, and other informational approximations to likelihoods.

One way to understand the Gaussian mixture model, which represents how the Bayesian model is coded and fitted to data in practice, is as a generative model:

$$x_i \sim \sum_{j=1}^{k} \pi_j N(\mu_j, \Sigma_j),$$
$$(\pi_1, \ldots, \pi_k) \sim Dir(\alpha/k, \ldots, \alpha/k), \tag{7.1}$$
$$\mu_j | \Sigma_j \sim N(m, \lambda \Sigma_j),$$
$$\Sigma \sim IW(q+2, q\Phi),$$

where each x_i is sampled according to a k-component Gaussian mixture model; $\{\pi_j, \mu_j, \Sigma_j\}$ is the set of parameters associated with the jth mixture component; $(\pi_1, \ldots, \pi_k)$ is the mixing proportions $\pi_j \geq 0$, for $j = 1, \ldots, k$, and $\sum_{j=1}^{k} \pi_j = 1$. The probability π_j also represents the prior probability that an event comes from each component j. The conjugate prior for $(\pi_1, \ldots, \pi_k)$ is the symmetric Dirichlet distribution $Dir(\alpha/k, \ldots, \alpha/k)$, where α is a positive constant that may be fixed or have its own prior distribution. The mean vector μ_j and covariance matrix Σ_j are jointly distributed according to a normal-inverse-Wishart distribution; m, λ, q, Φ are hyperparameters that may be fixed or have their own prior distributions. As discussed below, this basic probabilistic framework can be extended to incorporate additional structural information.

7.4.2 Dirichlet Process Models

Nonparametric Bayesian versions of the statistical mixture model can treat the number of components as another random variable to be estimated from data. Such models, often based on a Dirichlet process prior, are also known as *infinite mixture models,* and the number of components in such models grows as a function of the log of the number of events in the dataset. This is convenient, since the number of components necessary to fit the data is never known *a priori* in practice, and more efficient than fitting and selecting from a set of models with different numbers of components.

The Dirichlet process Gaussian mixture model (DPGMM) is a Bayesian nonparametric model that we have extensively used in cell subset identification. A DPGMM is a Gaussian mixture model with infinite components that can be construed as taking the limit of the finite mixture model (Equation 7.1) for k to infinity. This can be achieved by using the Dirichlet process (DP), which can be considered a "distribution of distributions," as a prior for the distribution of the mixture component parameters (μ_j, Σ_j):

$$x_i|\mu_i, \Sigma_i \sim N(\mu_i, \Sigma_i),$$
$$(\mu_i, \Sigma_i)|G \sim G, \quad\quad\quad (7.2)$$
$$G \sim DP(\alpha, G_0),$$

where we model the ith observation x_i by a Gaussian distribution with the observation-specific latent parameters μ_i and Σ_i, for $i = 1, \ldots, n$. Each pair of the parameters (μ_i, Σ_i) is independently and identically drawn from a distribution denoted by G, and DP is used as a prior over the distribution G, where DP is controlled by two parameters α and G_0. The concentration parameter α is a positive-valued scalar that affects the number of components of the mixture model—the larger the value of α, the more the components. The base distribution G_0 is where the random draws G will be centered. By the property of DP, the random distribution G is discrete, which can be expressed as $G = \sum_{j=1}^{\infty} \pi_j \delta_{(\mu_j^*, \Sigma_j^*)}$, where $\delta_{(\mu_j^*, \Sigma_j^*)}$ is a delta function equal to 1 if $(\mu, \Sigma) = (\mu_j^*, \Sigma_j^*)$ and 0 otherwise. Due to the discreteness of draws from the Dirichlet process, there is a nonzero probability that some (μ_i, Σ_i) will share the same value. This gives rise to the clustering property of the joint distribution of x_i.

To complete the model specification of Equation 7.2, both α and G_0 need to be prespecified. Typically, G_0 is chosen to be conjugate to the Gaussian likelihood as the normal-inverse-Wishart distribution, and α can be modeled by a Gamma distribution. In order to make actual draws from a DP, we use a constructive definition of the DP, which is called the *stick-breaking process* (Sethuraman 1994).

The constructive hierarchy of the conjugate DPGMM is formulated as

$$x_i \sim \sum_{j=1}^{\infty} \pi_j N(\mu_j, \Sigma_j),$$
$$\pi_j = V_j \prod_{l=1}^{j-1}(1 - V_l),$$
$$V_j \sim B(1, \alpha), \quad\quad\quad (7.3)$$
$$\alpha \sim G(e, f),$$
$$\mu_j|\Sigma_j \sim N(m, \lambda\Sigma_j),$$
$$\Sigma \sim IW(q+2, q\Phi),$$

for prespecified hyperparameters $(e, f, m, \lambda, q, \Phi)$. We let B denote the beta distribution, and G the gamma distribution. There are many algorithms for posterior sampling, including MCMC (e.g., Neal (2000); Jain and Neal (2004); Papaspiliopoulos and Roberts (2008)) and variational inference (e.g., Blei and Jordan (2006)). These computational algorithms are useful in analyzing small to moderate-sized data sets. However, for the large data sets generated by flow cytometry, a faster posterior inference algorithm is needed.

One way to reduce the computational complexity in fitting the DPGMM (Equation 7.2) is to adopt a version with an upper limit to the number of components, known as the *truncated DPGMM*. In particular, we use an encompassing Gaussian mixture model with a relatively large number J of components

$$x_i \sim \sum_{j=1}^{J} \pi_j N(\mu_j, \Sigma_j),$$

with prior hierarchically defined as in Equation 7.3:

$$\begin{aligned}
&\pi_1 = V_1, \quad \pi_j = (1 - V_1) \cdots (1 - V_{j-1}) V_j, \quad 1 < j < J, \\
&V_j \sim B(1, \alpha), \quad j = 1, \ldots, J-1, \quad V_J = 1 \\
&\alpha \sim G(e, f), \\
&\mu_j | \Sigma_j \sim N(m, \lambda \Sigma_j), \\
&\Sigma \sim IW(q + 2, q\Phi),
\end{aligned} \qquad (7.4)$$

with some fixed (large) upper bound J on the number of effective components to be prespecified before fitting the model. The truncated DPGMM (Equation 7.4) allows some of the mixture probabilities to be zero, so that the model can cut back to fewer components than the upper bound J as relevant for the data set at hand. The standard blocked Gibbs sampler (Ishwaran and James 2001; Ji et al. 2009) and Bayesian Expectation–Maximization algorithm (Lin et al. 2016) for this model is effective, widely used and implemented in efficient serial and parallel code (Suchard et al. 2010; Wang et al. 2010).

7.4.3 Hierarchical Dirichlet Process Models

We can also create a three-level model with events, clusters, and samples. By constraining mixture components to have the same location and covariance matrix across samples, such multilevel models enable identification of clusters across different samples for comparative analysis. Nonparametric Bayesian approaches, based now on two levels of Dirichlet process priors, can be used to estimate the number of model components as before, resulting in a hierarchical Dirichlet process (HDP) statistical mixture model (Cron et al. 2013; Teh et al. 2006). The HDP model represents a compromise between the extremes of no pooling (all samples treated as independent) and complete pooling (all samples assumed to come from the same distribution), allowing variation in the component weights across samples but shrinking the weight estimates towards the group mean. HDP facilitates the identification of cell subsets that are extremely rare in some samples but less so in others (e.g., positive control samples), which might otherwise be missed when fitting separate mixture models to each sample independently.

Explicitly, let j denote the sample index and i denote the event index within each group. Let $x_j = (x_{j1}, \ldots, x_{jn_j})$ represent all the events in sample j. The hierarchical model is defined by the one-way layout

$$x_{ji} | \mu_{ji}, \Sigma_{ji} \sim N(\mu_{ji}, \Sigma_{ji}),$$

$$(\mu_{ji}, \Sigma_{ji}) \sim G_j,$$

where we model the ith event from the jth sample x_{ji} by a Gaussian distribution with the observation and sample-specific latent parameters μ_{ji} and Σ_{ji}, for $i = 1, \ldots, n_j$, and j belongs to all the samples. Each pair of the parameters (μ_{ji}, Σ_{ji}) is independently and identically drawn from a sample-specific distribution denoted by G_j. The model is completed by the hierarchical specification $G_j | \alpha_j, G_0 \sim DP(\alpha_j, G_0)$, where G_0 is a global random probability measure distributed as $DP(\gamma, H)$. The α_j controls dispersion of the G_j around the global, underlying distribution G_0. The baseline distribution H provides the marginal prior distribution for (μ_{ji}, Σ_{ji}). The distribution G_0 varies around the prior H, with the amount of variability controlled by γ. The parameters in the stick-breaking representation of G_0 will be shared among all the G_j, whereas the parameters are also shared within each sample.

The sharing of information among all samples in the HDP model can be made more explicit via the stick-breaking construction:

$$x_{ji} \sim \sum_{k=1}^{\infty} \pi_{jk} N(\mu_k, \Sigma_k)$$

$$\pi_{jk} = \pi'_{jk} \prod_{l=1}^{k-1} (1 - \pi'_{jl}),$$

$$\pi'_{jk} \sim B\left(\alpha_j \beta_k, \alpha_j \left(1 - \sum_{l=1}^{k} \beta_l \right) \right), \tag{7.5}$$

$$\beta_k = \beta'_k \prod_{l=1}^{k-1} (1 - \beta'_l),$$

$$\beta'_k \sim B(1, \gamma),$$

$$(\mu_k, \Sigma_k) \sim H$$

where H is typically chosen as the normal-inverse-Wishart conjugate prior. The above model (Equation 7.5) implies that parameters are shared throughout the hierarchy. In this hierarchical model, each flow cytometry data sample can be thought of as a representative of the collection of data samples being simultaneously analyzed. The individual data samples then provide information on the properties of the collection, and this information in turn provides information on any particular data sample. In this way, an HDPGMM fitted to a single data sample "borrows strength" from all other samples in the collection being analyzed. In other words, if a rare cell subtype is found in more than one of the samples, we share this information across the samples in the collection to detect the subtype, even though the frequency in a particular data sample may be vanishingly small. HDPGMM thus increases sensitivity for clustering cell subsets that are of extremely low frequency in one sample but common to many samples or present in high frequency in one or more samples. In principle, there is no lower limit to the size of a cluster that can be detected in a particular sample. In practice, vanishingly small clusters (e.g., 3–5 events out of 100,000) require expert interpretation to distinguish background from signal, but it is not uncommon for biologically significant antigen-specific cells to be present at such frequencies.

As an example of the flexibility of multilevel probabilistic models, an alternative formulation of the HDP allows us to partition marker space for efficient quantification of multiple extremely rare antigen-specific T-cell subsets in *combinatorially encoded* samples. Combinatorial encoding expands the number of antigen-specific T cells that can be detected (Hadrup and Schumacher 2010). The basic idea is simple: by using multiple different fluorescent labels for any single epitope, we can identify many more types of antigen-specific T-cells by decoding the color combinations of their bound multimer reporters. For example, using r colors, we can in principle encode $2^r - 1$ different epitope specificities. In one strategy, all $2^r - 1$ combinations would be used to maximize the number of epitope specificities that can be detected (Newell et al. 2009). In a different strategy, only combinations with a threshold number of different multimers would be used to minimize the number of false positive events; for example, with $r = 5$ colors, we could set the restriction that only combinations using at least three colors be considered as valid encoding (Hadrup et al. 2009).

With such data sets, Lin et al. (2013) have shown that direct application of standard statistical mixture models, such as DPGMM, will typically generate imprecise if not unacceptable results due to the inherent masking of low probability subtypes. Hence, it is natural to seek hierarchically structured models that successively refine the focus into smaller, select regions of biological reporter space. The conditional specification of hierarchical mixture models now introduced does precisely this, and in a manner that respects the biological context and design of combinatorially encoded FCM.

Consider a sample of size n FCM measurements x_i, $i = 1, \ldots, n$, where now x_i contains both functional FCM phenotypic markers and the light emitted by the fluorescent reporters of multimers binding to specific receptors on the cell surface. In this experimental context, we typically seek to first identify specific T-cell subsets (e.g., CD4+ or CD8+) and then to distinguish antigen-specific clones within these subsets. To differentiate these two types of FCM measurements, we order the elements of x_i so that $x_i = (b_i, t_i)$, where b_i is the subvector of phenotypic marker measurements and t_i is the subvector of fluorescent intensities of each of the multimers being reported via the combinatorial encoding strategy. Let p_t and p_b denote the number of multimers and phenotypic markers, respectively, so that $p_t + p_b = p$.

In order to respect the phenotypic marker/reporter structure of the FCM data, each measurement x_i is modeled hierarchically:

$$x_i \sim f(b_i|\Theta)f(t_i|b_i, \Theta), \qquad (7.6)$$

where Θ represents all relevant and needed parameters, and $f(\cdot|\cdot)$ is a generic notation for any density function. The hierarchical likelihood (Equation 7.6) allows a natural hierarchical partition that integrates the combinatorial encoding experimental design. It allows the consideration of the distribution defined in the subspace of phenotypic markers first:

$$f(b_i|\Theta) = \sum_{j=1}^{J} \pi_j N(b_i|\mu_{bj}, \Sigma_{bj}), \qquad (7.7)$$

where the truncated DPGMM (Equation 7.4) is a natural choice to model Equation 7.7. The mixture model can be augmented by introducing the latent indicators z_{bi} for each b_i. That is, $z_{b_i} = j$ indicates that phenotypic marker b_i was generated from mixture component j, and with $P(z_{b_i} = j) = \pi_j$.

The distribution in Equation 7.7 allows understanding of substructure in the data reflecting differences in cell phenotypes. Then, given cells localized and differentiated at this first level, based on their phenotypic markers, $f(t_i|b_i, \Theta)$ facilitates the understanding of subtypes within that, now based on multimer binding that defines finer substructure among T-cell features. Specifically, we allow the distribution of t_i to depend on the latent classification indicator z_{bi}:

$$f(t_i|z_{bi} = j, b_i, \Theta) = \sum_{k=1}^{K} w_{jk} N(t_i|\mu_{tk}, \Sigma_{tk}), \qquad (7.8)$$

Hence the distribution of t_i is a set of J mixtures, each with K components. ω_{jk} reflects the relative abundance of cells differentiated by multimer reporters across these phenotypic marker subsets, and sums to 1 over $k = 1, \ldots, K$ for each j. The locations and shapes of these Gaussians (μ_{tk}, Σ_{tk}) reflect the localizations and local patterns of T-cell distributions in multiple regions of multimer. This second layer (Equation 7.8) models the multimer subspace by varying the mixture weights ω_{jk} but allowing the component Gaussians to be common across phenotypic marker subsets j, resulting in a sparse representation of the multimer subspace. HDP is a natural choice of prior for the parameters of the conditional density of multimer reporters given the phenotypic markers (Equation 7.8), as HDP is often used for model-based clustering of grouped data. In this example, where cells have been grouped by DPGMM (Equation 7.7) within their phenotypic marker subspaces, the conditional density (Equation 7.8) then defines a finer partitioning based on the localization of the cells based on their multimer markers.

7.5 Bayesian Models for Comparative Analysis of Count Data

Once cell subsets have been identified using automated analysis or other approaches, the natural next step is to perform statistical analysis and inference to assess the significance of variations in the cell subsets identified. In clinical studies, researchers are interested in understanding the association between cellular heterogeneity and disease progression or vaccine efficacy. For example, current vaccine development for major infectious diseases, including HIV/AIDS, has been targeted to induce protective T cells (Gilbert 2012; McMichael and Koff 2014).

The cellular adaptive immune response depends in part on the generation of antigen-specific T cells. T cells undergo selective pressure during maturation so that those that recognize their specific antigen on antigen-presenting cells become activated, undergo clonal expansion, transition into the blood, and eventually become a long-lived memory population. These antigen-specific cells are critical for antigen recall. T cells specific for a particular antigen represent a very small fraction of an individual's T-cell repertoire. Clinicians and immunologists often rely on flow cytometry to distinguish and identify rare antigen-specific T cells within heterogeneous cell samples such as blood. In many applications (e.g., finding tumor-specific T cells), the task is to identify subjects for whom the proportion of antigen-specific cytokine-producing T cells is significantly different between two experimental conditions (e.g., antigen stimulation vs. nonstimulation).

Polyfunctional T cells (De Rosa et al. 2004)—subsets of antigen-specific T cells that simultaneously produce multiple effector cytokines and other functional markers in response to activation—are believed to be of clinical relevance, and there is evidence linking their frequency to clinical outcome (Seder et al. 2008). They have been shown to be important in protective immunity and nonprogression of diseases (Ciuffreda et al. 2008; Li et al. 2008; Rodrigue-Gervais et al. 2010; Seder et al. 2008; Vordermeier et al. 2002). The intracellular cytokine staining (ICS) assay is an important tool to measure such polyfunctional T cells, and because these polyfunctional cell subsets are typically defined using Boolean combinations, the number of cell subsets to be tested is large.

To summarize, in the comparative analysis of cell subsets identified in flow cytometry, typically based on the relative frequency of cells, there are two key analytical challenges: (i) Most of the cell subsets are found at low frequencies (e.g., less than 0.1%); and (ii) the number of cell subsets that needs to be tested is large, typically increasing exponentially with the number of measured cell features.

Existing strategies for analyzing cytometry summary data include ad hoc rules based on fold-changes (Trigona et al. 2003), descriptive statistics (Roederer et al. 2011), Hotelling's T^2 statistics (Nason 2006), and simple analysis using Fisher's test of 2×2 contingency tables (Proschan and Nason 2009). These approaches do not robustly address the challenges of low frequency cell subsets and the need to adjust for multiple comparisons.

To address the first challenge of low cell subset frequencies, a Bayesian version of Fisher's 2×2 test (MIMOSA) (Finak et al. 2014b) was proposed. MIMOSA is a Bayesian hierarchical framework based on a beta-binomial mixture model. MIMOSA allows the inference to be subject specific, while borrowing strength across subject through common prior distributions. However, MIMOSA cannot jointly model all cell subsets. Hence, multiple comparisons across cell subsets have to be taken into account and can reduce statistical power.

To account for the remaining challenge of loss of power from multiple testing, a polyfunctionality index (Larsen et al. 2012) using empirical cell subsets proportions was proposed to summarize all observed cell subsets into a single number. However, empirical summaries are known to be extremely noisy when cell counts are small. Instead, a computational framework for unbiased combinatorial polyfunctionality analysis of antigen-specific T-cell subsets (COMPASS) (Lin et al. 2015a) was recently developed. COMPASS uses a Bayesian hierarchical framework to model all observed cell subsets and select those most likely to have antigen-specific responses.

To formally study the count data, let us assume that cell counts are observed from I subjects in two conditions: stimulated (s) and unstimulated (u). Let M denote the number of markers measured; then there are $K_M = 2^M$ possible Boolean combinations defining functional cell subsets, depending on whether the marker is expressed or not. In addition, let $K(K \leq K_M)$ denote the actual number of cell subsets considered for statistical analysis (i.e., after filtering empty and very sparse cell subsets). Let n_{sik} and n_{uik}, $k = 1, \ldots, K$, $i = 1, \ldots, I$, denote the observed counts for the K categories in the stimulated and unstimulated samples, respectively. In addition, let $n_{si} = (n_{si1}, \ldots, n_{siK})$, and $n_{ui} = (n_{ui1}, \ldots, n_{uiK})$. Then $N_{si} = \Sigma_k n_{sik}$ and $N_{ui} = \Sigma_k n_{uik}$ are the total numbers of cells measured for subject i in the stimulated and unstimulated samples, respectively. We arrange all K cell subsets in ascending order with respect to their degree of functionality (the number of cytokines the cell subset expresses), except for the Kth subset, which we set to be the null subset with zero degree of functionality.

For a given subject i, $i = 1, \ldots, I$, the K observed cell counts n_{si} and n_{ui} are jointly modeled by multinomial distributions:

$$(n_{si}|p_{si}) \sim MN\ (N_{si},\ p_{si}),\quad (n_{ui}|p_{ui}) \sim MN\ (N_{ui},\ p_{ui}),$$

where MN denotes the multinomial distribution, $p_{si} = (p_{si1}, ..., p_{siK})$ and $p_{ui} = (p_{ui1}, ..., p_{uiK})$ are the two unknown proportion vectors associated with the stimulated and unstimulated samples. To identify subjects for whom the proportion of antigen-specific cytokine-producing T cells is significantly different between stimulated and unstimulated conditions is equivalent to comparing the two proportion vectors ρ_{si} and ρ_{ui} for each subject i. A Bayesian latent variable model is a natural modeling strategy to perform such comparison. In particular, a binary indicator vector $\gamma_i = (\gamma_{i1}, ..., \gamma_{iK})$ can be introduced and defined as $\gamma_{ik} = 0$ if $p_{uik} = p_{sik}$, and $\gamma_{ik} = 1$ otherwise, for $k = 1, ..., K$. Figure 7.1 illustrates this Bayesian hierarchal model. More specifically, an individual p_{sik} disappears from the respective likelihood when the associated γ_{ik} is zero, and the dimensionality of the parameter space is reduced.

A natural prior for p_{ui} is the Dirichlet distribution, by its conjugacy to the multinomial distribution:

$$p_{ui} \sim Dir(\alpha_u), \tag{7.9}$$

where $\alpha_u = (\alpha_{u1}, ..., \alpha_{uK})$ is an unknown hyperparameter vector shared across all subjects under the unstimulated condition. This is given a vague exponential hyperprior: $\alpha_{uk} \sim \exp(\lambda_{uk})$, with λ_{uk} being predefined before fitting the model.

Special care is needed when defining priors for γ_i and p_{si}, $i = 1, ..., I$, as γ_i introduces dependencies between p_{si} and p_{ui}, and proportion vectors have to sum to 1. Therefore, both γ_i and p_{si} are modeled sequentially. For each γ_i, it is assumed that the first $K - 1$ elements of γ_i are independently distributed Bernoulli random variables with probability parameter ω_k. The independence assumption used is mainly for computational convenience, but it is not unrealistic given that there is no *a priori* information about the dependence among the subsets (if any). The parameter ω_k represents the proportion of responding subjects for subset k; and this parameterization allows information sharing across subjects when estimating values for γ_{ik}. Then the last element γ_{iK},

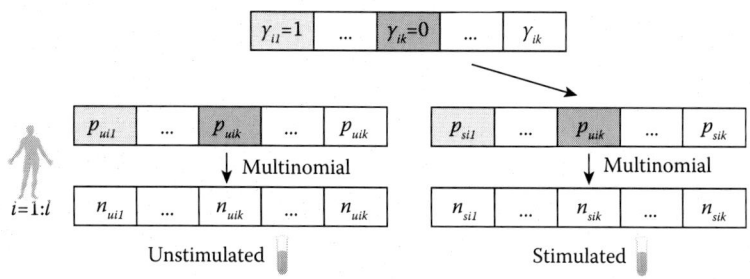

FIGURE 7.1
Graphical representation of COMPASS model.

conditioning on the information for all the first K elements, follows a mixture distribution that satisfies the constraint that the probability vector must sum to 1:

$$p(\gamma_i|\omega_{1:K}) = p(\gamma_{i,1:K-1})p(\gamma_{iK}|\gamma_{i,1:K-1})$$

$$= \prod_{k=1}^{K-1} Be(\gamma_{ik};\omega_k)\left\{\delta_1(\gamma_{ik})^{1\left[\sum_{k=1}^{K-1}\gamma_{ik}=1\right]}\right\}$$

$$\left\{\delta_0(\gamma_{ik})^{1\left[\sum_{k=1}^{K-1}\gamma_{ik}=0\right]}\right\}\left\{Be(\gamma_{iK};\omega_K)^{1\left[\sum_{k=1}^{K-1}\gamma_{ik}>1\right]}\right\},$$

(7.10)

where $\delta c(x)$ denotes a point mass distribution at c with $P(x = c) = 1$; $1[x]$ is the indicator function, equal to 1 if x is true and 0 otherwise. Let $Be(x; p)$ denote the Bernoulli distribution with probability p that x equals 1. By choosing a common conjugate prior for ω_k, the prior for γ by Equation 7.10 can be simplified by analytically integrating out ω.

Last, for each subject i, conditioning on p_{ui} and γ_i, p_{si} can be partitioned into two subvectors: $p_{si}^{\gamma_i^0}$ and $p_{si}^{\gamma_i^1}$, where the corresponding elements in γ_i are all c for $p_{si}^{\gamma_i^1}$, $c = 0, 1$. Therefore, we can write

$$p(p_{si}|\mathbf{p}_{ui},\gamma_i) = p\left(p_{si}^{\gamma_i^0}|p_{ui},\gamma_i\right)p\left(p_{si}^{\gamma_i^1}|p_{si}^{\gamma_i^0},p_{ui},\gamma_i\right),$$

(7.11)

where according to the definition of γ_i^0, $p(p_{si}^{\gamma_i^0}|p_{ui},\gamma_i)$ is a point mass at $p_{ui}^{\gamma_i^0}$. The conditional distribution $p(p_{si}^{\gamma_i^1}|p_{si}^{\gamma_i^0},p_{ui},\gamma_i)$ can be derived by applying the standard change-of-variable formula, which gives a scaled Dirichlet distribution. Because of the conjugate priors for p_u and p_s, a marginal likelihood can be obtained by analytically integrating out both p_u and p_s. This greatly facilitates MCMC computation and mixing.

In COMPASS, cell subset responses are quantified by the posterior probabilities of $\gamma_{ik} = 1$, which can be visualized using a heat map. Figure 7.2 illustrates the COMPASS analysis results on the ICS data generated through the RV144 HIV vaccine case-control study with 92TH023-Env peptide pool *ex vivo* stimulation, as described by Haynes et al. (2012) and Lin et al. (2015a). Columns in Figure 7.2 correspond to the different cell subsets modeled by COMPASS in the RV144 ICS data set, color-coded by the cytokines they express (white = off, shaded = on) and ordered by degree of functionality from one function on the left to five functions on the right. Rows correspond to subjects (226 vaccine recipients), who are ordered by their status: noninfected (top) and infected (bottom). Each cell of the heat map shows the probability that the corresponding cell subset (column) exhibits an antigen-specific response in the corresponding subject (row), where the probability is color-coded from white (zero) to black (one).

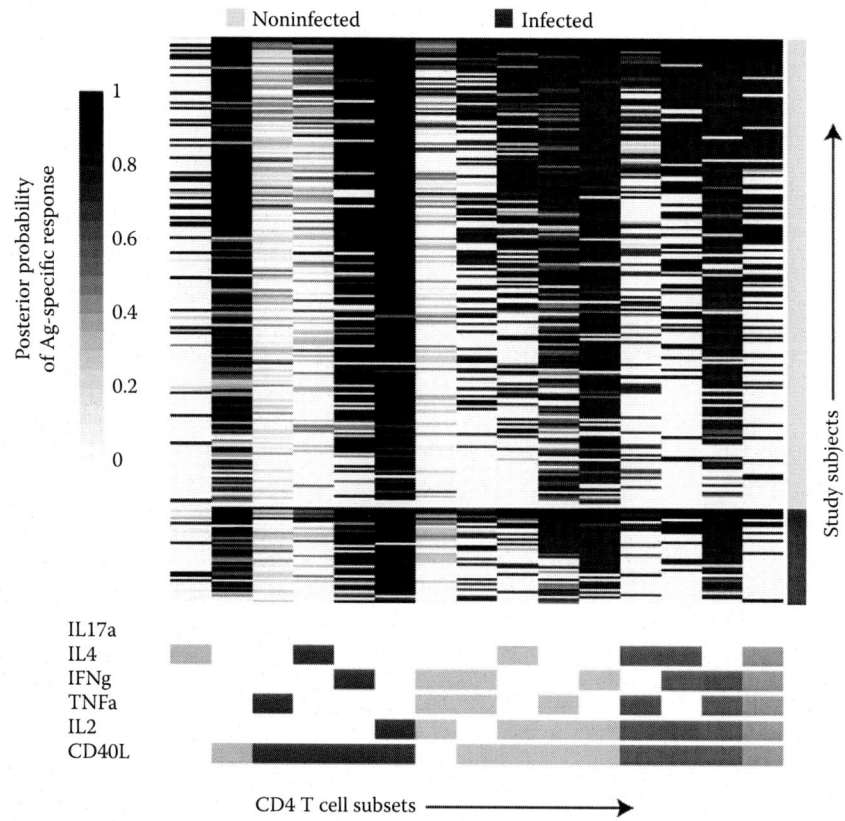

FIGURE 7.2
Heatmap of COMPASS posterior probabilities for the RV144 data set.

In addition to subject-level response probabilities, COMPASS defines two scores that summarize a subject's entire antigen-specific polyfunctional profile into a single numerical value. The functionality score is defined as the proportion of antigen-specific subsets detected among all possible ones. The polyfunctionality score is similar, but it weighs the different subsets by their degree of functionality, naturally favoring subsets with higher degrees of functionality, motivated by the observations that a higher-degree function has been correlated with better outcomes in certain vaccine studies (Attig et al. 2009; Ciuffreda et al. 2008; Rodrigue-Gervais et al. 2010). In the analysis of the RV144 vaccine efficacy trial data set, COMPASS improved characterization of antigen-specific T cells and revealed cellular "correlates of protection/immunity" missed by other methods. COMPASS is available as an R package on BioConductor.

7.6 Concluding Remarks

Flow cytometry has been with us for over 50 years and is still the most important technology to quantify multiparameter single-cell responses in HIV/AIDS research, with applications ranging from clinical monitoring of immune status to biomarker discovery for vaccine development. With rapid technological advancements pushing up the volume (e.g., robotics and multi-well plates), dimensionality (e.g., mass cytometry and new fluorescent dye families), and complexity (e.g., Phosflow and combinatorial encoding), the potential for flow cytometry to contribute to insights in HIV/AIDS is as great as ever. However, the increasing data volume, dimensionality, and complexity ensure that computational and statistical methods will have an increasing role to play in flow cytometry analysis in the future. We believe that Bayesian statistics will contribute significantly to improving methods for flow cytometry analysis and hope that the examples in this chapter convey some of the power and flexibility of Bayesian multilevel models.

References

Aghaeepour, N., Finak, G., Hoos, H., Mosmann, T. R., Brinkman, R., Gottardo, R., and Scheuermann, R. H. (2013). Critical assessment of automated flow cytometry data analysis techniques. *Nature Methods*, 10(3):228–238.

Aghaeepour, N., Nikolic, R., Hoos, H. H., and Brinkman, R. R. (2011). Rapid cell population identification in flow cytometry data. *Cytometry Part A*, 79(1):6–13.

Amir, el-A. D., Davis, K. L., Tadmor, M. D., Simonds, E. F., Levine, J. H., Bendall, S. C., Shenfeld, D. K., Krishnaswamy, S., Nolan, G. P., and Pe'er, D. (2013). viSNE enables visualization of high dimensional single-cell data and reveals phenotypic heterogeneity of leukemia. *Nature Biotechnology*, 31(6):545–552.

Attig, S., Hennenlotter, J., Pawelec, G., Klein, G., Koch, S. D., Pircher, H., Feyerabend, S., et al. (2009). Simultaneous infiltration of polyfunctional effector and suppressor T cells into renal cell carcinomas. *Cancer Research*, 69(21):8412–8419.

Azad, A., Khan, A., Rajwa, B., Pyne, S., and Pothen, A. (2013). Classifying immunophenotypes with templates from flow cytometry. In *Proceedings of the International Conference on Bioinformatics, Computational Biology and Biomedical Informatics*, pp. 256–265, New York, NY: ACM.

Azad, A., Pyne, S., and Pothen, A. (2012). Matching phosphorylation response patterns of antigen-receptor-stimulated T cells via flow cytometry. *BMC Bioinformatics*, 13(2):1–8.

Bashashati, A., and Brinkman, R. R. (2009). A survey of flow cytometry data analysis methods. *Advances in Bioinformatics*, 2009:1–19.

Blei, D. M., and Jordan, M. I. (2006). Variational inference for Dirichlet process mixtures. *Bayesian Analysis*, 1(1):121–143.

Boedigheimer, M. J., and Ferbas, J. (2008). Mixture modeling approach to flow cytometry data. *Cytometry Part A*, 73(5):421–429.

Carpenter, B., Gelman, A., Hoffman, M., Lee, D., Goodrich, B., Betancourt, M., Brubaker, M. A., Guo, J., Li, P., and Riddell, A. (2015). Stan: A probabilistic programming language. *Journal of Statistical Software*, 76(1):1–32.

Chan, C., Feng, F., Ottinger, J., Foster, D., West, M., and Kepler, T. B. (2008). Statistical mixture modeling for cell subtype identification in flow cytometry. *Cytometry Part A*, 73(8):693–701.

Chan, C., Lin, L., Frelinger, J., Hrbert, V., Gagnon, D., Landry, C., Skaly, R.-P., et al. (2010). Optimization of a highly standardized carboxyfluorescein succinimidyl ester flow cytometry panel and gating strategy design using discriminative information measure evaluation. *Cytometry Part A*, 77(12):1126–1136.

Ciuffreda, D., Comte, D., Cavassini, M., Giostra, E., Bhler, L., Perruchoud, M., Heim, M. H., et al. (2008). Polyfunctional hcv-specific T-cell responses are associated with effective control of hcv replication. *European Journal of Immunology*, 38(10):2665–2677.

Cron, A., Gouttefangeas, C., Frelinger, J., Lin, L., Singh, S. K., Britten, C. M., Welters, M. J. P., van der Burg, S. H., West, M., and Chan, C. (2013). Hierarchical modeling for rare event detection and cell subset alignment across flow cytometry samples. *PLoS Computational Biology*, 9(7):e1003130.

De Rosa, S. C., Lu, F. X., Yu, J., Perfetto, S. P., Falloon, J., Moser, S., Evans, T. G., Koup, R., Miller, J., and Roederer, M. (2004). Vaccination in humans generates broad T cell cytokine responses. *The Journal of Immunology*, 173(9):5372–5380.

Finak, G., Bashashati, A., Brinkman, R., and Gottardo, R. (2009). Merging mixture components for cell population identification in flow cytometry. *Advances in Bioinformatics*, 2009: Article ID 247646.

Finak, G., Jiang, W., Krouse, K., Wei, C., Sanz, I., Phippard, D., Asare, A., De Rosa, S. C., Self, S., and Gottardo, R. (2014a). High-throughput flow cytometry data normalization for clinical trials. *Cytometry Part A*, 85(3):277–286.

Finak, G., McDavid, A., Chattopadhyay, P., Dominguez, M., De Rosa, S., Roederer, M., and Got-tardo, R. (2014b). Mixture models for single-cell assays with applications to vaccine studies. *Biostatistics*, 15(1):87–101.

Gelman, A., Hill, J., and Yajima, M. (2012). Why we (usually) don't have to worry about multiple comparisons. *Journal of Research on Educational Effectiveness*, 5(2): 189–211.

Gilbert, S. C. (2012). T-cell-inducing vaccines: What's the future. *Immunology*, 135(1):19–26.

Hadrup, S. R., Bakker, A. H., Shu, C. J., Andersen, R. S., van Veluw, J., Hombrink, P., Castermans, E., et al. (2009). Parallel detection of antigen-specific T-cell responses by multidimensional encoding of MHC multimers. *Nature Methods*, 6(7):520–526.

Hadrup, S. R., and Schumacher, T. N. (2010). Mhc-based detection of antigen-specific CD8+ T cell responses. *Cancer Immunology, Immunotherapy*, 59(9):1425–1433.

Hahne, F., Khodabakhshi, A. H., Bashashati, A., Wong, C.-J., Gascoyne, R. D., Weng, A. P., Seyfert-Margolis, V., et al. (2010). Per-channel basis normalization methods for flow cytometry data. *Cytometry Part A*, 77(2):121–131.

Haynes, B. F., Gilbert, P. B., McElrath, M. J., Zolla-Pazner, S., Tomaras, G. D., Alam, S. M., Evans, T., et al. (2012). Immune-correlates analysis of an HIV-1 vaccine efficacy trial. *New England Journal of Medicine*, 366(14):1275–1286.

Herzenberg, L. A., Tung, J., Moore, W. A., Herzenberg, L. A., and Parks, D. R. (2006). Interpreting flow cytometry data: A guide for the perplexed. *Nature Immunology*, 7(7):681–685.

Hyrkas, J., Clayton, S., Ribalet, F., Halperin, D., Virginia Armbrust, E., and Howe, B. (2015). Scalable clustering algorithms for continuous environmental flow cytometry. *Bioinformatics*, 32(3):417–423.

Ishwaran, H., and James, L. F. (2001). Gibbs sampling methods for stick-breaking priors. *Journal of the American Statistical Association*, 96:161–173.

Jain, S., and Neal, R. M. (2004). A split-merge Markov chain Monte Carlo procedure for the Dirichlet process mixture model. *Journal of Computational and Graphical Statistics*, 13(1):158–182.

Ji, C., Merl, D., Kepler, T. B., and West, M. (2009). Spatial mixture modelling for unobserved point processes: Application to immunofluorescence histology. *Bayesian Analysis*, 4:297–316.

Kvistborg, P., Gouttefangeas, C., Aghaeepour, N., Cazaly, A., Chattopadhyay, P. K., Chan, C., Eckl, J., et al. (2015). Thinking outside the gate: Single-cell assessments in multiple dimensions. *Immunity*, 42(4):591–592.

Larsen, M., Sauce, D., Arnaud, L., Fastenackels, S., Appay, V., and Gorochov, G. (2012). Evaluating cellular polyfunctionality with a novel polyfunctionality index. *PLoS One*, 7(7):e42403.

Li, W., Murthy, A. K., Guentzel, M. N., Seshu, J., Forsthuber, T. G., Zhong, G., and Arulanandam, B. P. (2008). Antigen-specific CD4+ T cells produce sufficient IFN-gamma to mediate robust protective immunity against genital Chlamydia muridarum infection. *The Journal of Immunology*, 180(5):3375–3382.

Lin, L., Chan, C., Hadrup, S. R., Froesig, T. M., Wang, Q., and West, M. (2013). Hierarchical Bayesian mixture modelling for antigen-specific T-cell subtyping in combinatorially encoded flow cytometry studies. *Statistical Applications in Genetics and Molecular Biology*, 12(3):309–331.

Lin, L., Chan, C., and West, M. (2016). Discriminative variable subsets in Bayesian classification with mixture models, with application in flow cytometry studies. *Biostatistics*, 17(1):40–53.

Lin, L., Finak, G., Ushey, K., Seshadri, C., Hawn, T. R., Frahm, N., Scriba, T. J., et al. (2015a). COMPASS identifies T-cell subsets correlated with clinical outcomes. *Nature Biotechnology*, 33(6):610–616.

Lin, L., Frelinger, J., Jiang, W., Finak, G., Seshadri, C., Bart, P.-A., Pantaleo, G., McElrath, J., DeRosa, S., and Gottardo, R. (2015b). Identification and visualization of multidimensional antigen-specific T-cell populations in polychromatic cytometry data. *Cytometry Part A*, 87(7):675–682.

Lo, K., Brinkman, R. R., and Gottardo, R. (2008). Automated gating of flow cytometry data via robust model-based clustering. *Cytometry Part A*, 73A(4):321–332.

McMichael, A. J., and Koff, W. C. (2014). Vaccines that stimulate T cell immunity to hiv-1: The next step. *Nature Immunology*, 15(4):319–322.

Naim, I., Datta, S., Rebhahn, J., Cavenaugh, J. S., Mosmann, T. R., and Sharma, G. (2014). SWIFT-scalable clustering for automated identification of rare cell populations in large, high-dimensional flow cytometry datasets, part 1: Algorithm design. *Cytometry Part A*, 85(5):408–421.

Nason, M. (2006). Patterns of immune response to a vaccine or virus as measured by intracellular cytokine staining in flow cytometry: Hypothesis generation and comparison of groups. *Journal of Biopharmaceutical Statistics*, 16(4):483–498.

Neal, R. M. (2000). Markov chain sampling methods for Dirichlet process mixture models. *Journal of Computational and Graphical Statistics*, 9(2):249–265.

Newell, E. W., Klein, L. O., Yu, W., and Davis, M. M. (2009). Simultaneous detection of many T-cell specificities using combinatorial tetramer staining. *Nature Methods*, 6(7):497–499.

O'Neill, K., Aghaeepour, N., Spidlen, J., and Brinkman, R. (2013). Flow cytometry bioinformatics. *PLoS Computational Biology*, 9(12):e1003365.

Papaspiliopoulos, O., and Roberts, G. O. (2008). Retrospective Markov chain Monte Carlo methods for Dirichlet process hierarchical models. *Biometrika*, 95(1): 169–186.

Proschan, M. A., and Nason, M. (2009). Conditioning in 2 x 2 tables. *Biometrics*, 65(1): 316–322.

Pyne, S., Hu, X., Wang, K., Rossin, E., Lin, T.-I., Maier, L. M., Baecher-Allan, C., et al. (2009). Automated high-dimensional flow cytometric data analysis. *Proceedings of the National Academy of Sciences*, 106(21):8519–8524.

Qiu, P., Simonds, E. F., Bendall, S. C., Gibbs Jr, K. D., Bruggner, R. V., Linderman, M. D., Sachs, K., Nolan, G. P., and Plevritis, S. K. (2011). Extracting a cellular hierarchy from high-dimensional cytometry data with SPADE. *Nature Biotechnology*, 29(10): 886–891.

Rodrigue-Gervais, I. G., Rigsby, H., Jouan, L., Sauv, D., Skaly, R.-P., Willems, B., and Lamarre, D. (2010). Dendritic cell inhibition is connected to exhaustion of CD8+ T cell polyfunctionality during chronic hepatitis C virus infection. *The Journal of Immunology*, 184(6):3134–3144.

Roederer, M., Nozzi, J. L., and Nason, M. C. (2011). SPICE: Exploration and analysis of post- cytometric complex multivariate datasets. *Cytometry A*, 79(2):167–174.

Sarkar, D., Le Meur, N., and Gentleman, R. (2008). Using flowviz to visualize flow cytometry data. *Bioinformatics*, 24(6):878–879.

Seder, R. A., Darrah, P. A., and Roederer, M. (2008). T-cell quality in memory and protection: Implications for vaccine design. *Nature Reviews Immunology*, 8(4): 247–258.

Sethuraman, J. (1994). A constructive definition of Dirichlet priors. *Statistica Sinica*, 4(2): 639–650.

Sörensen, T., Baumgart, S., Durek, P., Grtzkau, A., and Hupl, T. (2015). immunoClust— An automated analysis pipeline for the identification of immunophenotypic signatures in high-dimensional cytometric datasets. *Cytometry Part A*, 87(7): 603–615.

Staats, J. S., Enzor, J. H., Sanchez, A. M., Rountree, W., Chan, C., Jaimes, M., Chan, R. C.-F., Gaur, A., Denny, T. N., and Weinhold, K. J. (2014). Toward development of a comprehensive external quality assurance program for polyfunctional intracellular cytokine staining assays. *Journal of Immunological Methods*, 409:44–53.

Suchard, M. A., Wang, Q., Chan, C., Frelinger, J., Cron, A., and West, M. (2010). Understanding GPU programming for statistical computation: Studies in massively parallel massive mixtures. *Journal of Computational and Graphical Statistics*, 19(2):419–438.

Teh, Y. W., Jordan, M. I., Beal, M. J., and Blei, D. M. (2006). Hierarchical Dirichlet processes. *Journal of the American Statistical Association*, 101(476):1566–1581.

Trigona, W. L., Clair, J. H., Persaud, N., Punt, K., Bachinsky, M., Sadasivan-Nair, U., Dubey, S., Tussey, L., Fu, T.-M., and Shiver, J. (2003). Intracellular staining for HIV-Specific ifn-γ production: Statistical analyses establish reproducibility and criteria for distinguishing positive responses. *Journal of Interferon and Cytokine Research*, 23(7):369–377.

Verschoor, C. P., Lelic, A., Bramson, J., and Bowdish, D. M. (2015). An introduction to automated flow cytometry gating tools and their implementation. *Frontiers in Immunology*, 6:380.

Vordermeier, H. M., Chambers, M. A., Cockle, P. J., Whelan, A. O., Simmons, J., and Hewinson, R. G. (2002). Correlation of ESAT-6-specific gamma interferon production with pathology in cattle following Mycobacterium bovis BCG vaccination against experimental bovine tuberculosis. *Infection and Immunity*, 70(6): 3026–3032.

Wang, Q., Cron, A. J., Chan, C., Frelinger, J., Suchard, M. A., and West, M. (2010). CPU and GPU code for Bayesian mixture modelling. Department of Statistical Science, Duke University. http://www.stat.duke.edu/research/software/west/gpu/.

Wiecki, T. (2013). Bayesian data analysis with pymc3. http://www.citeulike.org/group/4221/article/12844591.

8

The Immunoglobulin Variable-Region Gene Repertoire and Its Analysis

Thomas B. Kepler

Boston University School of Medicine, Boston, MA
Boston University, Boston, MA

Kaitlin Sawatzki

Boston University School of Medicine, Boston, MA

CONTENTS

8.1 Introduction

Immunoglobulin (Ig) is a protein that binds to molecular determinants (antigens) on pathogenic microbes, infected cells, and dysregulated self. It serves as the recognition element of the B-cell receptor (BCR) and as secreted antibody, one of the key effectors of immunity. The domain of the Ig gene responsible for these functions is called the *immunoglobulin variable region gene* (IgVRG). The IgVRG repertoire—the collection of all IgVRGs simultaneously present in an individual organism—is diverse and dynamic. This diversity is due to the assembly of IgVRG by stochastic recombination of gene-segment libraries early in B-cell ontogeny and to somatic hypermutation subsequent to antigen exposure. B cells are activated by engagement of their BCR and proliferate, forming clones that undergo affinity maturation by somatic hypermutation and differentiate into long-lived plasma or memory cells. Affinity maturation is essential to effective humoral immunity; its induction is a primary goal of much vaccine design and in particular of vaccine design against human immunodeficiency virus 1 (HIV-1) disease.

Breakthroughs in DNA sequencing have made it possible to sequence millions of IgVRGs at once, providing a view of the instantaneous state of the IgVRG repertoire. This approach, referred to as *Ig-seq*, was accomplished first in the zebra fish [1] and soon afterward in humans [2]. By longitudinal sampling, investigators were able to comprehend the dynamical characteristics of the repertoire. These methods have rapidly become pervasive (reviewed in [3–6]) and have provided novel insights into immune senescence [7], autoimmunity [8], leukemia [9], the postvaccination humoral response [10,11], and the coevolution of antibodies and viruses in chronic HIV-1 infection [12,13].

Repertoire sequencing has shown great promise, the full realization of which depends on the development and use of specialized statistical methods. The data-analytic tasks are to infer [1] the component gene segments and other parameters of each original recombination, [2] the clonal structure of the population, [3] the common ancestor of each clonal lineage, and [4] the natural history of each clonal lineage. These tasks are not independent of each other and require an integrated approach for their joint accomplishment.

In this chapter, we review the essential components of B-cell biology and the role of antibodies in contemporary HIV-1 vaccinology and describe an approach to the statistical analysis of antibody repertoire sequence data. In contrast to the biological material, the analytical material is not intended as a broad review of methods. It is instead a self-contained introduction to the methods we have ourselves developed.

8.2 Brief Review of B-Cell Biology

8.2.1 Antibodies

Each antibody or BCR molecule is a homodimer of heterodimers. Each heterodimer is made up of one heavy chain and one light chain. IgG, the most common secreted antibody, is ~150 kDa, where each heavy chain is ~50 kDa and each light chain is ~25 kDa. The structure of the molecule resembles a droopy-armed Y. The stem corresponds to the Fc ("fraction crystallizing") domain, which binds to receptors on phagocytes and to other effector molecules of innate immunity. The arms correspond to the two identical antigen-binding domains, Fab ("fraction antigen binding"), which bind to the antigenic determinants.

The structure of the variable region comprises four relatively conserved framework regions (FR1–4) and three intervening hypervariable loops, known as *complementarity determining regions* (CDR1–3), which fold together to make up the antigen-binding domain. Invariant cysteine residues are found within FR1 and at the 3' end of FR3 and form a disulfide bond that stabilizes the β-sheet structure of the FRs [14]. CDR3, which begins at the second invariant cysteine, terminates at an invariant tryptophan in the heavy chain or an invariant phenylalanine in the light chain. These residues are important markers for sequence analysis. The length of the heavy-chain variable region is typically between 115 and 130 amino acids.

The variable region is encoded by the IgVRG, which is not encoded in the genome but assembled from genomic segments in a manner unique to vertebrate immunity. There are several distinct Fc domains representing different *isotypes*—IgM, IgD, IgG, IgA, and IgE—that can be recombined with any given variable region. Each isotype has its own specialized set of effector functions; isotype switching allows antigen specificity (contributed by the variable region) to pair with any function. All naïve mature B cells first express IgM and IgD isotypes. After antigen stimulation, most B cells switch to a more mature isotype.

The antigenic determinants that should be recognized by the immune system may come from an enormous number of organisms across all kingdoms of life and are not known to the immune system in advance. The strategy of adaptive immunity is to generate an enormous diversity of binding proteins to provide substantial probability that some antibody will bind whatever antigen appears. As a consequence, antibody Fabs (and the related T-cell receptors) display more diversity within an individual than all of the rest of the proteome. The entirety of this collection is referred to as the *immunoglobulin variable region repertoire*.

8.2.2 B-Cell Development

The strategy adopted by adaptive immunity makes it imperative that the population of IgVRGs be large enough and diverse enough to cover the enormous chemical space of potential foreign antigens. In young adult humans, it has been estimated that there are approximately 10^{11} total B cells, implying that one out of every 50 cells is a B cell [15], and known mechanisms of antibody diversity have been estimated to be capable of producing >10^{14} unique Igs.

B cells, like T cells and all other white blood cells, originate from multipotent hematopoietic stem cells in the bone marrow [16]. In the initial stages of development, before emigration from the bone marrow, the pro-B cell produces an IgVRG through recombination. There are no mechanisms enforcing a condition of frame-consistency through the junctions: two of every three recombinations will be out of frame and therefore nonproductive. In this case, recombination is initiated on the corresponding locus on the other chromosome. If the recombination is productive and makes an intact protein, recombination on the other allele is blocked. This phenomenon is known as *allelic exclusion* and ensures that most B cells express a single antibody specificity. If neither allele is rearranged productively, the cell undergoes apoptosis [17–19].

After productive heavy-chain recombination, the pro-B cell becomes a pre-B cell, where the rearranged heavy chain is temporarily paired with a surrogate light chain and expressed at the cell surface as the pre-BCR. Signals transduced through this pre-BCR activate light-chain recombination, starting with the kappa light chain genes (IGκ) and proceeding to lambda light chain genes (IGλ) if no productive kappa recombinations occur [19]. If no signal is transduced, the pre-B cell dies apoptotically. After productive heavy and light chain recombinations have occurred, the mature BCR is expressed on the surface of the cell, which progresses to the immature B-cell stage.

The effector functions of humoral immunity are very potent and must be prevented from acting on the host's own tissues. Presumably for that reason, immature B cells are exquisitely sensitive to antigen binding and die by apoptosis, become anergic (nonresponsive), or are rescued by receptor editing if bound avidly at this stage [20–22]. After emigration from the bone marrow, most B cells die within a few days. Those that survive complete their maturation into naïve B cells and circulate throughout the lymphatic system, through lymphoid follicles within the spleen and lymph nodes (referred to as the *secondary lymphoid tissues*—bone marrow is primary). Naïve peripheral B cells have a half-life of 3–8 weeks in the absence of antigenic stimulation [23,24].

8.2.3 Development of the IgVRG Ig Repertoire

Adult humans have approximately 10^{11} total B cells, representing one in every 300 human cells [15]. Several estimates of the total number of distinct

IgVRG that can be produced by gene segment (VDJ) recombination have been offered; values of 10^{12}–10^{14} sequences are typical. These numbers are not, by themselves, entirely meaningful, because they are demonstrably too small if meant to include all possible genes. However, they are not altogether misleading because the vast majority of the possible genes have an extremely small probability of being produced in any individual's lifetime. Current estimates of total B-cell diversity by capture–recapture methods estimate the individual diversity of unique binding sites to be 3.5×10^{10} in naïve IgM$^+$ B cells, the most common subset [2].

Each heavy chain gene is constructed from the recombination of one each of variable (IGHV), diversity (IGHD), and joining (IGHJ) genes. In humans and mice, these germline genes are arrayed along a single locus. In humans there are 46–54 IGHV genes (there is copy number polymorphism among individuals), followed by 23 IGHD genes, and then by 6 IGHJ genes. The light chain genes come in two types on two distinct genomic loci, kappa and lambda, and are recombined using two components rather than three (variable and joining). The stochastic selection of these germline genes constitutes antibody *combinatorial diversity*.

In addition to combinatorial diversity, IgVRG exhibits *junctional diversity*. The enzymatic complex consisting of the recombination activating genes RAG1 and RAG2 binds to a recombination signal (RS) adjacent to each of the V, D, and J genes, bringing the genes into close proximity. Proper ordering of the genes is enforced by the so-called 12/23 rule. There are two different types of RS, one with a 12-nucleotide spacer and one with a 23-base spacer. Synapsis occurs only between heterogeneous pairs. The recombinase nicks the DNA at the start of each RS, resulting in a DNA hairpin on each gene, which is then cleaved stochastically by the Artemis complex, resulting in variable recombination points. Because of the hairpin structure, this cleavage may occur beyond the end of the coding region into the noncoding strand, resulting in the appearance of p-nucleotides (*p* for *palindromic*). Terminal deoxynucleotidyl transferase may then add several n-nucleotides (*n* for *nontemplated*), which are yet another source of stochasticity. The strands then pair in complementary regions, and unpaired nucleotides are removed and filled in to form the final junction region [19,25,26]. The site of RAG-mediated cleavage and n-nucleotides together supply the junctional diversity of the antibody repertoire.

8.2.4 Affinity Maturation

There is yet another source of IgVRG diversification. This mechanism, somatic hypermutation, is activated after engagement with antigen activation of the B cell. B-cell activation with nonmultivalent antigens requires co-stimulation by so-called cognate T cells as well as ligation of the BCR. The T-cell antigen cognate to a B-cell antigen is a peptide derived by proteolytic processing from the latter [27]. The structure of the lymph nodes and spleen, where the majority of lymphocytes reside, facilitates these otherwise rare interactions at the interface between T-cell–rich and B-cell–rich zones.

Once a B cell has been activated, it divides several times; its progenies differentiate into several different cell types, including plasmacytes, which continually secrete antibody for the few days that they are alive [28]. The key to this system is that this antibody is encoded by the same IgVRG that encodes the BCR and thus retains the same antigen specificity. Other progenies differentiate into germinal center cells and undergo *affinity maturation*, eventually becoming the memory cells and long-lived plasmacytes that provide protection against subsequent encounters with the pathogen from which the antigen was derived. Affinity maturation is an extraordinary encapsulation of Darwinian evolution in microcosm. Somatic hypermutation generates variety in the IgVRG; a proliferative advantage is gained by the B cell that happens to acquire a BCR that binds the eliciting antigen more avidly. All B-cell progenies that are produced from a shared, unmutated common B-cell progenitor are in a biological clonal lineage, called a *clone*.

Immunizations work by introducing controlled doses of foreign antigen to the body to induce these protective responses and establish long-term, antigen-specific memory. Germinal centers (GC) can be observed as early as 4 days after primary immunization and typically reach maximum size within a few days. These transient anatomical structures consist of the *dark zone*, containing rapidly dividing B cells, centroblasts, and the *light zone*, containing specialized antigen-presenting cells known as *follicular dendritic cells* (FDC), T cells, and nondividing B cells called *centrocytes*.

Centroblasts undergo somatic hypermutation (SHM) of their IgVRG, accumulating point mutations at a rate of 10^{-4}–10^{-3} mutations per nucleotide per cell division (orders of magnitude higher than is observed in typical genome replication) [29–31]. The enzyme activation-induced cytidine deaminase (AID) is responsible for the initial lesions in the DNA, which are followed by error-prone repair by the enzyme polymerase eta (polη). Centroblasts eventually differentiate into centrocytes and migrate to the light zone, where they interact with FDC and T cells and receive signals to survive, divide, or differentiate. Some surviving cells leave the GC as memory B cells, while others return to the dark zone and undergo further rounds of proliferation and mutation. At this stage, B cells may also undergo *class switch recombination*, which swaps out the constant region genes (IGHC) encoding the Fc portion of the antibody, changing the effector function of the antibody [29,30].

The mutation rate under SHM at any particular nucleotide depends on the state of the nucleotide itself and on the local nucleotide neighborhood. These biases are induced by the binding preferences of both polη and AID, and they have an interesting biological consequence. IgVRG have codon preferences that increase the mutation frequency in the CDR relative to the FR, perhaps to enhance plasticity under affinity maturation [32,33]. Furthermore, these biases are important to bear in mind when analyzing repertoire data.

Finally, very recently an entirely novel form of IgVRG diversification was apparently discovered [34]. These investigators observed the interchromosomal transposition of a stretch of DNA into the IgVRG genes of two malaria-infected individuals, whereby a 100 amino acid collagen-binding protein domain was introduced in the IgVRG. Instead of critically disabling this Ig, it gained mutations such that the gene segment's collagen-binding function was lost while gaining affinity for malaria-infected red blood cells [34]. It is unlikely that this mechanism is widespread, but the prospect of such surprises is intriguing and suggests that more excitement awaits the analysis of IgVRG repertoires.

8.2.5 B-Cell Response Kinetics

The earliest peripheral B-cell response to novel antigen exposure is typically observed in 4–5 days, when short-lived plasmacytes can differentiate and exit the lymph node. Plasmacytes are terminally differentiated antibody secreting cells, and early responders tend to secrete IgM with relatively low antigen affinity. The primary effector of protective humoral immunity is through antibody secreted by affinity matured plasmacytes. These antibodies are generally high affinity IgG and are observed in the periphery 7 or more days after primary exposure, or after 3–4 days upon subsequent exposure(s) [28]. Whereas plasmacytes cannot reenter the GC or survive for long-term memory, they are quickly differentiated from proliferating memory B-cell populations. Some memory B cells are capable of reentering the GC to undergo additional proliferation, affinity maturation, and differentiation, further enhancing affinity maturation potential [35,36].

Circulating mature B-cell subsets can be grouped into naïve, long-lived, and short-lived plasma cell and memory B cells. In peripheral blood mononuclear cells, 5%–20% is comprised of B cells. Although new B cells are produced throughout one's life, there are characteristic changes in the repertoire. The majority of peripheral B cells consistently express a naïve phenotype, but 0%–20% express a memory phenotype, increasing with age. Plasmablasts make up 0%–5% and remain steady with increasing age [37]. Long-lived plasma cells primarily reside in splenic and bone marrow survival niches that provide appropriate survival signals and only rarely circulate. Long-lived memory B cells also persist in these survival niches but are commonly found in circulation [38,39]. It is clear that even in a sequestered state, these cells are capable of constant antibody secretion [40,41]. Most impressively, long-lived antibody memory is capable of lasting a lifetime, up to 89 years in one subject over 100 years old [40].

8.3 IgVRG Repertoire Sequencing

The analysis of the IgVRG repertoire was made possible in large part by advances in DNA sequencing technologies that have collectively come to be called *next-generation sequencing* (NGS) and which greatly improve the throughput of Sanger (last-generation) sequencing.

NGS involves the binding of sample DNA molecules to a solid surface followed by cluster amplification to increase the independent molecule readout signal (fluorescence, light, pH). Massive parallel sequencing is conducted by covering the surface in a specific nucleotide and making a call for that base if there is a resulting chemical or physical signal indicating an incorporation event. The nucleotide solution is washed off and the process is repeated, resulting in a large number of sequencing reads for analysis. This process is termed *sequencing by synthesis*. The most dominant platforms for NGS and Ig-seq are currently the Illumina-based HiSeq and MiSeq sequencers. Similar platforms include the Roche 454 GS series and Ion Torrent PGM. Other NGS approaches include nanopore-based (MinION, Oxford Nanopore Technologies), sequencing by ligation (SOLiD, Life Technologies) and single molecule real-time sequencing (PacBio RS, Pacific Biosciences).

Before sequencing commences, the library of IgVRG to be sequenced must be prepared. There are several variations of library preparation. Libraries may be produced from genomic DNA or from mRNA, bearing in mind the fact that different subsets of B cells have widely varying numbers of Ig mRNA, but each cell has exactly one functional genomic Ig. Fluorescence activated cell sorting (FACS) may be used to isolate specific subsets, or unsorted peripheral blood mononuclear cells may be used (only B cells will have recombined IgVRG). Libraries may be performed on bulk samples or on individual B cells isolated by FACS, emulsion-based methods, or microfluidics. Unique nucleotide identifiers, or bar codes, may be incorporated to identify IgVRG from individual cells or to identify individual molecules. These molecular identifiers are essential for mitigating the "jackpot" effect inherent in polymerase chain reaction (PCR) amplification. [42–44].

Because of the large number of different V genes, one can multiplex pools of 5′ primers that together cover the V genes, or one may use 5′ RACE (rapid amplification of cDNA ends), which adds a known template switch primer to the 5′ end of mRNA during cDNA synthesis by template-switching reverse transcriptase. In either case, one would use a more modest multiplexed pool of 3′ primers to the constant-region genes.

While NGS has offered remarkable new capabilities, compromises on error rates and read length have been necessary, and there remains room for improvement. For example, the Illumina 300 bp paired-end chemistry has not yet proven to be as high quality over the full read length as the 50 and 100 bp chemistries, and it characteristically drops precipitously in quality score early in Read 2 [45–47]. This is problematic for Ig-seq because (1) the total sequence length can be up to 500 bp with the primer additions and untranslated regions, (2) the consistently low quality regions are at the end of each read, where they are computationally aligned and joined in reverse complement, and (3) the area of read overlap used for joining is also in the most variable, mutated region. That is, it is essentially impossible to join and make a confident base call where there is a conflict between two low quality reads, and library information cannot be reliably used to fill in the gaps. Similarly, the sequencing by synthesis platforms share a flaw in accurate base calling in homopolymer and long repeat regions, both of which are possible in IgVRG. The observed error rate for the Illumina MiSeq is 0.8%, or an expected ~2.8 nt errors in a 350 nt IgVRG sequence. Single molecule sequencers do not have increased error rates at specific patterns but do have much higher rates of random error, making Ig-seq a challenge [48,49].

8.4 Broadly Neutralizing Antibodies against HIV

HIV, the retrovirus that causes acquired immunodeficiency disease syndrome (AIDS), infects an estimated 36.7 million people globally and has caused over 35 million deaths since it was identified in 1983. Retroviruses replicate using RNA-dependent RNA polymerases that lack proofreading functions, resulting in very high viral mutation rates (3.4×10^{-5} mutations per bp per replication cycle) and very rapid in-host diversification. This tremendous diversity poses a significant challenge to the humoral immune response [50,51]. The immune system has no trouble identifying and expanding B cells that bear BCR capable of binding the envelope (Env) glycoproteins on the surface of virions, and thereby it neutralizes them by blocking their entry into uninfected target cells. However, once the humoral response begins to exert pressure on the viral population, viral variants arise that bear glycoproteins unrecognized by these B cells. The viral population remains consistently one step ahead.

There are, however, antibodies that exhibit neutralization capacity against a wide variety of viral strains. These are known as *broadly neutralizing antibodies*, or BNAbs. BNAbs are especially promising as potential effectors against pathogens with high mutation rates, which allow pathogen escape from other treatments and therapeutics [52]. The most commonly studied BNAbs are those against influenza virus and HIV-1. For both viruses, it is desirable to develop a single immunization strategy that elicits BNAbs that protect against any strain of the pathogen, as in a pan-influenza or cross-subtype HIV immunization.

In the case of HIV, BNAbs develop in 10%–30% of infected persons, with the earliest appearances generally 2 years after initial infection. BNAbs target highly conserved domains that are shielded by hypervariable components of Env. BNAbs are not typically protective against persistent infection by the time they have arisen naturally [53–57]. Some HIV-1 BNAbs, however, have been proven to provide effective prophylaxis against SHIV infection in rhesus macaques, and it is widely believed that BNAbs established prior to viral transmission would be protective [58,59].

8.4.1 Functional and Genetic Characteristics of BNAbs

The most common feature of the known BNAbs is their extraordinarily high mutation frequency. The mean IgVRG percent mutation for these BNAbs is 16%; several have mutation frequencies exceeding 30% and the smallest is 10% [57]. For comparison, in heavy chains responding to anthrax immunization over 18 months, 10% mutation frequency is at the 90th percentile of such heavy chains; 16% is at the 98th percentile (unpublished data). The development of highly mutated IgVRGs from unmutated germline antibodies is positively correlated to increasing neutralization breadth, and large sites of insertions and deletions are much more common than elsewhere. One phenotypic feature common among BNAbs is their autoreactivity, first observed in 2005 by Haynes et al. [60].

For BNAb research, one successful NGS-based approach has been in analyzing known BNAb sequences with Ig-seq data from the same donor; sequences that are inferred to be clonally related to the BNAb can then be synthesized, tested, and functional mutations identified [61]. Figure 8.1 illustrates this method, showing a set of sequences isolated by single-memory B-cell cultures together with the additional sequences obtained by NGS on the same donor. Impressively, cross-donor analysis with known BNAbs has also resulted in the identification of novel BNAbs [12,62–64]. In this approach, Ig-seq repertoires are investigated by (1) broad phylogenetic analysis or (2) restricting the dataset to sequences with broad shared characteristics such as V and J usage or CDR3 motifs followed by clonal inference with relaxed restrictions. The high hit rate of this method suggests that there are many unknown BNAbs yet to be discovered, and this relatively simple approach is an appropriate tool for significant data expansion.

One of the most promising recent strategies in HIV-1 vaccine research has been to devise a sequence of immunogens that first elicit antibodies capable of maturing into BNAbs and then drive that maturation [65]. Recent work in mice shows that it is possible to direct BNAb-associated mutations *in vivo* by designing and boosting with immunogens appropriate to the BCRs elicited after priming [66]. It still remains a challenge to specifically prime and boost B cells expressing BCR with the IgVRG segments associated with the target BNAb from the total repertoire.

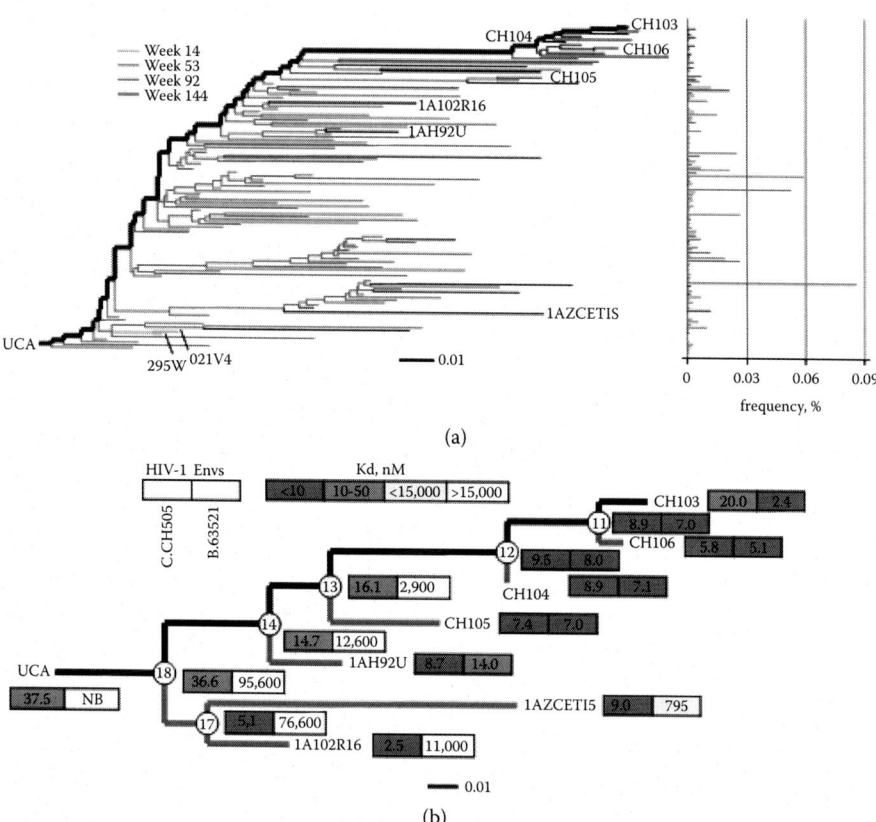

FIGURE 8.1
(a) The estimated phylogram for the broadly neutralizing antibody (BNAb) clone CH103. The immunoglobulin variable region genes (IgVRGs) labeled CH103-6 were isolated from sorted single memory B cells; the others were isolated through high-throughput IgVRG repertoire sequencing. The sizes of groups of identical sequences are shown in the panel on the right. (b) Binding affinities, measured by surface plasmon resonance biosensor assay, of the indicated antibodies against an HIV isolate from the same individual as the antibodies (autologous virus) and against a divergent HIV isolate from a different individual (heterologous virus). (Adapted from Liao et al., *Nature*, 496, 469–476, 2013. With permission.)

8.5 Analysis of IgVRG Repertoires

Generally, there are two approaches that can be used for the analysis of VRG sequences: discriminative modeling and generative modeling. In generative modeling, the goal is to produce a model that is in principle capable of generating data indistinguishable from that to be analyzed. One utilizes all of the information available regarding the processes giving rise to the data and incorporates it into the model. A generative model represents an attempt to accurately represent the biology underlying the data and provides the framework within which inferences may be conducted. A discriminative model, by contrast, seeks to identify those features of the data that will prove informative in a given analytical task, without reference to the underlying mechanism of their generation. If the generative model is sufficiently accurate, it will provide the more effective inferential tool. However, model misspecification can cause bias and lead to erroneous inferences. A discriminative model is less susceptible to misspecification but requires substantial labeled data to serve as training sets for learning. Such datasets, however, are not available for the analyses of interest in the present context. In what follows, therefore, we focus exclusively on generative models and their applications.

We describe methods to carry out three analyses: (1) the inference of the unmutated (preaffinity maturation) form of the VRG, (2) the determination of clonal kinship between two VRGs, and (3) the partitioning of a set of VRGs into clones.

8.5.1 Stochastic Generative Models for VDJ Recombination and Affinity Maturation

Our model for VRG repertoire analysis comprises two submodels: one for the generation of VDJ recombinations and the other for affinity maturation. As described above, the complete recombination of an Ig heavy-chain VRG is specified completely by the three categorical variables V, D, and J (which should be thought of as pointers to DNA sequences that are known in advance), the four integer variables RV, RD1, RD2, and RJ (the recombination points), and two short DNA sequences NVD and NDJ (the nontemplated nucleotides). Negative recombination points correspond to the use of p-nucleotides. For example, RV = −1 indicates the presence of a single p-nucleotide at the 3′ end of the V gene. Figure 8.2 illustrates the definitions of recombination points and their relationship to n-nucleotide regions, as well as the possible uncertainty inherent in estimating them. Sequence c7067 in this figure was isolated using Atreca's proprietary Immune Repertoire Capture™ technology in our laboratory's study of the response to the anthrax vaccine (unpublished data). The expected error (Figure 8.2) is also shown. Note that the uncertainty is greatest around the recombination junctions and n-nucleotides.

The starting point for our approach is a model for the generation of unmutated VDJ recombinations. Each such recombination is determined by the vector θ of recombination parameters. Many different model families may be considered, differing in the assumptions made about independence among the recombination parameters. The default recombination model in

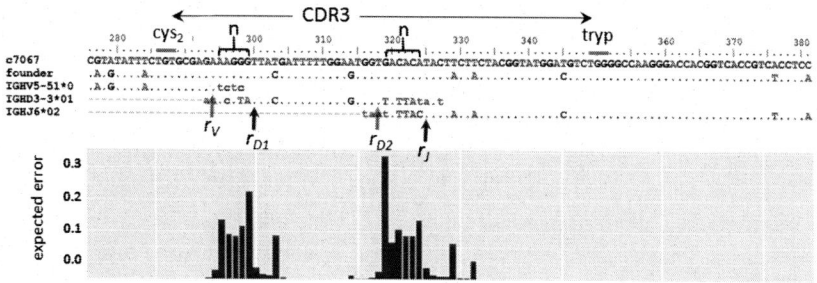

FIGURE 8.2
Alignment of human heavy-chain variable region gene c7067 against the maximum-likelihood gene segments. The codon for the second invariant cysteine cys₂ is indicated, as is the codon for the invariant tryptophan tryp. Dots indicate identity with c7067. The recombination points are indicated; n-nucleotides are indicated by curly braces and the letter *n*. The bar plot below indicates the expected error from the marginal posterior probability mass function (pmf) for the founder at each nucleotide position.

our system assumes that each recombination point depends on the relevant germline gene but that all other parameters are mutually independent, giving

$$p_\Theta(v,d,j,r_V,r_{D1},r_{D2},r_J,n_{VD},n_{DJ}) = p_V(v)p_D(d)p_J(j)p_N(n_{VD})p_N(n_{DJ})$$
$$\times p_{R|V}(r_V|v)p_{R|D}(r_{D1},r_{D2}|d)p_{R|J}(r_J|j) \qquad (8.1)$$

The first factor on the right, for example, is the probability that a recombination chosen at random uses *v* for its germline IGHV gene. The middle three factors are the probabilities on recombination points conditional on germline gene. All of the probabilities are estimated empirically using Bayesian estimation procedures. The last factors are the probabilities on n-region sequences, for which we assume that the individual n-nucleotides are independent of each other.

The other submodel is that for affinity maturation. In spite of some obvious oversimplifications, described below, we use conventional nucleotide substitution models borrowed from statistical phylogenetics [67]. The initial state of the nucleotide at the position of interest is denoted *f* for *founder* and takes any of the four nucleotide values $f \in \{A,G,T,C\}$. The nucleotide state after evolving over time *t* is a random variable *S* with probability mass function (pmf) $p_S(s|\alpha,t) = \text{Prob}(S=s|f,t)$. The default model in our analyses is the venerable Kimura80 model [68].

We generalize from the evolution of individual nucleotides to that of whole sequences by assuming that nucleotides at different sequence positions evolve independently; the pmf over sequences is then the product of the pmfs of the individual nucleotide positions. This assumption is, strictly speaking, invalid. First, it ignores selection and, specifically relevant for somatic hypermutation, it ignores the sequence specificity of the mutation rate. It is known, for example, that the mutation rates of the G and C nucleotides in the motif AGCT are substantially greater than when found in other contexts. We can, and do, make a zeroth-order correction by using different starting values for the mutation rate at each position. However, if the G in the motif above changes, say to A, making the motif AACT, the mutation rate at C decreases as a result. This is a first-order effect that breaks the position independence. This a problem on which investigators are currently working. However, the methods appear to work very well and to provide consistent results in spite of this and other shortcomings. In the following, we will use Greek letters for sequences and roman letters for nucleotides.

The first step in all of this computing is to align the sequencing read (or *contig*) to the gene segments. This step provides the starting point for assigning likelihoods to each gene segment. The pairwise alignment of reads to gene segments is performed using a scoring function that corresponds to the log of the likelihood, so that maximizing the alignment score by dynamic programming also gives the maximum likelihood. The match/mismatch score for the alignment of S_j (the *j*th nucleotide in the observed read) against f_i (the nucleotide state at the founder's *i*th position) is $\mu_{ij} = \log(p_S(s_j | f_i, t))$. Insertion and deletion scores are given by affine gap penalties with distinct *open* and *continue* scores corresponding to the zero-inflated negative binomial distributions.

However, we also need to specify scores for n-nucleotides—the unmatched nucleotides in the gaps between the aligned gene segments. The score for placing an n-nucleotide against observed nucleotide S_j is $v_j = \log(\sum_{n \in \{A,G,T,C\}} p_S(s_j | n, t) \pi_N(n))$, where π_N is the prior pmf for n-nucleotides. Each pairwise alignment provides a likelihood score for the gene segment/recombination point pair. Once we have these pairwise alignments, we incorporate the prior pmf on rearrangement parameters and perform the Bayesian average.

Although not contributing to the diversity of any individual IgVRG repertoire, allelic diversity (among individuals) poses a few special challenges for the analysis of the repertoire. It is rare that the expressed alleles in any subject are known prior to analysis. Therefore, it is not evident what database of germline gene segments should be used. First, the total allelic diversity in a population or species is difficult to capture in genetic databases. This is particularly true in animals with less individual sequencing data. For instance, while several thousands of sequenced human Igs have contributed to 273 alleles among 53 IGHV genes, just 10 sequenced macaque genomes have resulted in 215 alleles IGHV alleles, indicating the population is likely to have many more as yet unidentified variants. Second, standard alignment methods against a library of known genes are not sufficient to differentiate between alleles that may have as few as 1 base pair (bp) difference [69]. New methods are currently in development to mitigate these challenges by performing intra-individual gene and allele library building, which is expected to improve correct gene inference.

8.5.2 Inference of the Founder

With this machinery we infer the ancestor for a mature IgVRG. The posterior pmf on recombination parameters is

$$p_{\Theta|\Sigma}(\theta|\sigma, t) \propto p_{\Sigma}(\sigma|g(\theta), t)p_{\Theta}(\theta) \tag{8.2}$$

where I function and $g(\theta)$ is the gene sequence obtained under VDJ recombination with parameters θ.

The evolution time t appears in the evolution model and must be estimated. Somatic mutation operates discontinuously on any clonal lineage, with some branches experiencing a greater effective mutation time than others. For this reason, we cannot use any estimated "real" time. The time must be estimated from the mutation frequency itself, as is done in conventional methods in molecular evolution. Our method differs from the existing methods in that the root sequence—the founder—is itself estimated and the estimated time depends on the estimated founder. We proceed iteratively starting with some initial estimate $\hat{t}_0$. Obtain the initial estimated founder $\hat{\varphi}_0$ by computing $\hat{\theta}_0 = \text{argmax}_\theta\, p_{\Theta|\Sigma}(\theta|\sigma, \hat{t}_0)$. Now fix $\hat{\varphi}_0 = g(\hat{\theta}_0)$ and compute $\hat{t}_1 = \text{argmax}_t\, p_{S|\Phi}(\sigma|\hat{\varphi}_0, t)$. Substitute $t = \hat{t}_1$ into Equation 8.2 and obtain the posterior pmf on φ,

$$p_{\Phi|S}(\varphi|\sigma, t) = \sum_\theta I\Big(\varphi = g(\theta)\Big)p_{\Phi|\Sigma}(\theta|\sigma, t) \tag{8.3}$$

where I is the indicator function.

The advantage of having the posterior pmf is that we are able to assess the uncertainty of the inferred ancestor. Figure 8.3 illustrates the inference of the

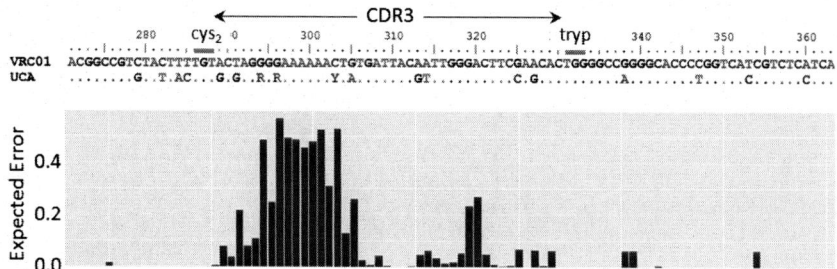

FIGURE 8.3
The BNAb VRC01 and its unmutated common ancestor (UCA) from VRC01 alone. The codons for the invariant amino acids are indicated. The bar plot below shows the expected error from the marginal posterior pmf for the founder at each nucleotide position.

founder of the VRC01 BNAb and the expected error obtained from the marginal posterior pmf at each nucleotide position.

8.5.3 Inference of the Founder from a Clonal Alignment

The methods outlined above are generalizable to alignments of IgVRG by using a tree T in place of the time t. To make this generalization more transparent, note that the case of a single IgVRG corresponds to a simple tree with the founder at the root and the observed sequence at the only leaf. The topology is invariable so this tree is completely determined by the branch time, t. Let σ be an alignment of IgVRGs, assumed to derive from a single (unknown) founder φ and thus to be members of the same clone. We use bold-face Greek letters to indicate collections of sequences. The evolution model now takes the form $p_{\Sigma|\Phi}(\sigma|\varphi, T)$; the procedures are remarkably similar to those for individual IgVRGs. In particular, the tree T is estimated iteratively in the same manner as the time t in the foregoing description. The marginal probability for each clone

$$p_\Sigma(\sigma|T) = \sum_\theta p_{\Sigma|\Phi}(\sigma|g(\theta), T)p_\Theta(\theta). \tag{8.4}$$

plays a key role in the assessment of clonal kinship and in the partitioning of IgVRG collections into clones, discussed below. Figure 8.4 shows how much more information about the founder can be gained by using a whole clone to infer the founder. Heavy chain sequence c4469 has a mutation frequency of 20% per nucleotide and is a member of a clone with 123 members.

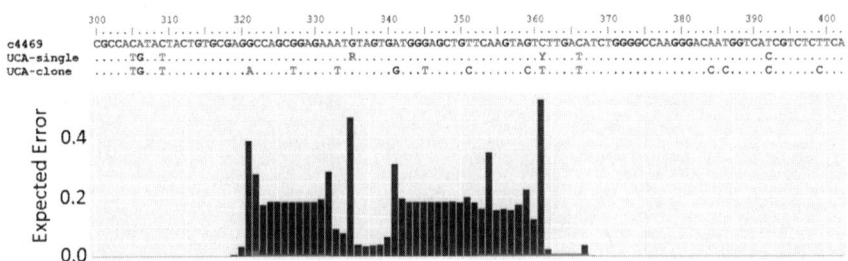

FIGURE 8.4

An alignment of heavy chain c4469 against two versions of its unmutated common ancestor (UCA). UCA-single is the UCA inferred using c4469 alone; UCA-clone is the UCA inferred using all of the members of the clone containing c4469. The bar plot below shows the corresponding expected errors: dark gray indicates the error associated with UCA-single; light gray indicates that associated with UCA-clone.

8.5.4 Determination of Clonal Kinship

To determine whether two IgVRGs are clonally related, we compare two hypothesized tree topologies (Figure 8.3). That is, we compute the two marginal probabilities

$$p_1 = \sum_{\varphi} p(\sigma_1, \sigma_2, \varphi | \hat{T}) \tag{8.5}$$

and

$$p_2 = \sum_{\varphi_1} p(\sigma_1, \varphi_1 | \hat{t}_1) \sum_{\varphi_2} p(\sigma_2, \varphi_2 | \hat{t}_2) \tag{8.6}$$

and base our inference of clonal kinship on the Bayes' factor p_1/p_2. The first model corresponds to a single clonal history underlying both sets of sequences, the second to independent histories and independent ancestors. Note that that we may evaluate the clonal relatedness of two sets of sequences by generalizing from sequences to sequence alignments as we have done above.

8.5.5 Clonal Partitioning

An important component of the large-scale analysis of VRG repertoire data is the partitioning of the sequences into sets that are intended to represent clonal kinship. Suppose we have a set S of IgVRG; these may be heavy chains, light chains, or paired heavy–light genes. A partition is a nonoverlapping and complete set of clones $P = \{\sigma_1, \sigma_2, ..., \sigma_k\}$, where k, the number of clones, is not known in advance. Every IgVRG in S belongs to exactly one clone. Clones may have only one member. We have developed several methods for producing clonal partitions, differing among themselves in their error rates, need for manual intervention, and required computational effort. The first method, *Clonogenetic Partitioning*, is premised on the goal of maximizing the likelihood over all clones. The log likelihood for a partition is the sum over marginal log likelihoods

$$\log p(P) = \sum_{i=1}^{k} \log p(\sigma_i | \hat{T}_i) \tag{8.7}$$

When practical, this is the preferred method for clonal partitioning, in our experience. However, it does require estimating a maximum-likelihood phylogenetic tree for each clone. When clones become large, in the several hundreds of sequences, this inference can get quite expensive in computing effort. Furthermore, having a function to maximize is important, but the maximization itself is not trivial. There are several algorithms that can be used for this task. The one we use starts with no clones and proceeds taking each IgVRG in turn, testing it for kinship in each existing clone, by the criterion that the marginal likelihood of the thus-incremented clone is larger than the product of the marginal likelihoods of the singlet and original clone. If the likelihood is not improved placing the sequence into an existing clone, the sequence is assigned to a new clone and becomes its first member.

In cases where the complete method is impractical, we compute pairwise clonal kinship. This eliminates the need to compute maximum-likelihood phylogenetic trees and provides the opportunity to relax some of the unrealistic assumptions about somatic hypermutation that the tree models thus far require. Once kinship pairs have been identified, we construct an undirected graph where the IgVRG at two nodes are joined by links if and only if they are estimated to be clonally related. We then find the connected components of the graph and take these to be the estimated clones. This is a purely heuristic method and may require manual adjustment, particularly if any of the IgVRGs have unusually low connectivity within the connected component.

8.6 Software Availability

The methods described herein have been implemented in software and are available as a Microsoft Windows installer at http://www.bu.edu/computationalimmunology/research/software.

Source code is available at Codeplex, at https://lplib.codeplex.com.

Acknowledgments

This work was supported by the National Institute of Immunology, Allergy, and Transplantation under cooperative agreement 1 U19 AI117892-01.

References

1. J. A. Weinstein, N. Jiang, R. A. White, D. S. Fisher, and S. R. Quake. High-throughput sequencing of the zebrafish antibody repertoire. *Science* 324, 807–810 (2009).
2. J. Glanville, W. Zhai, J. Berka, D. Telman, G. Huerta, G. R. Mehta, I. Ni, et al. Precise determination of the diversity of a combinatorial antibody library gives insight into the human immunoglobulin repertoire. *Proceedings of the National Academy of Sciences* 106, 20216–20221 (2009).
3. J. A. Finn, and J. E. Crowe, Jr. Impact of new sequencing technologies on studies of the human B cell repertoire. *Current Opinion in Immunology* 25, 613–618 (2013).

4. H. Robins. Immunosequencing: Applications of immune repertoire deep sequencing. *Current Opinion in Immunology* 25, 646–652 (2013).
5. P. Mathonet, and C. Ullman. The application of next generation sequencing to the understanding of antibody repertoires. *Frontiers in Immunology* 4, 265 (2013).
6. G. Georgiou, G. C. Ippolito, J. Beausang, C. E. Busse, H. Wardemann, and S. R. Quake. The promise and challenge of high-throughput sequencing of the antibody repertoire. *Nature Biotechnology* 32, 158–168 (2014).
7. S. D. Boyd, Y. Liu, C. Wang, V. Martin, and D. K. Dunn-Walters. Human lymphocyte repertoires in ageing. *Current Opinion in Immunology* 25, 511–515 (2013).
8. W. H. Robinson. Sequencing the functional antibody repertoire—Diagnostic and therapeutic discovery. *Nature Reviews Rheumatology* 11, 171–182 (2015).
9. A. C. Logan, H. Gao, C. Wang, B. Sahaf, C. D. Jones, E. L. Marshall, I. Buño, et al. High-throughput VDJ sequencing for quantification of minimal residual disease in chronic lymphocytic leukemia and immune reconstitution assessment. *Proceedings of the National Academy of Sciences* 108, 21194–21199 (2011).
10. N. Jiang, J. He, J. A. Weinstein, L. Penland, S. Sasaki, X.-S. He, C. L. Dekker, et al. Lineage structure of the human antibody repertoire in response to influenza vaccination. *Science Translational Medicine* 5, 171ra119 (2013).
11. J. D. Galson, A. J. Pollard, J. Trück, D. F. Kelly. Studying the antibody repertoire after vaccination: Practical applications. *Trends in Immunology* 35, 319–331 (2014).
12. X. Wu, T. Zhou, J. Zhu, B. Zhang, I. Georgiev, C. Wang, X. Chen, et al. Focused evolution of HIV-1 neutralizing antibodies revealed by structures and deep sequencing. *Science* 333, 1593–1602 (2011).
13. H. X. Liao, R. Lynch, T. Zhou, F. Gao, S. M. Alam, S. D. Boyd, A. Z. Fire, et al. Co-evolution of a broadly neutralizing HIV-1 antibody and founder virus. *Nature* 496, 469–476 (2013).
14. G. M. Edelman. Antibody structure and molecular immunology. *Science* 180, 830–840 (1973).
15. F. Trepel. Number and distribution of lymphocytes in man. A critical analysis. *Klinische Wochenschrift* 52, 511–515 (1974).
16. R. Somasundaram, M. A. Prasad, J. Ungerback, and M. Sigvardsson. Transcription factor networks in B-cell differentiation link development to acute lymphoid leukemia. *Blood* 126, 144–152 (2015).
17. E. ten Boekel, F. Melchers, and A. Rolink. The status of Ig loci rearrangements in single cells from different stages of B cell development. *Internal Immunology* 7, 1013–1019 (1995).
18. E. Meffre, and M. C. Nussenzweig. Deletion of immunoglobulin beta in developing B cells leads to cell death. *Proceedings of the National Academy of Sciences of the United States of America* 99, 11334–11339 (2002).
19. M. S. Naradikian, J. L. Scholz, M. A. Oropallo, and M. P. Cancro. *Drugs Targeting B-Cells in Autoimmune Diseases.* (Springer, New York, 2014), pp. 11–35.
20. D. Gay, T. Saunders, S. Camper, and M. Weigert. Receptor editing: An approach by autoreactive B cells to escape tolerance. *Journal of Experimental Medicine* 177, 999–1008 (1993).
21. H. Wardemann, S. Yurasov, A. Schaefer, J. Young, E. Meffre, and M. Nussenzweig. Predominant autoantibody production by early human B cell precursors. *Science* 301, 1374–1377 (2003).

22. E. Gaudin, Y. Hao, M. M. Rosado, R. Chaby, R. Girard, and A. A. Freitas. Positive selection of B cells expressing low densities of self-reactive BCRs. *Journal of Experimental Medicine* 199, 843–853 (2004).

23. A. G. Rolink, J. Tschopp, P. Schneider, and F. Melchers. BAFF is a survival and maturation factor for mouse B cells. *European Journal of Immunology* 32, 2004–2010 (2002).

24. Y. X. Fu, and D. D. Chaplin. Development and maturation of secondary lymphoid tissues. *Annual Review of Immunology* 17, 399–433 (1999).

25. M. Nishana, and S. C. Raghavan. Role of recombination activating genes in the generation of antigen receptor diversity and beyond. *Immunology* 137, 271–281 (2012).

26. D. G. Schatz, and Y. Ji. Recombination centres and the orchestration of V(D)J recombination. *Nature Reviews Immunology* 11, 251–263 (2011).

27. J. M. den Haan, R. Arens, and M. C. van Zelm. The activation of the adaptive immune system: Cross-talk between antigen-presenting cells, T cells and B cells. *Immunology Letters* 162, 103–112 (2014).

28. C. A. Janeway, Jr., P. Travers, M. Walport, and M. Schlomchik. *Immunobiology: The Immune System in Health and Disease.* 6th edn. (Garland Science, New York, 2005), pp. 369–383.

29. N. S. De Silva, and U. Klein. Dynamics of B cells in germinal centres. *Nature Reviews Immunology* 15, 137–148 (2015).

30. G. D. Victora, and M. C. Nussenzweig. Germinal centers. *Annual Review of Immunology* 30, 429–457 (2012).

31. A. Tanaka, H. M. Shen, S. Ratnam, P. Kodgire, and U. Storb. Attracting AID to targets of somatic hypermutation. *Journal of Experimental Medicine* 207, 405–415 (2010).

32. S. D. Wagner, C. Milstein, and M. S. Neuberger. Codon bias targets mutation. *Nature* 376, 732–732 (1995).

33. T. B. Kepler. Codon bias and plasticity in immunoglobulins. *Molecular Biology and Evolution Society* 14, 637–643 (1997).

34. J. Tan, K. Pieper, L. Piccoli, A. Abdi, M. Foglierini, R. Geiger, C. M. Tully, et al. A LAIR1 insertion generates broadly reactive antibodies against malaria variant antigens. *Nature* 529, 105–109 (2016).

35. M. Seifert, M. Przekopowitz, S. Taudien, A. Lollies, V. Ronge, B. Drees, M. Lindemann, et al. Functional capacities of human IgM memory B cells in early inflammatory responses and secondary germinal center reactions. *Proceedings of the National Academy of Sciences of the United States of America* 112, E546–555 (2015).

36. L. J. Mcheyzer-Williams, P. J. Milpied, S. L. Okitsu, and M. G. Mcheyzer-Williams. Class-switched memory B cells remodel BCRs within secondary germinal centers. *Nature Immunology* 16, 296–305 (2015).

37. H. Morbach, E. M. Eichhorn, J. G. Liese, and H. J. Girschick. Reference values for B cell subpopulations from infancy to adulthood. *Clinical & Experimental Immunology* 162, 271–279 (2010).

38. M. P. Cancro. The persistence of memory: A unique niche for IgG memory B cells. *Proceedings of the National Academy of Sciences of the United States of America* 107, 12737–12738 (2010).

39. R. A. Manz, A. Thiel, and A. Radbruch. Lifetime of plasma cells in the bone marrow. *Nature* 388, 133–134 (1997).

40. X. Yu, T. Tsibane, P. A. McGraw, F. S. House, C. J. Keefer, M. D. Hicar, T. M. Tumpey, et al. Neutralizing antibodies derived from the B cells of 1918 influenza pandemic survivors. *Nature* 455, 532–536 (2008).

41. M. K. Slifka, R. Ahmed. Long-lived plasma cells: A mechanism for maintaining persistent antibody production. *Current Opinion in Immunology* 10, 252–258 (1998).
42. J. A. Weinstein, X. Zeng, Y. H. Chien, and S. R. Quake. Correlation of gene expression and genome mutation in single B-cells. *PLoS One* 8, e67624 (2013).
43. C. E. Busse, I. Czogiel, P. Braun, P. F. Arndt, and H. Wardemann. Single-cell based high-throughput sequencing of full-length immunoglobulin heavy and light chain genes. *European Journal of Immunology* 44, 597–603 (2014).
44. B. J. DeKosky, G. C. Ippolito, R. P. Deschner, J. J. Lavinder, Y. Wine, B. M. Rawlings, N. Varadarajan, et al. High-throughput sequencing of the paired human immunoglobulin heavy and light chain repertoire. *Nature Biotechnology* 31, 166–169 (2013).
45. J. L. Duke, C. Lind, K. Mackiewicz, D. Ferriola, A. Papazoglou, O. Derbeneva, D. Wallace, and D. S. Monos. Towards allele-level human leucocyte antigens genotyping—Assessing two next-generation sequencing platforms: Ion Torrent Personal Genome Machine and Illumina MiSeq. *International Journal of Immunogenetics* 42, 346–358 (2015).
46. M. Schirmer, U. Z. Ijaz, R. D'Amore, N. Hall, W. T. Sloan, and C. Quince. Insight into biases and sequencing errors for amplicon sequencing with the Illumina MiSeq platform. *Nucleic Acids Research* 43, e37 (2015).
47. J. J. Kozich, S. L. Westcott, N. T. Baxter, S. K. Highlander, and P. D. Schloss. Development of a dual-index sequencing strategy and curation pipeline for analyzing amplicon sequence data on the MiSeq Illumina sequencing platform. *Applied and Environmental Microbiology* 79, 5112–5120 (2013).
48. M. Quail, M. E. Smith, P. Coupland, T. D. Otto, S. R. Harris, T. R. Connor, A. Bertoni, H. P. Swerdlow, and Y. Gu. A tale of three next generation sequencing platforms: Comparison of Ion torrent, Pacific Biosciences and Illumina MiSeq sequencers. *BMC Genomics* 13, 1 (2012).
49. M. Jain, I. T. Fiddes, K. H. Miga, H. E. Olsen, B. Paten, and M. Akeson. Improved data analysis for the MinION nanopore sequencer. *Nature Methods* 12, 351–356 (2015).
50. World Health Organization. (2016, November) *HIV/AIDS* [Fact Sheet]. Retrieved from http://www.who.int/mediacentre/factsheets/fs360/
51. L. M. Mansky, and H. M. Temin. Lower in-vivo mutation-rate of human-immunodeficiency-virus type-1 than that predicted from the fidelity of purified reverse-transcriptase. *Journal of Virology* 69, 5087–5094 (1995).
52. J. F. Koellhoffer, C. D. Higgins, and J. R. Lai. Protein engineering strategies for the development of viral vaccines and immunotherapeutics. *FEBS Letters* 588, 298–307 (2013).
53. D. R. Burton, R. Ahmed, D. H. Barouch, S. T. Butera, S. Crotty, A. Godzik, D. E. Kaufmann, et al. A blueprint for HIV vaccine discovery. *Cell Host and Microbe* 12, 396–407 (2012).
54. N. A. Doria-Rose, R. M. Klein, M. G. Daniels, S. O'Dell, M. Nason, A. Lapedes, T. Bhattacharya, et al. Breadth of human immunodeficiency virus-specific neutralizing activity in sera: Clustering analysis and association with clinical variables. *Journal of Virology* 84, 1631–1636 (2010).
55. L. M. Walker, M. D. Simek, F. Priddy, J. S. Gach, D. Wagner, M. B. Zwick, S. K. Phogat, P. Poignard, and D. R.Burton. A limited number of antibody specificities mediate broad and potent serum neutralization in selected HIV-1 infected individuals. *PLoS Pathogens* 6, e1001028 (2010).

56. M. D. Simek, W. Rida, F. H. Priddy, P. Pung, E. Carrow, D. S. Laufer, J. K. Lehrman, et al. Human immunodeficiency virus type 1 elite neutralizers: Individuals with broad and potent neutralizing activity identified by using a high-throughput neutralization assay together with an analytical selection algorithm. *Journal of Virology* 83, 7337–7348 (2009).

57. J. R. Mascola, and B. F. Haynes. HIV-1 neutralizing antibodies: Understanding nature's pathways. *Immunological Reviews* 254, 225–244 (2013).

58. A. J. Hessell, P. Poignard, M. Hunter, L. Hangartner, D. M. Tehrani, W. K. Bleeker, P. W. Parren, P. A. Marx, and D. R. Burton. Effective, low-titer antibody protection against low-dose repeated mucosal SHIV challenge in macaques. *Nature Medicine* 15, 951–954 (2009).

59. A. J. Hessell, E. G. Rakasz, P. Poignard, L. Hangartner, G. Landucci, D. N. Forthal, W. C. Koff, D. I. Watkins, and D. R. Burton. Broadly neutralizing human anti-HIV antibody 2G12 is effective in protection against mucosal SHIV challenge even at low serum neutralizing titers. *PLoS Pathogens* 5, e1000433 (2009).

60. B. F. Haynes, J. Fleming, E. W. St Clair, H. Katinger, G. Stiegler, R. Kunert, J. Robinson, et al. Cardiolipin polyspecific autoreactivity in two broadly neutralizing HIV-1 antibodies. *Science* 308, 1906–1908 (2005).

61. R. Diskin, J. F. Scheid, P. M. Marcovecchio, A. P. West, F. Klein, H. Gao, P. N. P. Gnanapragasam, et al. Increasing the potency and breadth of an HIV antibody by using structure-based rational design. *Science* 334, 1289–1293 (2011).

62. J. Zhu, G. Ofek, Y. Yang, B. Zhang, M. K. Louder, G. Lu, K. McKee, et al. Mining the antibodyome for HIV-1-neutralizing antibodies with next-generation sequencing and phylogenetic pairing of heavy/light chains. *Proceedings of the National Academy of Sciences of the United States of America* 110, 6470–6475 (2013).

63. J. Zhu, X. Wu, B. Zhang, K. McKee, S. O'Dell, C. Soto, T. Zhou, et al. De novo identification of VRC01 class HIV-1-neutralizing antibodies by next-generation sequencing of B-cell transcripts. *Proceedings of the National Academy of Sciences of the United States of America* 110, E4088–4097 (2013).

64. J. Zhu, S. O'Dell, G. Ofek, M. Pancera, X. Wu, B. Zhang, Z. Zhang, et al. Somatic populations of PGT135-137 HIV-1-neutralizing antibodies identified by 454 pyrosequencing and bioinformatics. *Frontiers in Microbiology* 3, 315 (2012).

65. B. F. Haynes, G. Kelsoe, S. C. Harrison, and T. B. Kepler. B-cell-lineage immunogen design in vaccine development with HIV-1 as a case study. *Nature Biotechnology* 30, 423–433 (2012).

66. A. Escolano, J. M. Steichen, P. Dosenovic, D. W. Kulp, J. Golijanin, D. Sok, N. T. Freund, et al. Sequential immunization elicits broadly neutralizing anti-HIV-1 antibodies in Ig knockin mice. *Cell* 166, 1445–1458. e12 (2016).

67. Z. Yang. *Molecular Evolution: A Statistical Approach.* (Oxford University Press, Oxford, UK, 2014).

68. M. Kimura. Estimation of evolutionary distances between homologous nucleotide sequences. *Proceedings of the National Academy of Sciences* 78, 454–458 (1981).

69. Ramesh A. Immunogenetics of the Rhesus Macaque, an Animal Model for HIV Vaccine Development (Doctoral dissertation, Boston University School of Medicine), (2017).

9

Probability-Scale Residuals in HIV/AIDS Research: Diagnostics and Inference

Bryan E. Shepherd
Vanderbilt University School of Medicine, Nashville, TN

Qi Liu
Merck & Co., Rahway, NJ

Valentine Wanga
University of Washington, Seattle, WA

Chun Li
Case Western Reserve University, Cleveland, OH

CONTENTS

9.1 Introduction

There is a wide variety of data in HIV/AIDS research. In clinical studies, common variables include CD4 cell count, HIV-1 RNA (viral load), demographics, World Health Organization or Centers for Disease Control and Prevention disease stage, and time-to-event variables such as time from antiretroviral therapy (ART) initiation to an AIDS-defining event, viral failure, or death. Biomarker data are common in both clinical and basic studies of HIV; these may include markers of inflammation, pharmacokinetics, drug use, or metabolism, and may be biomarkers commonly used in other disease settings (e.g., diabetes or hepatitis). Genomic data, both human and viral, are also important.

Of course, the characteristics of these and other variables used in HIV research are extremely diverse. The distribution of some are fairly symmetric (e.g., age at ART initiation), somewhat skewed (e.g., CD4 count), or highly skewed (e.g., viral load).

Many variables are left censored at detection limits (e.g., viral load and other biomarkers) or right censored due to finite follow-up (e.g., time to death). Many are ordered categorical (e.g., stage of disease and single nucleotide polymorphisms [SNPs]). Much of the statistical work in the analysis of HIV data involves finding proper models for these variables to assess associations, to predict outcomes, and hopefully in the end to improve patient and public health. Given the diversity of variables, a wide variety of statistical models are used.

There are benefits to having statistical methods that are robust and efficient across a wide variety of data types. Such methods can be quickly applied with confidence in many different situations and may be useful as a first pass in big data settings (e.g., data sets with many variables of interest). Such methods may also be useful in smaller analyses because they provide nice, simple summaries. Spearman's rank correlation is one such example: its simplicity, validity, and utility across a wide variety of orderable variables make it popular in practice.

We have developed a new type of residual, the probability-scale residual (PSR), which is remarkably useful and well defined across a wide variety of variable types and models (Li and Shepherd 2010, 2012; Shepherd et al. 2016). As a residual, it can be used for model diagnostics and for inference. We have proposed to use the correlation of PSRs to adjust Spearman's rank correlation for covariates (Liu et al. 2017). The goal of this chapter is to introduce the PSR to HIV researchers to describe a few of its important properties, and to demonstrate its utility across a diverse set of analyses with HIV data.

We first introduce the PSR and describe some of its properties (Section 9.2). We then illustrate its use for model diagnostics (Section 9.3) and inference (Section 9.4). Several data sets that we have encountered in our collaborative HIV/AIDS research will be used to illustrate the methods. The final section discusses a few points and proposes directions for future research. Analysis code for all of the data examples is available at our website, biostat.mc.vanderbilt.edu/ArchivedAnalyses.

9.2 Probability-Scale Residual

In linear regression, a residual is defined as $y - \hat{y}$, where y is an observed value and $\hat{y}$ is a fitted value, typically the estimated expectation of the outcome conditional on covariates. This observed-minus-expected residual (OMER) is simple and has many desirable properties, but it is not easily extendable to outcomes where conditional expectations are difficult to calculate or are not meaningful. For example, for ordinal outcomes there is no natural definition of difference or conditional expectation unless scores are assigned to the ordered categories; for right censored outcomes with partially defined fitted distributions, one may not be able to calculate the conditional expectation. Furthermore, the OMER may be misleading with models where one is fitting a nonsymmetric distribution to data.

The OMER can be thought of as the expectation of the difference between the observed value, y, and a random variable, Y^*, from the fitted distribution with cumulative distribution function (CDF) F^*: $E(y - Y^*) = y - \hat{y}$. Instead of using the difference to contrast y and Y^*, one could use the sign function, specifically, sign(y, Y^*), where sign(a, b) is -1, 0, and 1 for $a < b$, $a = b$, and $a > b$, respectively. The PSR is simply the expectation of this contrast, $r(y, F^*) = E\{\text{sign}(y, Y^*)\}$, which can be written in terms of probabilities as $P(Y^* < y) - P(Y^* > y)$ or equivalently $F^*(y-) + F^*(y) - 1$.

A few benefits of the PSR are immediately apparent. First, the sign function is more generally applicable than the difference, so by contrasting variables with the sign function we are able to define a residual for more types of outcomes. Second, the PSR does not require estimation of conditional expectation but rather estimation of the conditional distribution itself. Note that it is not necessary to estimate the entire distribution, but the distribution only needs to be estimated at the observed value, y. Hence, the residual is flexible for a wide range of outcome variables (including ordered categorical) and models (including semiparametric), while still providing information on model fit.

We originally introduced the PSR for use with ordered categorical variables (Li and Shepherd 2010, 2012). In that setting, the residual has several nice properties including the following:

1. The PSR captures order information without assigning arbitrary numbers to the ordinal categories.
2. The PSR yields only one value per observation regardless of the number of categories of the ordinal variable.
3. The PSR has expectation zero with a correctly specified model; that is, for a random variable Y with distribution F, $E\{r(Y, F^*)\} = 0$ if $F^* = F$.

In addition to the above, the PSR is the only residual that satisfies several natural properties for ordinal outcomes such as the branching property

(Brockett and Levine 1977), reversibility, and monotonicity with respect to the observed value. Details are in Li and Shepherd (2012). For proportional odds models, the PSR sums to 0.

The PSR is also well defined for other types of orderable data, including binary, count, continuous, and censored outcomes (Shepherd et al. 2016). In all cases, the PSR has zero expectation under correctly specified models. With continuous data, the PSR equals zero at the median of the fitted distribution. In addition, with continuous data the random variable $r(Y, F^*)$ is uniformly distributed between -1 and 1 if the fitted distribution is correctly specified, suggesting that with sufficiently large sample sizes, one can approximately assess model fit by comparing the distribution of PSRs with a uniform $(-1, 1)$ distribution. With binary data, the PSR is simply the OMER, or the unscaled Pearson residual. With right censored data, the PSR is a function of the observed minimum of the censoring and event times, y, and the indicator that an event occurred, δ: $r(y, F^*, \delta) = F^*(y) - \delta\{1 - F^*(y-)\}$. Given δ, the PSR with time-to-event data is a one-to-one function of the martingale, deviance, and Cox–Snell residuals. The PSR can also be written for current status data. Details are in Shepherd et al. (2016), where we also demonstrated the calculation and the utility of the PSR in a variety of settings including normal linear models, least-squares regression, exponential regression models, median or quantile regression, semiparametric transformation models, Poisson and negative binomial regression, Cox regression, and the analysis of current status data.

Although novel, the PSR is related to other methods proposed in the statistical literature. The PSR was part of a test statistic in genetic analysis of ordinal traits (Zhang et al. 2006). The PSR is closely related to ridits (Bross 1958) and can be thought of as a linear transformation of an observed value's adjusted rank (see Section 9.4). With continuous data, the PSR is simply a rescaling of the probability integral transformation, which has been previously proposed for assessing goodness of fit (Pearson 1938; David and Johnson 1948) and as a component of a residual (Cox and Snell 1968; Davison and Tsai 1992; Dunn and Smyth 1996). One of the strengths of the PSR is its unification of several of these concepts into a single residual.

9.3 Model Diagnostics

As a residual, the PSR can be useful for model diagnostics. In this section, we introduce a few HIV data sets and demonstrate the residual's use in these settings.

9.3.1 Stage of Cervical Lesions: Proportional Odds Models

Cervical specimens from 145 HIV-infected women in Zambia were examined using cytology and categorized into five ordered stages; 10 specimens were normal, 26 atypical squamous cells of undetermined significance (ASCUS), 35 low-grade intraepithelial lesions, 49 high-grade intraepithelial lesions, and 30 suspicious for cancer (Parham et al. 2006). Other data were collected from the women including age, CD4 count, education, and frequency of condom use (never, rarely, almost always, and always). There is interest in modeling the association between these variables and stage of cervical lesions. To this end, we fit proportional odds models with stage of cervical lesions as the outcome and various combinations of the other variables as predictors.

Figure 9.1a shows a residual-by-predictor plot with the x-axis showing age and the y-axis showing PSRs from a proportional odds model with age and CD4 included as linear predictors; a lowess curve demonstrating the smoothed relationship between the residuals and age is also included. When age is included in the proportional odds model as a linear variable, there appears to be a quadratic relationship between the PSRs and age: the model tends to overpredict severity of lesions at low and high ages. For example, a 23-year-old woman in the data set with a CD4 count of 309 cells/mm^3 had predicted probabilities of 0.10, 0.25, 0.27, 0.27, and 0.11 for cytology being normal, ASCUS, low, high, and cancerous, respectively. This suggests that her observed cytology of ASCUS was less severe than predicted by the model—resulting in a residual of $0.10 - (0.27 + 0.27 + 0.11) = -0.55$ (left-most residual in Figure 9.1a). If both linear and quadratic terms of age are included in the proportional odds model, the quadratic relationship between the residuals and age is no longer seen (Figure 9.1b), suggesting a better model fit.

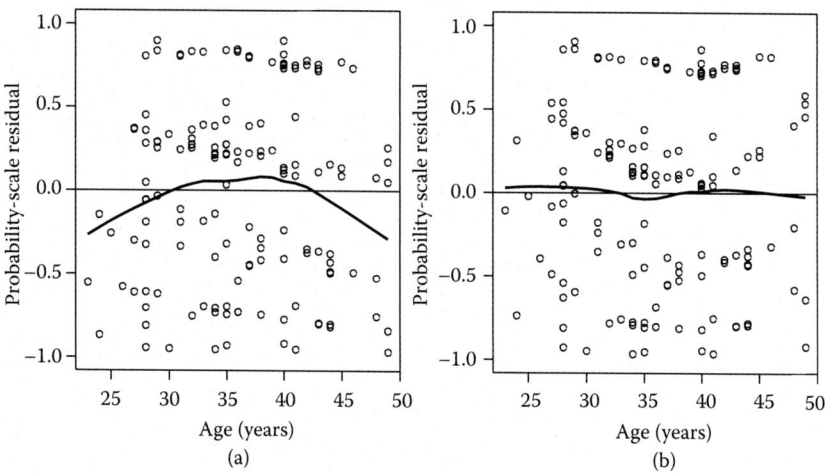

FIGURE 9.1
Probability-scale residual-by-predictor plots with age included in a proportional odds model (a) as a linear term and (b) as a linear and quadratic term. (Reproduced from Li, C. and Shepherd, B. E., *Biometrika*, 99:473–480, 2012. With permission.)

The observed ASCUS cytology for the 23-year-old woman is now more consistent to what the model predicts (probability of normal, ASCUS, low, high, and cancerous estimated as 0.26, 0.38, 0.21, 0.12, and 0.03, respectively), resulting in a PSR closer to zero: $0.26 - (0.21 + 0.12 + 0.03) = -0.11$.

9.3.2 Biomarker Study of Metabolomics: Semiparametric Transformation Models

HIV-positive individuals who have been on long-term ART appear to be at an increased risk of cardiometabolic diseases, including diabetes, compared to HIV-negative individuals. Plasma levels of amino acids and other small molecules reflective of impaired energy metabolism, such as acylcarnitines and organic acids, were measured with mass spectrometry to provide a detailed metabolic profile for 70 nondiabetic, HIV-infected persons who were on efavirenz, tenofovir, and emtricitabine with an undetectable viral load for over 2 years (Koethe et al. 2016).

There is interest in assessing associations between these biomarkers and demographic or clinical variables. In this section, we will focus on modeling a specific biomarker, 2-hydroxybutyric acid, which is thought to be an early indicator of insulin resistance in nondiabetic persons; elevated serum 2-hydroxybutyric acid has been seen to predict worsening glucose tolerance. 2-Hydroxybutyric acid is fairly skewed, ranging from 13 to 151 µM, median 34 µM in our data set. Even after a log transformation, the distribution remains slightly right skewed with some outlier levels. Predictor variables for our model include age, sex, race, body mass index (BMI), CD4 cell count, smoking status, and ART duration (log transformed).

Because of the skewness of the biomarker outcome, we favor fitting a semiparametric transformation model, specifically $Y = T(\beta Z + \epsilon)$, where $T(\cdot)$ is an unspecified monotonic increasing transformation and ϵ is a random error with a specified parametric distribution F_ϵ (Zeng and Lin 2007). The conditional distribution of Y given Z is therefore

$$
\begin{aligned}
F_{Y|Z}(y) &= P(T(\beta Z + \epsilon) \leq y) \\
&= P(\epsilon \leq T^{-1}(y) - \beta Z) \\
&= F_\epsilon(T^{-1}(y) - \beta Z).
\end{aligned}
$$

Hence, the semiparametric transformation model can be written in a manner similar to that of the ordinal cumulative probability model, $g[F_{Y|Z}(y)] = \alpha(y) - \beta Z$, with the link function $g(\cdot) = F_\epsilon^{-1}(\cdot)$ and the intercept $\alpha(y) = T^{-1}(y)$. Harrell (2015) has proposed using this fact to estimate parameters from the semiparametric transformation model with continuous data by maximizing an approximated multinomial likelihood, and he has implemented this procedure, denoted as orm, in R Statistical Software as part of his popular "rms" package.

In our biomarker analysis, we fit three models of 2-hydroxybutyric acid (denoted as Y) on covariates: (1) a multivariable linear regression model with Y untransformed; (2) a multivariable linear model with Y log transformed; and (3) a semiparametric transformation model fitted using orm with the link function $g(\cdot) = \log(-\log(\cdot))$, which corresponds to assuming F_ϵ follows an extreme value distribution. Figure 9.2 shows quantile–quantile (Q–Q) plots of PSRs from each of these models compared to quantiles from a uniform $(-1, 1)$ distribution. If the model is correctly specified, the residuals should be approximately uniformly distributed. Clearly, PSRs from the normal linear model are far from uniform, and although PSRs from the linear model after log transforming the biomarker are closer to being uniform, PSRs from the flexible, semiparametric transformation model are more uniform.

In this analysis, we could also have used OMERs to uncover lack of fit for the linear models. However, the OMER is difficult to calculate for the semiparametric transformation model because it requires computation of the conditional expectation, and even if we went through the process of estimating the conditional expectation for all observed covariate combinations, OMERs would still be skewed and not very good for model diagnostics because the semiparametric transformation model makes no assumptions of symmetry of the OMERs, equal variance, etc. In contrast, the PSR is easily and naturally calculated from the fitted semiparametric transformation model and makes no additional assumptions beyond that of the original model. Hence, the PSR is useful for comparing fit across the three different models because it is on the same scale for each.

Figure 9.3 shows residual-by-predictor plots for continuous covariates from the semiparametric transformation model using PSRs. There is some evidence of nonlinear relationships (top panel). The model was refit expanding age, BMI, and log-transformed ART duration using restricted cubic splines with 3 knots.

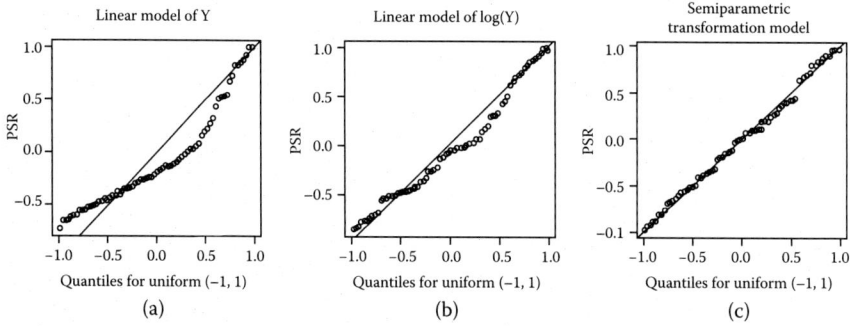

FIGURE 9.2
Q–Q plots of PSRs from (a) linear, (b) linear after log transformation, and (c) semiparametric transformation models of 2-hydroxybutyric acid compared to a uniform $(-1, 1)$ distribution.

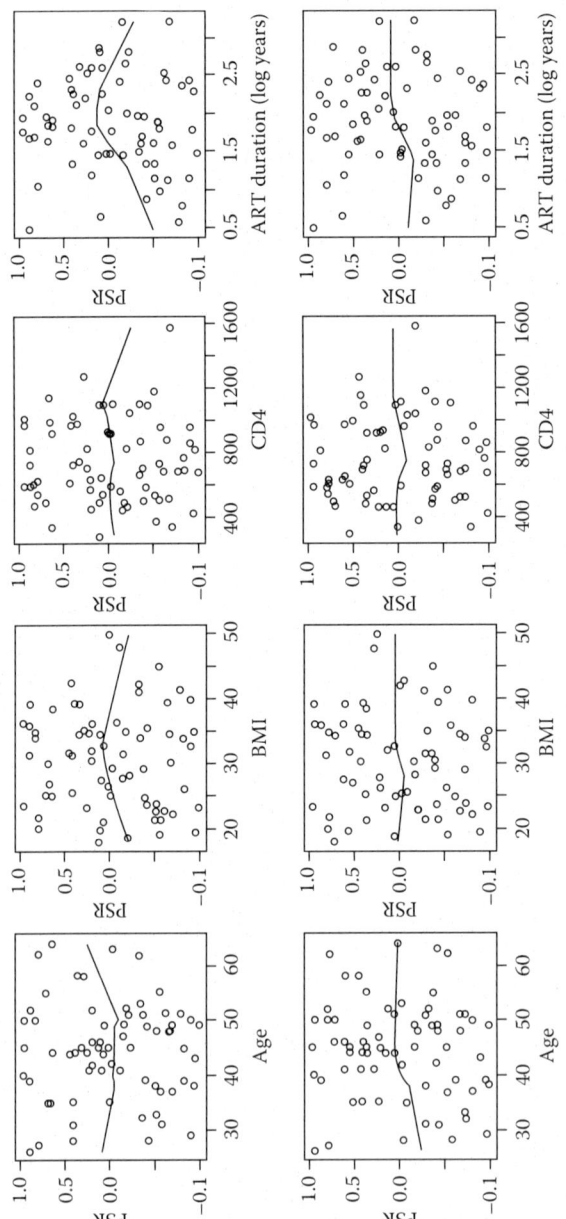

FIGURE 9.3
Residual-by-predictor plots. The smoothed relationship is shown using lowess curves. The top panel shows PSRs versus continuous predictors from an initial model fit without splines. The bottom panel shows PSRs versus continuous predictors after expanding age, BMI, and log-transformed ART duration using restricted cubic splines with 3 knots.

Residual-by-predictor plots from these models are given in the bottom panel of Figure 9.3. There is no longer evidence of nonlinear residual relationships. A likelihood ratio test confirms that the second model with the nonlinear terms is a better fit ($p = 0.010$); despite the added model complexity, the Akaike information criterion (AIC) for the model with the nonlinear terms is lower than that without them (599 vs. 605).

9.4 Inference

Because the PSR is applicable to and has a common scale across a wide variety of outcome types, it can be used to test for conditional associations using residual correlation. We describe these tests for residual correlation using PSRs in Section 9.4.1 and show their connection with Spearman's rank correlation in Section 9.4.2.

9.4.1 Tests of Residual Correlation

We initially developed the PSR as a component of an approach for testing the association between two ordinal variables, X and Y, while controlling for covariates Z (Li and Shepherd 2010). Our approach was to fit separate multinomial models (e.g., proportional odds models) of X on Z and Y on Z, obtain residuals from these models, and then test the association between residuals from these models. This is analogous to linear regression where the association between Y and X conditional on Z is captured by the correlation between OMERS from linear models of X on Z and of Y on Z. We could not find a good residual for ordinal outcomes that resulted in a single value per observation and captured the necessary residual information without imposing assumptions additional to those imposed by the original model—hence, we created the PSR. In Li and Shepherd (2010), we proposed three test statistics for testing the conditional association between X and Y, one of which was simply the sample correlation between PSRs from the two models. We showed that our test statistics equal zero under the null hypothesis of independence between Y and X conditional on Z, and we derived their large sample distributions. Collectively, we referred to our test statistics as COBOT (conditional ordinal by ordinal tests).

We found that these test statistics performed well in simulations, finding a nice balance between power and robustness. For example, if data were simulated from a proportional odds model with a linear relationship between the log odds of Y and the labels of the ordinal predictor X conditional on Z, then our COBOT methods resulted in minimal loss of power compared to the gold standard analysis of simply fitting a proportional odds model with X included as a continuous variable. Under this scenario, the power of COBOT was much higher than models treating ordinal X as a categorical variable that ignored the order information. And when data were generated such that the log odds of Y and the labels of the ordinal predictor X were nonlinear conditional on Z, then the power of COBOT was higher than that of approaches that included X in the proportional odds model as a continuous variable or a categorical variable. Details are in Li and Shepherd (2010).

It would be disingenuous to claim that COBOT always outperforms other approaches. For example, COBOT has poor power to reject the null of conditional independence when the relationship between X and Y conditional on Z is not monotonic. Also, subsequent simulations have suggested that the advantages of COBOT depend on the number of categories of the ordinal variable and the probability distribution of those categories. For example, if an ordinal variable, X, has few categories (i.e., 2 and 3) then there appears to be little advantage to using COBOT over simply treating X as a categorical predictor variable in a proportional odds model, whereas when there are lots of categories (i.e., >7), treating the ordinal variables as continuous seems to perform reasonably well, even with nonlinear relationships. These caveats noted, we believe that COBOT fills an important gap in the statistical literature regarding methods to test the conditional association between two ordinal variables while accounting for their ordinal nature.

Because of its applicability and common scale with a wide variety of outcomes, the correlation of PSRs can also be used to test for conditional associations in more general settings. For example, using the correlation of PSRs, one could test for association between continuous, count, or ordinal X and continuous, count, or ordinal Y conditional on Z.

9.4.2 Spearman's Partial and Conditional Rank Correlations

Consider a model of an ordinal outcome Y with a constant predictor for all subjects (i.e., a model with only an intercept). With such a model, the predicted probability for each category is simply its empirical distribution (n_j/n), and the PSR is therefore a linear transformation of the ranks of Y. As such, when there are no covariates, the correlation coefficient between PSRs from models for X and Y is equivalent to Spearman's rank correlation. When covariates are present, the PSR can be thought of as a linear transformation of the adjusted ranks of subjects and our test statistic can be thought of as an adjusted rank correlation. This also holds for continuous outcomes and other types of ordered discrete variables (e.g., count data) and suggests an approach for extending Spearman's rank correlation to account for covariates.

More formally, the population parameter of Spearman's rank correlation, denoted as γ_{XY}, is the scaled difference between the probability of concordance and the probability of discordance between (X, Y) and (X_0, Y_0), where X_0 and Y_0 have the same marginal distributions as X and Y, denoted

F and G, respectively, but $X_0 \perp Y_0$ and $(X_0, Y_0) \perp (X, Y)$ (Kruskal 1958). With continuous X and Y, the scaling factor is 3, which ensures that $-1 \leq \gamma_{XY} \leq 1$; for noncontinuous X and/or Y, the scaling factor is a function of the marginal distributions of the noncontinuous variables (Neslehova 2007). It can be shown that this difference between concordance and discordance probabilities is equal to the covariance of PSRs (from unconditional models), and the scaling factor is simply the inverse of the square root of the product of the variances of the PSRs (Liu et al. 2017). Specifically,

$$\gamma_{XY} = c\{P[(X - X_0)(Y - Y_0) > 0] - P[(X - X_0)(Y - Y_0) < 0]\}$$
$$= c\text{Cov}[r(X, F), r(Y, G)]$$
$$= \text{corr}[r(X, F), r(Y, G)].$$

Note, as highlighted in Section 9.2, that with continuous variables and correct model specification, the PSR is uniformly distributed from -1 to 1 and hence has variance $1/3$, leading to a scaling factor of $c = 3$; with discrete random variables, the variance of the PSR is $\text{Var}[r(X, F)] = (1 - \Sigma f_x^3)/3$, where $f_x = P(X = x)$, which leads to the scaling factor for Spearman's correlation with discrete variables. Therefore, Spearman's rank correlation can be written as the correlation of PSRs. Similarly, Spearman's rank correlation conditional on Z can be defined as

$$\gamma_{XY|Z} = c_Z\{P[(X - X_0)(Y - Y_0) > 0|Z] - P[(X - X_0)(Y - Y_0) < 0|Z]\}$$
$$= \text{corr}[r(X, F_{X|Z}), r(Y, G_{Y|Z})|Z],$$

the conditional correlation between PSRs from models conditional on Z. This expression is equivalent to Spearman's conditional rank correlation for continuous variables recently proposed by Gijbels et al. (2011). Unlike Gijbels et al. (2011), however, our conditional rank correlation using PSRs can also be easily applied to discrete variables. Such a statistic describes how the rank correlation between X and Y varies as a function of Z.

Finally, we define Spearman's partial rank correlation as

$$\gamma_{XY \cdot Z} = c^*\{P[(X - X_0)(Y - Y_0) > 0|Z] - P[(X - X_0)(Y - Y_0) < 0|Z]\}$$
$$= \text{corr}[r(X, F_{X|Z}), r(Y, G_{Y|Z})],$$

which is a weighted average of $\gamma_{XY|Z}$. Partial correlations describe the association between X and Y after adjusting for Z, but not as a function of Z. Details are in Liu et al. (2017).

These observations fill another gap in the literature. Pearson's partial correlation is derived as the correlation between OMERs from models of Y on Z and X on Z. When Z is a single variable, this is equivalently written as $(\rho_{XY} - \rho_{XZ}\rho_{YZ})/\sqrt{(1 - \rho_{XZ}^2)(1 - \rho_{YZ}^2)}$, where ρ_{XY} denotes Pearson's correlation between X and Y and so forth. The traditional Spearman's partial correlation has been proposed by substituting ρ_{AB} with the corresponding rank correlations, γ_{AB}. Although not a poor measure of association, this traditional

Spearman's partial correlation is ad hoc and does not correspond with a sensible population parameter (Kendall 1942; Gripenberg 1992). In contrast, Spearman's partial rank correlation defined as the correlation of PSRs directly corresponds to the population parameter of Spearman's rank correlation and is elegantly analogous to the definition of Pearson's partial correlation— instead of the correlation of OMERs; it is the correlation of PSRs.

The above arguments are made at the population level. In practice, one must fit models of Y on Z and X on Z to compute the partial Spearman's rank correlation.

Given the flexibility of the PSR to a wide variety of models, the choice of models for Y on Z and X on Z is almost unlimited. However, the choice of model is still important to ensure adequate fit for investigating residual correlation. For example, if a model of Y on Z poorly fits the data, then residual correlations from this model may be misleading. To be true to the robust nature of Spearman's rank correlation, yet to be efficient, we favor fitting semiparametric models that only use the order information of the outcomes for models of Y on Z and X on Z. Specifically, we favor using the semiparametric transformation model described in Section 9.3.2 with $Y = T(\beta Z + \epsilon)$, where $T(\cdot)$ is an unspecified monotonic increasing transformation and ϵ is a random error with a specified parametric distribution F_ϵ (Zeng and Lin 2007). A similar model is fit for X on Z. An advantage of the semiparametric transformation model is that it can be fit to binary, ordered categorical, and continuous variables. In practice, we have used orm, introduced in Section 9.3.2, to obtain maximum likelihood estimates based on the semiparametric transformation model. Extensive simulations have shown that Spearman's partial correlation using PSRs performs remarkably well with orm, even when models are misspecified (e.g., orm with a cloglog, instead of probit, link is fit to normal data) (Liu et al. 2017).

Computation of conditional Spearman's rank correlations can also be computed using PSRs from semiparametric transformation models. If Z is categorical, then this correlation can simply be calculated in each level of Z. With continuous Z, the conditional rank correlation can be computed either nonparametrically with, for example, kernal smoothers, or modeled with parametric functions (Liu et al. 2017).

9.4.3 Covariance of PSRs

In COBOT, we proposed three test statistics. One of them, the correlation between PSRs, has been described above as an extension of Spearman's rank correlation to account for covariates. A second COBOT test statistic was to compare the observed values of (X, Y) with the distribution of possible values under the null that X and Y are independent conditional on Z using the difference of concordance–discordance probabilities. It can be shown that this is equivalent to the expectation of the product of PSRs, $E[r(Y, F_{Y|Z}) \ r(X, G_{X|Z})]$, which with correctly specified models is simply the covariance of PSRs. Hence, not surprisingly, we could also use the covariance of PSRs as a test statistic. Although some interpretation is lost when using the covariance, it may have advantages over the correlation when modeling the rank association between X and Y as a function of Z because it only requires modeling $E[r(X, F_{X|Z})r(Y, G_{Y|Z})|Z]$. In contrast, models of Spearman's conditional rank correlation with discrete data also require modeling $Var[r(X, F_{X|Z})|Z]$ and $Var[r(Y, G_{Y|Z})|Z]$.

9.4.4 Examples

9.4.4.1 Stage of Cervical Lesions

Returning to the Zambia data set of Section 9.3.1, there is interest in assessing the association between stage of cervical lesions and condom use, after controlling for other variables. Stage of cervical lesions and condom use are both ordered categorical variables. The unadjusted Spearman's rank correlation is -0.057 (p-value = 0.50). Using the methods described above, Spearman's partial rank correlation was estimated to be -0.037 (95% confidence interval [CI] -0.196, 0.123; p-value = 0.65), adjusted for age, age^2, CD4, education, and marital status.

9.4.4.2 Biomarker Study of Metabolomics

Returning to the biomarker study of Section 9.3.2, there is interest in assessing the correlation between plasma levels of various metabolites to better understand how these molecules interact among persons infected with HIV who have been on long-term ART. There were 21 primary biomarkers measured on 70 HIV-infected patients. Data were complete except for a single patient who was missing a measurement of oral glucose insulin sensitivity (OGIS) 120. The distributions of the biomarkers are quite heterogenous (data not shown), many are right skewed (e.g., 2-hydroxybutyric acid highlighted in Section 9.3.2), some have several patients with values below assay detection limits, and pairwise associations are not expected to be linear. The biomarkers' scales vary and there is little interest in obtaining interpretable regression coefficients. For these reasons, Spearman's rank correlations between biomarkers would be ideal because of their robustness and their single number summary of the strength of association on a common scale between -1 and 1. However, other variables could be associated with various biomarkers that we would like to control for, including age, sex, race, BMI, CD4 cell count, smoking status, and ART duration. Hence, we also computed Spearman's partial rank correlation using the correlation of PSRs from models that adjusted for those variables. This was done by fitting a model for each biomarker using a semiparametric transformation model with the covariates listed above (with ART duration log transformed) and estimating via orm with a logit link. (Results were very similar when using a complementary log–log link, and are not shown.) As illustrated in Section 9.3.2, some of these models may have benefited from including nonlinear relationships between covariates

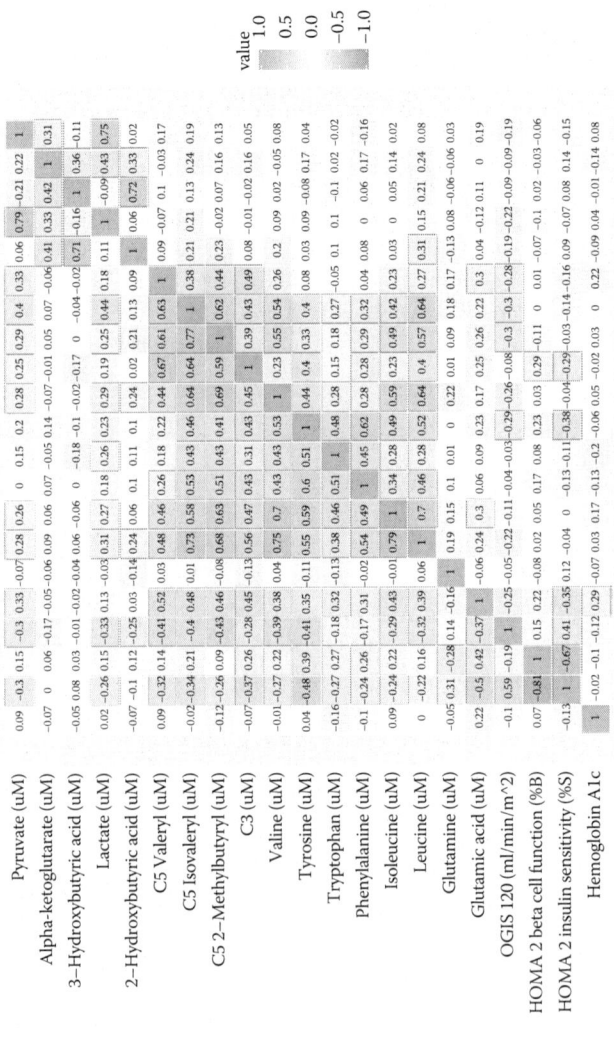

FIGURE 9.4

Heatmap showing the pairwise Spearman's rank correlations between 21 biomarkers. The upper-left correlations are unadjusted, the lower right correlations are partial correlations adjusted for age, sex, race, BMI, CD4, smoking status, and ART duration. Shades denote the strength of correlations with those closer to -1 and 1 being darker.

and biomarkers using splines; however, with only 70 patients, overfitting could be an issue. Also, these estimates are meant to be a first pass that could lead to further investigation, perhaps fine-tuning model fit using diagnostics as done in Section 9.3.2.

Figure 9.4 shows Spearman's rank correlation for all pairs of biomarkers; the quantities to the upper left of the diagonal are unadjusted, the quantities to the lower right of the diagonal are adjusted using the correlation of PSRs. Shading indicates stronger correlation and black boxes are drawn around those correlations that are significantly different from 0 (i.e., p-values < 0.05). The figure demonstrates that many of the correlations are reduced after adjusting for these additional variables. For example, homeostasis model assessment (HOMA)-2 insulin sensitivity appears to be correlated (positively or negatively) with many of the other biomarkers, with 15 of the 20 unadjusted pairwise correlations significantly different from 0. However, after controlling for covariates, the correlations generally weakened with point estimates closer to 0 and only 5 of 20 adjusted pairwise correlations significantly different from 0. A similar reduction in correlation is observed for the lactate biomarker. Although correlations generally weakened after controlling for other variables, this was not always the case. For example, the rank correlation between hemoglobin A1C and glutamic acid increased from 0.22 to 0.29 after controlling for covariates, and the rank correlation between alpha-ketogluterate and pyruvate increased from 0.22 to 0.31 in the presence of covariates.

9.4.4.3 Genome-Wide Association Study

As an additional illustration of our methods, we use the correlation of PSRs to examine the potential association between SNP and tenofovir clearance among patients randomized to the tenofovir or emtricitabine arm in AIDS Clinical Trials Group Protocol A5202. Tenofovir causes kidney toxicity in some patients and there is interest in identifying SNPs that may be associated with plasma tenofovir clearance, as these SNPs may in turn be associated with risk of kidney toxicity. An earlier genome-wide association study (GWAS) looked at the association between approximately 890,000 SNPs and tenofovir clearance using standard methods (Wanga et al. 2015). In these analyses, the association between SNPs and tenofovir clearance was modeled using linear regression adjusting for sex, age, BMI, other antiretrovirals (efavirenz or ritonavir-boosted atazanavir), baseline creatinine clearance, self-reported race (white, black, Hispanic, or other), and the first two principal components for genetic ancestry. SNPs were included in those models assuming additive effects; that is, for biallelic markers with alleles A and a, genotypes A/A, A/a, and a/a were coded as 0, 1, and 2.

Genotype can be thought of as an ordered categorical variable, and there may be benefits to treating it as such in a GWAS. In particular, genetic effects may be additive (as assumed by the analysis model given above), dominant, or recessive, and it would be desirable to have a single analysis that is robust for detecting monotone associations between SNPs and tenofovir clearance without specifically assuming effects are either additive, dominant, or recessive. To that end, we repeated the GWAS using the correlation of PSRs. Specifically, we regressed tenofovir clearance on the same covariates adjusted for in Wanga et al. (2015) with the exception that SNPs were not included in the model, and we also fit proportional odds models of SNPs based on these same covariates. PSRs were then derived from all models; for the linear model, we used an empirical estimate of the distribution of the residuals to compute PSRs (i.e., $PSR_i = \sum_{j=1}^{n} I(\hat{\epsilon}_j < \hat{\epsilon}_i)/n - \sum_{j=1}^{n} I(\hat{\epsilon}_j > \hat{\epsilon}_i)/n$, where $\hat{\epsilon}_i$ is the OMER for subject i). We then computed the correlation between PSRs from the tenofovir clearance model and PSRs from the SNP models (i.e., Spearman's partial rank correlation), and computed p-values under the null hypothesis of no residual correlation. Finally, for purpose of comparison, we repeated all analyses fitting linear models in a manner identical to that of Wanga et al. (2015) except using dominant, recessive, and categorical specifications for the SNPs. Specifically, this amounts to coding (A/A, A/a, a/a) as (0, 1, 1) for dominant, (0, 0, 1) for recessive, and using two (dummy) variables coded as (0, 1, 0) and (0, 0, 1) for categorical which therefore ignores the order information.

Table 9.1 shows a pairwise Spearman's correlation matrix of the approximately 890,000 p-values using the five different analysis models. P-values between the residual correlation and additive models were strongly correlated ($\gamma = 0.801$); results from the residual correlation model were also highly correlated with the dominant model ($\gamma = 0.709$), less so with the categorical model ($\gamma = 0.557$), and weakly correlated with the recessive model ($\gamma = 0.204$). Table 9.2 shows the top 10 SNPs under each analysis model, and their respective p-values. SNP rs12387850 was ranked first in the correlation of PSRs analysis (p-value $= 2.80 \times 10^{-7}$), additive (p-value $= 1.26 \times 10^{-6}$) and dominant models (p-value $= 5.63 \times 10^{-7}$), but ranked the 75th (p-value $= 1.07 \times 10^{-5}$) and 26th (p-value $= 3.71 \times 10^{-6}$) in the recessive and categorical models, respectively. Among the SNPs significantly associated with tenofovir clearance, SNP rs12082252 ranked first (p-value $= 2.28 \times 10^{-10}$) and second (p-value

TABLE 9.1

Tenofovir Clearance: Correlation Matrix of P-values in GWAS

	Corr(PSRs)	Additive	Dominant	Recessive	Categorical
Corr(PSRs)	1				
Additive	0.801	1			
Dominant	0.709	0.734	1		
Recessive	0.204	0.326	0.067	1	
Categorical	0.557	0.649	0.643	0.653	1

Note: PSR, probability-scale residual.

TABLE 9.2

Tenofovir Clearance: SNPs with the Smallest *p*-values in Combined Group Analysis

	corr(PSRs)			Additive			Dominant			Recessive			Categorical	
CHR	SNP	*p*	CHR	SNP	*p*	CHR	SNP	*p*	CHR	SNP	*p*	CHR	SNP	*p*
2	rs887829	7.08e-10	2	rs887829	2.24e-11	2	rs3755319	1.03e-07	2	rs887829	4.49e-12	2	rs887829	1.74e-12
2	rs4148325	2.54e-09	2	rs4148325	7.30e-11	19	rs4239638	3.74e-07	2	rs4148325	8.81e-12	2	rs4148325	4.60e-12
2	rs6742078	4.87e-09	2	rs6742078	1.32e-10	19	rs7257832	4.52e-07	2	rs6742078	5.13e-11	2	rs6742078	1.69e-11
2	rs4148324	1.04e-08	2	rs4148324	3.11e-10	2	rs4663333	4.68e-07	2	rs4148324	1.02e-10	2	rs929596	2.48e-11
2	rs10179091	1.63e-08	2	rs929596	3.39e-10	2	rs4663967	5.17e-07	2	rs4148324	1.05e-10	2	rs4148324	4.39e-11
2	rs3771341	3.07e-08	2	rs3771341	3.89e-10	2	rs4399719	8.00e-07	2	rs3771341	3.36e-10	2	rs3771341	6.07e-11
2	rs929596	3.63e-08	2	rs10179091	3.15e-09	2	rs4124874	1.03e-06	2	rs17862875	6.46e-09	2	rs17862875	2.92e-09
2	rs3755319	4.34e-08	2	rs17862875	1.56e-08	2	rs4663965	1.48e-06	2	rs10179091	2.48e-08	2	rs10179091	1.01e-08
2	rs4148326	6.53e-08	2	rs2221198	2.04e-08	2	rs6431628	2.17e-06	2	rs4148326	6.00e-08	2	rs4148326	5.80e-08
2	rs2221198	1.34e-07	2	rs4663969	2.24e-08	11	rs1560994	2.50e-06	2	rs2221198	1.86e-07	2	rs2221198	6.47e-08
2	rs4663969	1.93e-07	2	rs3755319	2.38e-08	2	rs17862866	2.77e-06	2	rs4663969	2.68e-07	2	rs3755319	7.48e-08
2	rs4663967	2.43e-07	2	rs4148326	2.73e-08	2	rs3806597	2.96e-06	2	rs16862202	2.69e-07	2	rs7604115	7.53e-08
2	rs4663333	2.81e-07	2	rs7604115	2.94e-08	2	rs2008595	3.90e-06	2	rs7556676	4.01e-07	2	rs4663969	7.94e-08
2	rs7556676	2.84e-07	2	rs7556676	3.05e-08	2	rs4294999	3.91e-06	2	rs7604115	4.46e-07	2	rs7556676	1.15e-07
2	rs871514	4.07e-07	2	rs871514	4.00e-08	10	rs7915217	4.02e-06	19	rs8111761	2.67e-06	2	rs4663967	2.53e-07
2	rs4294999	4.80e-07	2	rs4663967	5.55e-08	2	rs871514	4.12e-06	7	rs1395381	2.80e-06	2	rs4663333	2.58e-07
2	rs4663965	5.48e-07	2	rs4663333	5.97e-08	2	rs4663963	4.63e-06	3	rs9310867	4.57e-06	2	rs871514	2.87e-07
2	rs4399719	5.65e-07	2	rs4294999	6.26e-08	19	rs8108083	4.68e-06	12	rs7303705	4.87e-06	14	rs2353726	3.55e-07
2	rs3806597	6.46e-07	2	rs4663965	1.16e-07	6	rs199634	5.13e-06	4	rs3866838	5.14e-06	2	rs4294999	4.28e-07
2	rs7604115	6.46e-07	2	rs4663963	1.33e-07	19	rs2377572	5.64e-06	9	rs7847905	5.53e-06	2	rs4663965	5.99e-07

Note: CHR, chromosome; SNP, single nucleotide polymorphism.

= 1.69 × 10^{-9}) in the recessive and categorical Models, respectively, but was ranked much lower in the other model specifications (346688th using the correlation of PSRs, 1924th in additive, 90918th in dominant).

These results are fairly consistent with extensive simulations in which we generated data under different scenarios (additive, dominant, recessive, and nonlinear; and with different minor allele frequencies) and investigated the power of the correlation of PSRs to detect associations under the various scenarios (Wanga 2014). The correlation of PSRs had greater power to detect associations than the recessive and dominant models (except, of course, when the data were generated under these models). The correlation of PSRs did well when the true association was additive, resulting in only a slight loss of power when compared with models that were correctly specified as additive. However, the correlation of PSRs struggled to detect associations generated under the recessive model; categorical models were better at detecting these recessive associations and even additive models performed as well as the correlation of PSRs in the recessive case. Hence, although it is certainly reasonable to analyze GWAS data using the correlation of PSRs, the benefits of this approach are not as apparent in this setting as in some others. This is somewhat expected: with only three categories, the loss of power by treating ordinal SNP data as categorical is likely minimal.

9.5 Discussion

We have described a new residual, the probability-scale residual, and demonstrated its use for diagnostics and inference in several settings using actual HIV data. We believe the PSR should be the go-to residual for the analysis of ordered categorical data and semiparametric transformation models fit to continuous data. The PSR is also useful in many other settings that are illustrated elsewhere [see Shepherd et al. (2016)], including time-to-event outcomes. In some of these settings, existing residuals are available that offer similar information to the PSR. However, as seen in Section 9.3.2, there are advantages to having a residual that is defined across multiple classes of models, as residuals on the same scale become easier to directly compare fit across model classes. Because it is bounded between −1 and 1, the PSR is poor at detecting outliers. (It should be noted that in some analyses [e.g., semiparametric transformation models and quantile regression] the analysis model down weights the influence of outliers, so residual plots that are dominated by "outliers" are actually inconsistent with the model that was fit and may not be desirable.) If outlier detection is desired, a simple transformation of the PSRs (e.g., $\Phi^{-1}\{(PSR + 1)/2\}$ with $\Phi^{-1}(\cdot)$ denoting the inverse CDF of the standard normal distribution) allows their detection.

There are certainly other diagnostics for which residuals more specialized than the PSR might be more appropriate.

The extension of Spearman's rank correlation to adjust for covariates using the correlation of PSRs is an important development. In many settings, researchers are not interested in regression coefficients, but would like a simple, single-number summary of the strength of relationship between variables, after controlling for other variables, that is given in a constant scale regardless of the type of outcome. Our definition of Spearman's partial rank correlation provides such a summary measure, and it estimates a sensible population parameter.

The examples described in this chapter have focused on univariate outcomes. Of particular interest would be whether some of these approaches could be of value with multivariate data, for example, in the analysis of repeated measures data. We are also interested in examining the utility of Spearman's partial rank correlation using PSRs where at least one of the outcomes is a time-to-event. These represent areas of future research.

Acknowledgments

We would like to thank Vikrant Sahasrabuddhe, John Koethe, and the AIDS Clinical Trials Group for giving us permission to use their data. This work was funded in part by the National Institutes of Health, grant numbers R01 AI93234 and P30 AI110527.

References

Brockett, P. L. and Levine, A. (1977). On a characterization of ridits. *Annals of Statistics*, 5:1245–1248.

Bross, I. D. J. (1958). How to use ridit analysis. *Biometrics*, 14:18–38.

Cox, D. R. and Snell, E. J. (1968). A general definition of residuals. *Journal of the Royal Statistical Society: Series B*, 30:248–275.

David, F. N. and Johnson, N. L. (1948). The probability integral transformation when parameters are estimated from the sample. *Biometrika*, 35:182–190.

Davison, A. C. and Tsai, C. L. (1992). Regression model diagnostics. *International Statistical Review*, 60:337–353.

Dunn, P. K. and Smyth, G. K. (1996). Randomized quantile residuals. *Journal of Computational and Graphical Statistics*, 5(3):236–244.

Gijbels, I., Veraverbeke, N., and Omelka, M. (2011). Conditional copulas, association measures, and their applications. *Computational Statistics and Data Analysis*, 55:1919–1932.

Gripenberg, G. (1992). Confidence intervals for partial rank correlations. *Journal of the American Statistical Association*, 87:546–551.

Harrell, F. E. (2015). *Regression Modeling Strategies: With Applications to Linear Models, Logistic and Ordinal Regression, and Survival Analysis*. New York: Springer.

Kendall, M. G. (1942). Partial rank correlation. *Biometrika*, 32:277–283.

Koethe, J. R., Jenkins, C. A., Petucci, C., Culver, J., Shepherd, B. E., and Sterling, T. R. (2016). Superior glucose tolerance and metabolomic profiles, independent of adiposity, in HIV-infected women compared to men on antiretroviral therapy. *Medicine*, 95:e3634.

Kruskal, W. H. (1958). Ordinal measures of association. *Journal of the American Statistical Association*, 53:814–861.

Li, C. and Shepherd, B. E. (2010). Test of association between two ordinal variables while adjusting for covariates. *Journal of the American Statistical Association*, 105(490):612–620.

Li, C. and Shepherd, B. E. (2012). A new residual for ordinal outcomes. *Biometrika*, 99:473–480.

Liu, Q., Shepherd, B. E., Wanga, V., and Li, C. (2017). Covariate-adjusted Spearman's rank correlation with probability-scale residuals. *Submitted*.

Neslehova, J. (2007). On rank correlation measures for non-continuous random variables. *Journal of Multivariate Analysis*, 98:544–567.

Parham, G. P., Sahasrabuddhe, V. V., Mwanahamuntu, M. H., Shepherd, B. E., Hicks, M. L., Stringer, E. M., and Vermund, S. H. (2006). Prevalence and predictors of squamous intraepithelial lesions of the cervix in HIV-infected women in Lusaka, Zambia. *Gynecologic Oncology*, 103:1017–1022.

Pearson, E. S. (1938). The probability integral transformation for testing goodness of fit and combining independent tests of significance. *Biometrika*, 30:134–148.

Shepherd, B. E., Li, C., and Liu, Q. (2016). Probability-scale residuals for continuous, discrete, and censored data. *Canadian Journal of Statistics*, 44:463–479.

Wanga, V. (2014). *Residual-based Test of Conditional Association between Continuous and Ordinal Variables with Application to Genome-wide Association Studies*. Vanderbilt University Thesis.

Wanga, V., Venuto, C., Morse, G. D., Acosta, E. P., Daar, E. S., Haas, D. W., Li, C., and Shepherd, B. E. (2015). Genome-wide association study of tenofovir pharmacokinetics and creatinine clearance in AIDS Clinical Trials Group Protocol A5202. *Pharmacogenetics and Genomics*, 25:450–461.

Zeng, D. and Lin, D. (2007). Maximum likelihood estimation in semiparametric regression models with censored data. *Journal of the Royal Statistical Society: Series B*, 69:507–564.

Zhang, H., Wang, X., and Ye, Y. (2006). Detection of genes for ordinal traits in nuclear families and a unified approach for association studies. *Genetics*, 172(1):693–699.

Section III

Quantitative Methods for Dynamical Models and Computer Simulations

10

Simulation Modeling of HIV Infection—From Individuals to Risk Groups and Entire Populations

Georgiy Bobashev

Center for Data Science, RTI International, Research Triangle Park, NC

CONTENTS

10.1 Introduction

This chapter provides a brief overview of methods used for modeling HIV in human populations. It is not intended to be a comprehensive review of the models (which are numerous) but rather a description of major modeling approaches and illustrations of how each has been applied to HIV research.

Because of the chronic nature of HIV and the strong behavioral aspect associated with its spread, understanding and controlling HIV spread is complex. Two behavior-related HIV transmission pathways are most prominent: unprotected sexual contact and sharing injecting equipment.[1,2] These risky behaviors adapt to interventions in sometimes unexpected ways (e.g., the success of antiretroviral therapy [ART] can reduce the stigma of HIV and increase unprotected sex), and a straightforward causal relationship might not work as intended.[3,4]

Modeling is needed and is broadly used to forecast potential behavior outcomes and specific intervention impacts because natural experiments can be too long, costly, unethical, and often impossible to conduct. For example, to understand the impact of male circumcision it is necessary not just to estimate intervention efficacy but to understand how the intervention would be effective when implemented at the country level.[5]

The need for modeling goes beyond long-term forecasting at the population level. Modeling is often used to interpret data, understand the causal process, and develop and evaluate interventions.[6] The history of HIV research illustrates a long and controversial process of understanding the impact of the disease and ways to fight it. Decisions were sometimes made based on moral and nonscientific mental models. For example, the belief that HIV is a "punishment" for "sinful" behavior led to an erroneous mental model that was translated into public health inactivity, eventually resulting in thousands of premature and avoidable deaths.[7,8] Another example is AIDS denialism in South Africa, which was based on a flawed mental model of AIDS causality. As the biology and epidemiology of HIV/AIDS became better understood, mathematical models reflected and often summarized the current state of knowledge, from the first models developed by Kaplan for injecting drugs and Blower for sexual transmission[9,10] to current sophisticated agent-based models (ABMs) used to forecast HIV prevalence and incidence in the United States and around the world.[11,12] Models can influence policy by filling in evidence gaps that clinical trials cannot directly address, such as cost-effectiveness and long-term, population-level impact of interventions, including replacement of standard syringes with low dead space syringes, provision of free voluntary male medical circumcision, and the expansion of needle exchange programs.[5,13,14]

Modeling takes many forms, including mental and statistical models, system dynamics (SD), and microsimulations, and thus can be confusing. This chapter provides a distinction between these types of models and illustrates how they all can be used in HIV research.

The rest of the chapter consists of two parts and a discussion: The first part provides an overview of modeling methods and highlights the importance and advantages of each method. The second part provides examples of models that illustrate modeling utility. Finally, future trends and research directions are discussed.

10.2 Modeling Methodology

A number of approaches and methods have been used in modeling HIV. Because there is no firm classification of modeling methods, here we attempt to classify existing approaches, illustrate their application to a number of HIV problems, and describe the relative advantages of each approach. Specifically we consider statistical, Markov, SD, microsimulations (e.g., discrete events), and ABMs (Figure 10.1). At the higher level, statistical, Markov, and SD models do not distinguish between individuals in populations and describe populations (or subpopulations) as a whole. As the names suggest, microsimulation models and ABMs describe each individual in the population and thus can be averaged across specific characteristics to obtain population-level estimates.

Each subsequent approach in the sequence adds more capabilities and complexity to the implementation. More complex approaches also require more parameters and more data to back them.

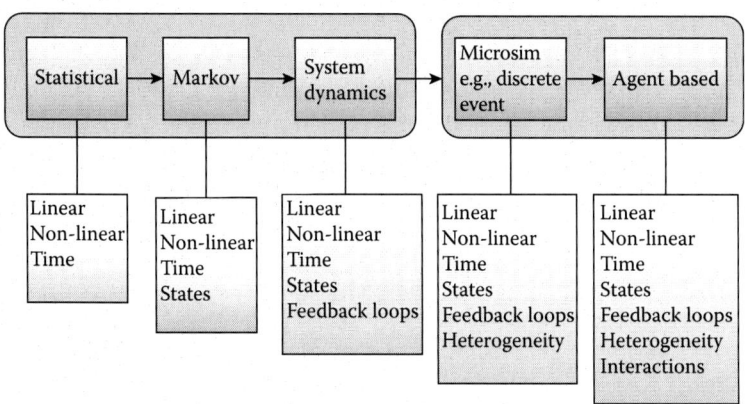

FIGURE 10.1
Predictive modeling approaches.

10.3 Statistical Models

Statistical models commonly focus on three major tasks:

1. Estimation of some quantity (e.g., prevalence, incidence, size of an association)
2. Hypothesis testing (e.g., test of association)
3. Prediction/forecast (e.g., given the effect of the intervention, how many lives could be saved)

Although the tasks can be different in nature, statistical models are based on a fundamental set of assumptions that are quite common and often ignored in model description. The key assumption is that individuals are independent and identically distributed following some often-known distribution. This assumption is convenient because it allows one to use well-established statistical theory.

In reality, however, individuals are often not independent from each other, are not identically distributed, and sometimes the distributions are quite complex and multimodal. A number of methods have been used to address these issues, for example, generalized estimating equations and hierarchical linear models to address within-cluster correlations.[15–17] Mixture models are used to address multimodal distributions,[18] and nonparametric methods are used to deal with nonstandardized distributions.[19]

Another common assumption is linearity, which means that the sum of two independent variables will result in the sum of the proportional (linear) sum of the dependent variable or effects. This assumption is extremely useful and leads to elegant theories but is often wrong and misleading. For example, the effect of age on sexual risk is nonlinear because humans are mostly active during certain age intervals. Nonlinearly shaped effects are commonly seen in pharmacology. As a drug dose gradually increases, the therapeutic effect is improved, but as the dose gets too high, toxicity and other effects start overweighing the positive effect of the drug. Similar effects can be observed with public health interventions (e.g., increased taxation on tobacco products). Statistical method can deal with nonlinearity by either explicitly adding interactions or high-order terms[19] or by the use of nonparametric models such as smoothing splines.[19]

Statistical models can handle changes in time and describe dynamically changing effects. This can be achieved by either explicitly including time as a covariate in the model or by using time series modeling tools such as auto-regressive integrated moving average to describe temporal relationships and project into the future.[20]

Modeling tasks used in estimation deal with past, existing data and usually make inferences about the population from a given sample. The results of these tasks are usually parameter estimates obtained from the data. A prediction task focuses on the opposite problem: given the model and estimated parameters, what would future data look like? In this sense predictions made by models are based on some form of "what if" and "what is likely" scenarios. Because it is not possible to predict the future exactly, each prediction contains a certain degree of uncertainty. This uncertainty is larger than that associated with the estimation of model parameters. Below we illustrate this in an example of a linear regression.

Consider a hypothetical association model with the outcome y (e.g., number of unprotected sex acts per month) and an independent variable x, such as the amount of funds spent on a successful intervention in many experimental regions.

The strength of the association will be measured by fitting an ordinary regression with normally distributed error terms (ignore nonlinearities for now).

$$y \sim N(\hat{\beta}_0 + \hat{\beta}_1 x_1, \sigma^2)$$

The variance of the residual (unexplained variation) in this model is denoted by σ^2.

This model can now be used to predict (simulate) a new number of unprotected sex acts after the intervention has been broadly implemented with increased funds x^*. The new mean estimated number $\hat{y}$ then is predicted as

$$\hat{y} = \hat{\beta}_0 + \hat{\beta}_1 x_1{}^*$$

The variance of the prediction $y = \hat{y} + \varepsilon$ will now become

$$Var(\hat{y} + \varepsilon) = Var(\hat{\beta}_0 + \hat{\beta}_1 x_1{}^* + \varepsilon) = \sigma^2 + \sigma^2 \left(\frac{1}{n} + \frac{(x^* - \bar{x})^2}{S_{xx}} \right)$$

The total variance of the prediction now consists of three components: (1) model uncertainty obtained from the fitted equation σ^2, (2) the uncertainty associated with the imperfect estimate of the association coefficient, and (3) the uncertainty associated with distance from the mean. This third term is a critical component of model-based prediction. The best prediction is achieved around the mean; the further one moves from that mean, the less accuracy is achieved.

In this exercise we made another implicit assumption: that the model will remain correct forever and for all values of x and y. This assumption might be justifiable for models in biology where biological processes remain relatively stable (within the evolutionary scale), but it is often not the case in social science because the governing rules of society and behavior change over time. Thus when presenting and discussing predictive models, it is important to keep in mind that uncertainty is *model-based* (i.e., assumes that the model is correct). One should consider a critical view when "trusting" the model; this is relevant to all predictive models described here.

When simulating potential outcomes from a statistical model, a traditional approach is first to estimate the model parameters and then to generate new data using the predicted values of the mean and estimated uncertainty. The type of distribution depends on the modeling assumptions and physical limitations. For example, a normal approximation can be used when estimating nonnegative outcomes; however, simulated data cannot be negative, and thus some adjustments (e.g., considerations of Poisson or Gamma distribution) are necessary. A new simulated dataset thus can be of an arbitrary size and used for further analysis.

Traditionally, the quality of predictive models is assessed by validating them on a dataset not used in model building. This could be done through cross-validation (a popular one is k-fold), splitting the sample into training and test sets, and validating on a completely new dataset (e.g., from a different study, population). In k-fold cross-validation, a dataset is randomly split into k equal subsets, then the model is sequentially fitted to $k - 1$ of them and validated on the remaining subset. Thus the model never uses the same data for fitting and validation, but all observations are used in validation. Model building is often an iterative process that has to address overoptimism (i.e., overfitting) when a model well fitted to one dataset provides poor prediction of independent data. Regularization methods (e.g., ridge regression, least absolute shrinkage and selection operator [LASSO]) provide ways to reduce such overoptimism.[19]

Although statistical models can be quite powerful, they contain a number of limitations that require the use of different types of models. One limitation is that statistical models do not consider multiple states in which an individual can exist. Using an example from HIV, an individual can be not infected, be infected in the acute stage, be infected in the latent stage, have AIDS, or be partially recovered if on ART. A single statistical model cannot describe the dynamics of transition between stages, and thus special models describing such transitions are needed.

10.4 State Transition and Markov Models

When an individual can be in different states (e.g., not infected, infected, partially recovered), probabilities of being in specific states and times until transition to a different stage are described by dynamic transition models. A simple form of such models is a Markov model, which assumes that the transition to a different state only depends on the state in which a person is and does not depend on the history (i.e., how the person got to that stage).

When there is only one direction of transition (e.g., from being not infected to infected/acute stage, latent stage, and end stage, i.e., AIDS),[21–23] each transition can be described by a sequence of survival models. However, when stages can recur, such as with the introduction of ART, an individual can move from being on ART to not on ART and thus from being partially recovered back to the latent or end stage.[24] A common example of a Markov model is a change in sexual partnership. For example, an individual can have zero, one, two, or more partners at any time, which can define specific states and the transitions between them.[25] A transition process can be defined at the individual level (e.g., an individual is passing through the stages) and at the population level. The former is used in microsimulations including ABMs, which are described later in this chapter. In the latter case the population is divided into compartments, each containing individuals in a specific state. As individuals move between states, the number of individuals (and thus population proportions) in each compartment also changes. If the model considers N states, then there can be maximum $N^*(N - 1)$ transitions (i.e., from each state to each other state). Each transition is usually described by a probability of transition within a given time interval, which can be interpreted as a proportion of individuals making such a transition. Some proportion of individuals does not leave the state during the given time interval, and the sum of probabilities of leaving and staying has to be equal to 1. As can be shown mathematically, transition probabilities over time can be translated into average waiting times in each of the states.[26] As an example, consider a hypothetical population at risk in which individuals can be in three states: not injecting drugs, injecting but not sharing syringes, and injecting and sharing. Each stage is associated with different risks of HIV, and there are six transitions between each of the states. Each month individuals can move between stages. Transition probabilities between states are defined in terms of a unit of time (e.g., a month). After the states, time interval, and transitions are defined, the model can be used to simulate trajectories of injecting and sharing by starting with initial population proportions and then iterating the model many times. In the simplest case the transition probabilities do not change and do not depend on history. At each time step, a Markov model that simulates the population proportions at time n + 1 can be written in a matrix form as

$$X_{n+1} = AX_n$$

where n denotes the proportion of the population in each of the states to be described by a three-component vector X_n and A is a 3 x 3 matrix of transition probabilites.

Assume that weekly transition probabilities between the states are represented by the following matrix:

$$A = \begin{bmatrix} 0.9 & 0.075 & 0.25 \\ 0.15 & 0.8 & 0.05 \\ 0.25 & 0.25 & 0.5 \end{bmatrix}.$$

Under general conditions such Markov models asymptotically reach the steady state (i.e., further iterations do not change the population proportions). The steady state for this population becomes X_∞ = [0.63, 0.31, 0.06] (i.e., 63% will not inject, 31% will inject but not share, and 6% will inject and share syringes with others).

More complex models would describe each of the transitions as a function of demographics and other factors. Interventions are modeled as modifications to the transition probabilities that in turn change the dynamics of population proportion and alter the steady state.

Markov models can be described in continuous time (i.e., rather than modeling transition probabilities over a prespecified time interval, the probabilities change continuously and the rate of change is used instead of actual probabilities). A good summary of the different forms of Markov models and the relationships between them may be found in Tuckwell.[26]

Although modeling states and transitions are an improvement over statistical models, these models are not well equipped to deal with adaptive behavior that changes the structure of the transition matrices. For example, with the increase in ART, quality of life among HIV patients can increase, reducing the stigma of HIV, which in turn can lead to an increase in risky behavior, leading to higher incidence. An SD approach to modeling accounts for various potential responses.

10.5 System Dynamics

SD models provide a flexible approach to modeling population processes. As with Markov models, SD models consider states and population flows between states. However, SD models additionally consider events that can affect each other in sequence or simultaneously, thus creating "feedback." SD models are represented with differential equations when time is considered continuous or with difference equations for discrete time. For example, the dynamics of HIV infection in a network of injectors could be described with a simple difference equation, with the time unit considered a month:[13]

$$I(t+1) = I(t) + \Delta I(t)_{inside} + \Delta I(t)_{outside} - r^* I(t)$$

where ΔI_{inside} and $\Delta I_{outside}$ are the numbers of newly infected individuals who were infected by sharing a syringe with a "buddy" from the same network or with a stranger from another network, respectively, and $r^* I(t)$ is the number of infected individuals who have been removed either because of death or other reasons. Assuming that all members of the cluster have an equal chance to share, the equation for newly infected injecting drug users who get infected by their buddies becomes:

$$\Delta I(t)_{inside} = S(t)^* G^* \left(1 - (1-P)^{C_{inside}}\right)$$

where $S(t)$ is the number of susceptible individuals in the network, G is the proportion of the network participating in sharing at each particular sharing event, P is the probability of HIV transmission through a sharing episode, and C_{inside} is the number of times a susceptible individual shared with an HIV-infected person in a month. Introduction of affordable ART increases the survival of infected individuals (which increases $I(t)$ because of the lower mortality) but also reduces viral load and thus reduces the probability of transmission P, which in turn reduces the incidence $\Delta I(t)$.

SD models explicitly describe relationships between events that are usually represented with SD diagrams (see Figure 10.2).[27]

SD models can consider how history affects future transitions and feedback loops. For example, the introduction of ART to treat HIV can lead to the emergence of resistant traits. ART also leads to the reduction in stigma, which in turn can lead to an increase in risky behavior and, as a consequence, an increase in incidence.[4]

An SD model can contain a number of models linked to each other. For example, in Granich et al.,[24] the model contains states associated with HIV-related epidemiological states (susceptible, HIV infected in acute, latent,

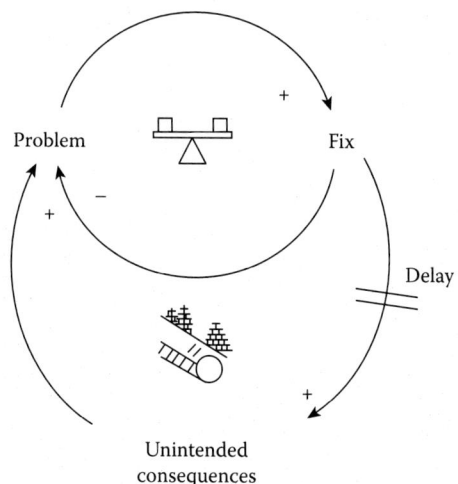

FIGURE 10.2
A system dynamics (SD) process where a mitigating solution to a problem (balancing process) can also lead to delayed unintended consequences that in turn aggravate the problem (problem reinforcing process).

and AIDS states) but also with the state of government support to specific interventions: ART availability, condom distribution, prevention education, needle exchange, and so on. Transitions between stages depend on state support for specific interventions.[24]

As comprehensive as they can be, SD models become very cumbersome when the population is highly heterogeneous (structured) and each subgroup requires its own model. For example, HIV transmission can be different in heterosexual versus homosexual versus bisexual subgroups. Different dynamics can also occur among sex workers, drug users (separate for injecting drug users and non-injecting users), geographic locations, and so on. As the number of factors to consider grows, the granularity of SD models increases and the models become very cumbersome. When the number of subgroups becomes large, the number of parameters that require estimation grows geometrically, and it becomes more and more difficult to obtain or find parameter estimates for all subgroups and between them, especially when some subgroups become very small.

Another limitation is that individuals within each compartment are considered homogeneously mixed. Often interactions between individuals are critical to the correct description of the process, and other, individual-level, models are needed.

10.6 Individual-Based (Microsimulation, Agent-Based) Models and Synthetic Populations

The language defining individual-based models is not consistent, with the terms *multi-agent model*, *individual-based model*, and *microsimulation* often used interchangeably. In this chapter we call any model that tracks individuals rather than populations an *individual-based model* or, interchangeably, a *microsimulation*. The term *ABM* often implies an interaction between entities. For example, in a microsimulation model for colorectal cancer,[28] life trajectories are modeled for each individual in a cohort. Because these trajectories are independent, there is no statistical difference, regardless of whether a cohort of 10,000 subjects is run simultaneously or a single-subject model is run 10,000 times, with each run corresponding to a different individual in a cohort. Such models are often used to simulate chronic diseases.[28] When simulating an infectious process, such as HIV spread, it is necessary to consider interactions between infected and uninfected subjects such as an unprotected sexual act or an act of syringe sharing. In the gray area remain models where interaction between subjects is implicit (e.g., when subjects do not interact with each other explicitly but rather their activity is controlled by a limiting resource). For example, consider a cohort of noninteracting HIV patients, each experiencing an individual course of the disease. Such a model can be considered a non–agent-based microsimulation. However, if the amount of ART is limited, and the distribution depends on individual needs and actions, it would be incorrect to run the model one person at a time. Whether such a model should be called an *agent-based* or *discrete event* or something else is a matter of semantics.[29] The personal choice of the author is to call such a model an *ABM*; however, these are all individual-based or microsimulation models.

A central part of an ABM is an individual agent, which can be in specific states and move between states. These states are usually described by state diagrams, which can look exactly like a corresponding Markov model for the population. The major difference is that at each point in time an individual is only in one state, whereas in the population-level Markov model each state can contain a number of individuals. An individual can belong to a number of independent state diagrams, for example, one related to sexual partnership (no sexual partners, having enough partners, looking for more partners, etc.) and another related to disease progression (e.g., not infected, infected non-AIDS, AIDS) (Figure 10.3a and b).

Bershteyn et al.[30,31] present an individual-based epidemic model called *EMOD* with age-specific sexual mixing patterns. These patterns were configured to match those observed in a rural, HIV-hyperendemic region of KwaZulu-Natal, South Africa. Recently, a validation study showed self-reported partner ages in this setting to be relatively accurate, with 72% of

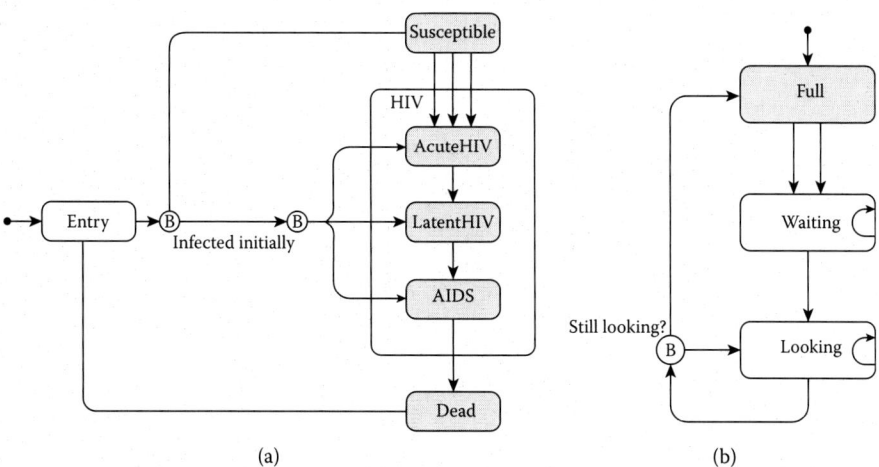

(a)   (b)

FIGURE 10.3
Individual state transition diagrams. (a) Disease diagram: A person can acquire HIV in three ways: through unprotected vaginal or anal sex with an infected individual or by injecting with the same syringe after an infected person. (b) State diagram describing partner change: An individual can have enough partners (full) or break up with a partner and after waiting for some time start looking for another partner until finding enough partners.

self-reported estimates falling within 2 years of the partner's actual date of birth.[32] Such data and validations are relatively rare in HIV research because of the sensitive nature of the subject and cost associated with collecting and validating such data.

Another important feature of ABMs is that they can explicitly account for heterogeneous migration patterns and different ways migrants can get involved in the HIV transmission process within and between countries and regions. A model of migration in the EMOD ABM model[30,31] is depicted in Figure 10.4.

Agents can interact with each other and with the environment and pass infection (e.g., HIV) and information (word-of-mouth spread of a preventive message). Although a number of simulation techniques exist,[29] a commonly used approach in HIV simulation is to update the status of each individual at each time step. Another approach is to calculate the time that the next dynamically relevant event will occur in the model (such as a coital act, death, or uptake of an intervention that could modify transmission rates), increment the simulation clock by the precise time elapsed until the event, and then simulate the event. However, this approach is not widely used. When the population size is large (e.g., the entire country) one needs to consider computational burden. Even with the advantages of modern technologies, the increased complexity and scale of ABM can create new computational challenges.

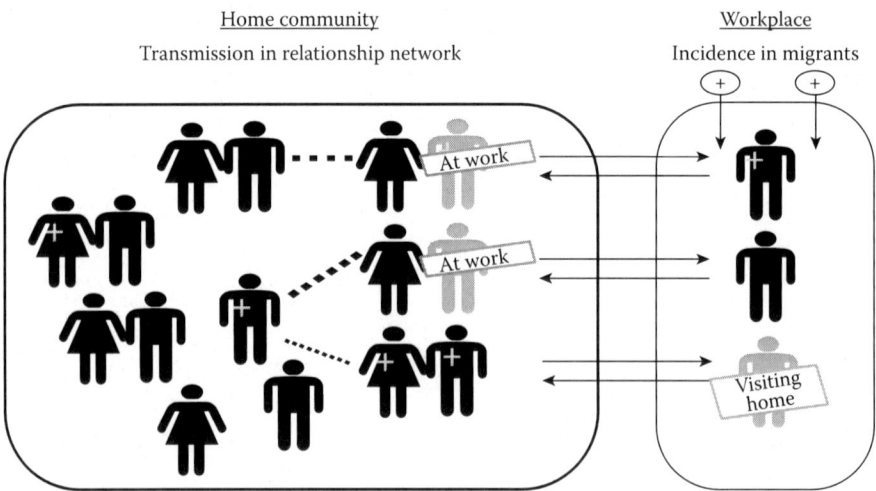

FIGURE 10.4

Migration diagram describing heterosexual HIV transmission among migrant workers and their partners. (Adapted from Bershteyn A, et al., *Int. Health,* 2016;8(4):277–285; Bershteyn A, et al., Description of the EMOD-HIV Model v0.7, http://arxiv.org/pdf/1206.3720.pdf. Accessed October 17, 2016.)

ABMs have at least three major advantages. First, they allow for a description of local dynamics. Policy is defined globally, but it is realized locally. Using synthetic populations to describe neighborhoods and local dynamics is a rapidly developing area. An example and details of such synthetic populations may be found at RTI's synthetic population viewer portal,[33] described later in the chapter. Second, ABMs allow one to add social network structures (sexual, injecting, support, and others). Third, they allow for a more correct representation of nonlinear relationships than population-averaged models. This feature is well known in mathematics as *Jensen's inequality* (i.e., the mean of the nonlinear function is likely to be different from the nonlinear function of the mean). Depending on whether the function is concave or convex, the inequality goes in one direction or another. Consider a variable X distributed normally with the mean zero and standard deviation 1 and consider a quadratic function $Y = X^2$. The square of the variable's mean will remain zero (as zero squared), whereas the mean of the squared function Y has to be positive. In fact, it follows a chi-square distribution with the mean equal to 1. A simple illustration is reproduced in Figure 10.5.

Compartmental SD models first estimate the values of the population-level parameters and then apply them to potentially nonlinear functions that simulate population flows. Individual-based models conversely track each individual first and then average over the population of simulated individuals to obtain a result. This latter approach thus more correctly describes the real-life process.

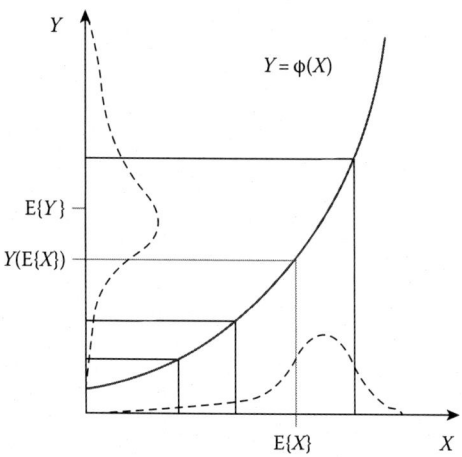

FIGURE 10.5
Illustration of Jensen's inequality for a probabilistic case. The dashed curve along the x-axis is the hypothetical distribution of X, whereas the dashed curve along the y-axis is the corresponding distribution of Y values. The convex mapping $Y(X)$ increasingly "stretches" the distribution for increasing values of X. (From Wikipedia, Jensen's Inequality, https://en.wikipedia.org/wiki/Jensen's_inequality.)

A good overview of individual-based simulation models is provided in Abuelezam et al.[35] This paper also attempts to provide guidance to reporting of HIV-specific individual-based models. A more general protocol to design and report individual-based models was developed by Grimm et al.[36,37] and is widely accepted as a good practice standard. The protocol is called *overview, design concepts, and detail* (ODD) and contains checklists of reportable items within the respective ODD subsections. The ODD protocol provides a way to standardize model reporting, review, and reproducibility. This becomes especially important when the models contain a large number of interrelated components, making them difficult to reproduce.

Individual-based models, however, pose a number of serious and often impossible challenges for researchers. The biggest challenge is usually the lack of appropriately measured behavioral parameters. For individual-based models, each individual's behavior is governed by a set of parameters. Often these parameters are assumed to come from some distribution, which is estimated from the population sample. For multiple parameters it is also critical to understand whether they are independent or correlated to each other. For example, in a model of the impact of different syringe types of HIV spread,[13] knowledge of the actual network structure would probably change the actual numerical values of the results. However, the qualitative assessment might remain very similar. Depending on the purpose of the models and the results of sensitivity analysis, one should make decisions about spending large amounts of money to improve the model's numerical values, as opposed to conducting inexpensive qualitative assessment of a simple model.

Another challenge is model validation. Many models can only be validated at the macro level, which means that with a large number of parameters many models, even those that have opposite assumptions, can be calibrated to the same set of data. In this sense models only provide suggestive plausible solutions and should not be taken as the ultimate truth.

━━━━━━━

10.7 Synthetic Populations

Synthetic populations are representations of every household and person in a population and provide a way to understand local models and the dynamics of local and global disease. They are produced in a dataset with each individual's coordinates and characteristics. Synthetic populations can be considered as a "scrambled" census. Specifically, at the aggregate level a statistic matches that of the census; however, at the household and individual levels, the data are drawn from a complex multivariate distribution. Besides demographics, individuals are probabilistically assigned characteristics such as job availability and distance to clinics, schools, and ART treatment. One of the first and most comprehensive synthetic populations was developed at RTI

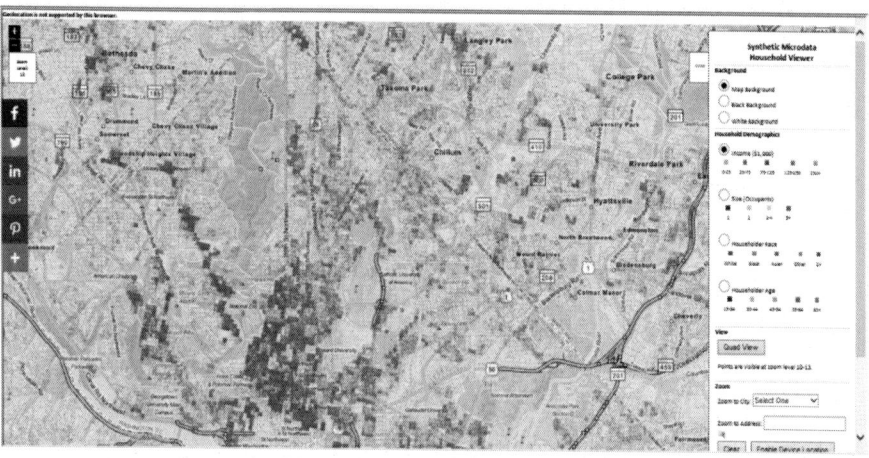

FIGURE 10.6
A synthetic population is a geospatial dataset that maps the highly heterogeneous nature of human population distributions. The figure shows distributions of households by income in the Washington, DC, area (see RTI's synthetic population viewer portal 2016 at synthpopviewer.rti.org).[33]

to represent the United States (Figure 10.6), with subsequent development representing Indonesia, China, India, Mexico, Pakistan, and more.[33] Because synthetic populations provide a rich source of realistic (e.g., matching census data) microdata, they are used to initiate the "agents" in agent-based (individual-based) models and have been used by government and academia, for example, the Framework for Reconstructing Epidemiological Dynamics.[38]

10.7.1 Future Population Projections

The US Census is run about every 10 years, and information about demographics can change over time. Thus, the synthetic population needs to be adjusted during the between-census years. Future Population Projections (FPOP) serves this purpose and is a dynamic, discrete-time microsimulation that incorporates linkages between life events, changes in household structure, and changes in the attributes of individuals and their location as part of the aging process. The life events that modify households and populations include aging, mortality, birth, marriage/union formation and dissolution, and migration. The occurrence of life events for each individual at each discrete time step is determined stochastically by transition probabilities that subsequently can be modified during the course of the simulation. With FPOP running in conjunction with a disease model and annually updating the synthetic population, the resulting public tool will enable us and other researchers to forecast the HIV status of individuals in local communities and entire populations under different intervention scenarios.

10.8 Uncertainty in Simulation Models

When analyzing the results of simulations it is necessary to understand the many sources of uncertainty. Figure 10.7 presents a diagram representing the sources of uncertainty in ABMs, which are selected for this example because they contain the most uncertainty components. Uncertainty in input parameters includes uncertainty from the data collected for the study (e.g., surveys). Uncertainty associated with surveys is often known and quantified based on statistical sampling theory.[39] Other parameters can be based on the *published literature* (e.g., meta-analysis), with the levels of uncertainty not as clearly addressed as in surveys but nevertheless quantifiable; on *big data* when data are available but without reference population, sampling frame, or other rigorous ways to estimate representativeness; and finally, when no other information is available, on *educated guesses* ("common sense," anecdotal evidence). To represent uncertainty, a parameter value is often drawn from a distribution; thus, formalism becomes inherently Bayesian even if the estimation methodology is frequentist.

Simulation models use random number generators to represent stochasticity and thus introduce internal model uncertainty. Distribution assumptions and the choice of simulator type can have an effect on overall uncertainty. The impact of this uncertainty can be addressed by repeating the simulations many times and analyzing the variability of the outcomes.

Structural uncertainty refers to the assumptions and implementation of the model. In addition to uncertainty in the choice of assumptions, the same assumptions can be implemented using slightly different computational algorithms. In this sense two modelers can develop differently performing models, even when following the same conceptual model.

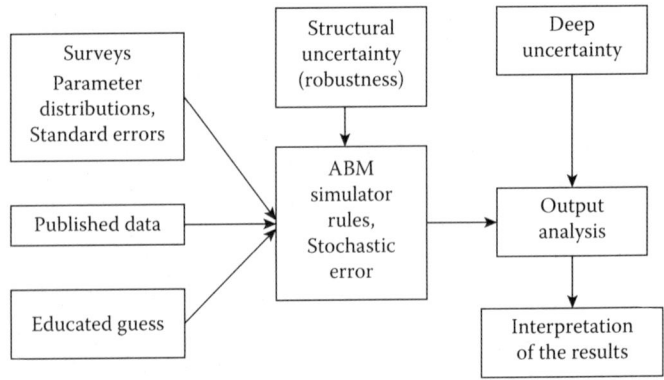

FIGURE 10.7
Sources of uncertainty in simulation models.

Deep uncertainty refers to the fact that no one can truly predict the future, and every model is just a simplification of human cognition of reality based on past experience. Thus, there are factors that one cannot foresee and model. Validation on an independent dataset is considered the gold standard for predictive models, but even such validation does not guarantee future performance. Numerous models exist to forecast stock markets, with legal disclaimers that past performance does not guarantee future returns on investment. A good illustration of such uncertainty in HIV modeling is presented in Eaton et al. 2015[12] and discussed later in this chapter.

The uncertainty associated with output analysis is related to various interpretations of measurements. For example, a Likert scale can be interpreted as continuous, ordinal, or categorical, and depending on the interpretation the results can differ. Finally, the interpretation of the same results and their presentation to policy makers (glass half full vs. half empty) can have an effect on the resulting action.

Acknowledgment of underlying uncertainties guards against blind trust in model results but also summarizes the state of knowledge and critical thinking paradigms. A high-quality model would not necessarily provide the "truth" but the best evidence- and knowledge-based assessment of the problem.

10.9 The Use of Simulation Models in Forecasting

One of the most common uses of simulation models is forecasting. It is, however, important to clearly understand all assumptions behind the forecast to interpret the results correctly. Although it is not possible to predict the future, it is possible to reduce uncertainty or to explore potential outcomes of specific actions. Simulation modeling can also allow one to explore the HIV risk of specific behaviors in a population where some individuals have HIV and others are at risk for eventual acquisition of HIV. An approach to such modeling is presented in Figure 10.8.

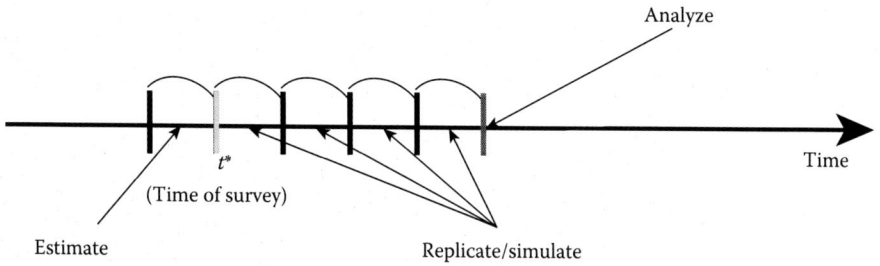

FIGURE 10.8
Simulation models in forecasting.

At time t data are collected about behavior over a past period of time (e.g., past 90 days). From that assessment, behavior and risk parameters are estimated. These parameters can include number of sex partners, rate of partner change, or network characteristics. Each individual in the simulation is then assigned an estimated behavior and either assumed to continue the same behavior or to change it according to a specific intervention. Simulation can take this projection as far as one needs (e.g., 5 years), during which period an individual can acquire HIV or die. At the end of that period, all individuals are assessed and HIV prevalence and incidence are estimated.

The advantage of this approach is that in real life it is difficult and often unethical to control behavior and require that it not change over time. This simulation allows one to evaluate behavior risk through computerized experiments. It can be used as an argument in counseling when encouraging an individual to change to a less risky behavior. By contrast, the same assumption makes the model impractical for predicting *actual* incidence and prevalence at the population level, because in real life behavior changes and often in unpredictable ways.

These arguments make the validation of HIV population models problematic. Models are often validated by predicting some independent past data. However, when the models produce long-term forecasts, the only true validation is to wait and see how well the forecast compares to new data. Even that does not guarantee the accuracy of future predictions.[12] Over a long period of time, initial assumptions that were valid when the model was built could become obsolete. For example, advances in economic development, nutrition, health care, and travel patterns can change the ways disease spreads. Nevertheless, the models provide very useful insights into epidemiology, interventions, and potential response, especially when several models are built with different assumptions and aim to forecast the same event, as was done in a comparison of 12 HIV forecasting models.[6,12]

10.10 Model Parameterization, Calibration, and Validation

A large body of literature is dedicated to the topics of parameterization, calibration, and validation. Depending on the discipline, definitions can be confusing. For example, some would use the terms *verification and validation* or *validations of first, second, and third type,* and so on. Here we provide a simple distinction between terms that could be more relevant to policy and health researchers than to computer scientists and programmers. *Parameterization* provides the model with all required parameter values accompanied by their uncertainty (ranges). It is often an iterative process and involves literature reviews, analysis of available data, and consultations with experts. When multiple sources of information are available, it is customary to present the ranges of parameter values.[40] Bayesian approaches allow one to combine information about parameters from multiple sources. For example, a prior distribution could be formed by using the means and standard errors from published studies. A posterior distribution will then be derived from updating the prior with the likelihood function from the available data using Bayesian methodology.[41] *Calibration* serves the purpose of searching the uncertainty bounds of parameters to find values that achieve best fit to known outcomes (calibration targets). Calibration allows one to estimate *working* parameter values when uncertainty is high. This stage often requires the identification of most sensitive parameters (i.e., parameters for which a small change in values can produce large changes in outcome). Validation is probably the most contested term of the three, but it commonly implies that the model has reasonably reproduced outcomes that were not used in model calibration. This approach is often viewed as a necessary rather than sufficient condition for model "trustworthiness" (i.e., if the model cannot reproduce past observation, it is not likely to be a good tool to predict future data). At the same time, if it does reproduce the past well, good future performance is not guaranteed. In many policy cases, however, a carefully developed model is the best tool available to predict future outcomes.

10.11 Modeling Applications to HIV Research Problems

10.11.1 Within-Person HIV Dynamics

Detailed models of within-person dynamics of HIV and immune response are influential in therapeutic areas for drug development and clinical purposes (e.g., Perelson & Ribeiro 2013,[43] Rivadeneira et al. 2014,[44] other chapters in this book) but go beyond the scope of this chapter. Nevertheless, the overall transition models between the stages of HIV (acute, latent, end stage) are often used in individual and population-level models.

10.11.2 Individual Behavior Risks

Mechanistically, the majority of HIV transmission from one person to another occurs through sexual contact or syringe sharing.[1] As risky behaviors accumulate so does the overall probability of transmission. Denoting the probability of HIV transmission per unprotected sex act as p, the cumulative probability P of seroconversion after N such sex acts with an HIV-positive individual becomes

$$P = 1 - (1 - p)^N$$

The model can also accommodate different probabilities of transmission for a variety of unprotected sexual activities (e.g., oral and anal sex) and syringe sharing.[45]

$$P = 1 - \prod_{i=1}^{K}(1-p_i)\prod_{j=1}^{M}(1-p_j)$$

Here M and K indicate the number of unprotected sex acts and the number of times syringes were shared. For each individual act i or j, a corresponding probability p_i or p_j would vary depending on the type of sex act, use of condoms, rinsing the syringe with bleach, and so on. A number of statistical models have been used to estimate individual risks of HIV transmission.[40,46] An example of projection of behavior into the future is presented in Figure 10.9. These estimates were used to develop a simulation model that calculates the probability of becoming HIV infected over time (e.g., in 2 years).[45] The model was applied to a cohort of discordant couples and used to identify individuals at highest risk. These models can be expanded more generally for any behavior that can potentially lead to HIV. Such a model was developed for a sample of at-risk individuals in North Carolina. Individuals at the highest risk of acquiring HIV not surprisingly either had a large number of concurrent sexual

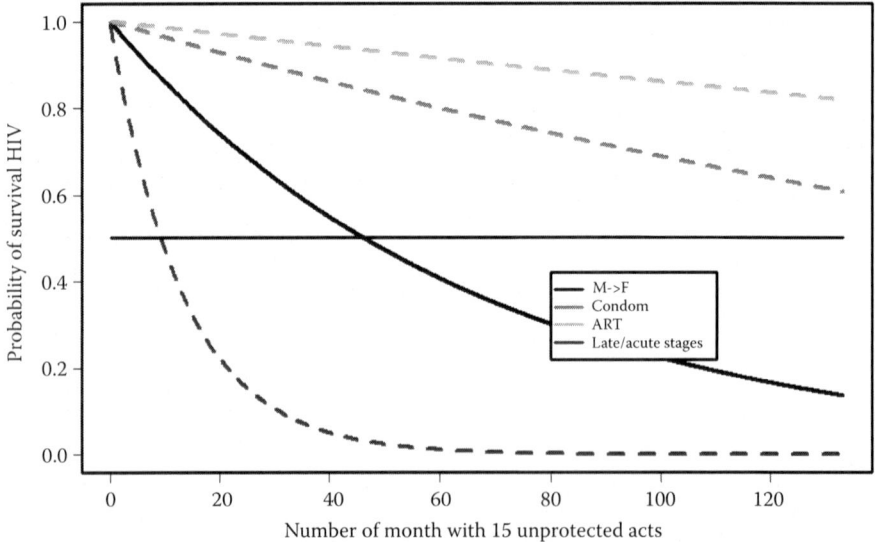

FIGURE 10.9
Projections of specific behavior into the future for male-to-female transmission in a discordant couple assuming having two unprotected sex acts per week. The model emphasizes the need for the partner to be on antiretroviral therapy (ART) to reduce the chances of HIV transmission. When a couple wants to conceive a child, having unprotected sex is critical and the main protective measures become ART and Pre-Exposure Prophylaxis (PrEP).

partners or often shared syringes with strangers.[47] Recently the CDC published a statistical risk calculator[2,48] that uses this approach to estimate the risk of HIV if the behavior does not change and the possible effects of behavior changes.

Simulations can also be used to suggest possible behavioral conditions under which certain incidence is observed. For example, when high incidence is observed in a sample but little risky behavior is reported, the question becomes one of which behaviors are not being reported.[49]

10.11.3 Risk Groups

HIV spread within risk groups has been extensively studied and modeled since the early 1990s.[10,50,51] Modeling often focuses on men who have sex with men, injecting drug users, sex workers, and prison populations in various cultural and environmental settings. The majority of these models are SD in nature, which considers mixing within and between groups. Although it has been shown that sexual and drug-using networks play an important role[52–57] in disease transmission, actual data on the structure of sexual networks and especially for drug-injecting networks are rare.[58] These structures are imposed from egocentric networks (i.e., information provided by an individual about his or her injecting and sexual partners).[52,59]

Among specific risk groups such as injecting drug users, simulation models predict the impact of high dead-space syringes on the spread and sustainability of HIV. These models allow us to estimate the impact of low dead-space syringes and potential interventions when direct measurement is not possible.[13]

The impact of interventions has been estimated in a number of ways. The most popular is to estimate the reduction in risk factors such as sex without condoms, syringe sharing, or number of sex partners. When incidence data are available in the intervention and control groups, the impact of interventions can be evaluated by projecting them into the future and modeling average time to seroconversion. Although such models are similar to traditional survival analysis, they can expand it by considering a mix of trajectories and risk models, thus relaxing restrictive assumptions of proportionality of hazard.

10.11.4 Population Models

As the name suggests, population-level models aim to make projections to the general population often including the entire country. In countries where HIV is concentrated in specific groups, the estimation of risk group size is usually sufficient to project prevalence and incidence to entire populations. Whenever HIV expands to the general population such as in South Africa, a large portion of the population becomes at risk; thus focusing on specific subpopulations is insufficient.

A number of population-level models have been developed since the 1980s. Most were of the SD type and covered the entire world, the United States, sub-Saharan Africa, Europe, China, and so on.[6,51,60–62] Model objectives included (1) forecasting incidence, (2) forecasting prevalence, but mostly (3) estimating the potential impact of interventions on prevalence with the overall goal of eventual disease elimination. Although the majority of the models are compartmental (SD) models, more models developed in recent years are of individual-based microsimulation types that account for sexual and injecting networks.

For example, in Lasry et al.,[51] the compartmental model projected HIV infections over time in the US population given a specific allocation scenario. The entire population was divided into 15 compartments defined by sex, race/ethnicity, and HIV transmission risk groups, including high-risk heterosexuals, men who have sex with men, and injection drug users. HIV transmission rates within and between compartments were dependent on the amount of risky behavior, which was controlled by HIV screening and risk-reduction interventions. The model used an optimization algorithm to provide the best allocation of limited funds to specific risk groups. Such models, although they use oversimplifying assumptions about individual behaviors, are of high importance to policy makers because government-supported prevention funds are generally allocated to large governing bodies such as states or regions, and corresponding policies thus affect large population subgroups.

Another example is the use of modeling to evaluate and expand the provision of ART to reduce the spread of HIV in generalized epidemics in sub-Saharan Africa.[6,30] These models consider the relatively new concept of *HIV treatment as prevention*, which implies that ART treatment and subsequent reduction in viral load would have a preventive effect (i.e., would reduce HIV transmissions) and as a result prevent new infections. The challenge in modeling such interventions is in connecting multiple components describing the reduction of viral load because of ART efficacy, real-world compliance with ART treatment link between an infected individual's viral load and HIV transmissibility, description of the contact network, and change in the network associated with social intervention, treatment, and reduction of stigma.[6] High-quality models provide state-of-the-art knowledge about the subject matter and a "best knowledge-based guess" about the future. At the same time, depending on assumptions and available, often partial, information, there is a potential to create different models that provide competing forecasts and public policy debates. As summarized by Eaton et al.,[6] models developed by Granich and colleagues[24] suggest possible elimination of HIV by 2050. Conversely, models by Wagner and Blower[63] suggest that such elimination is not possible, whereas subsequent papers examined various assumptions about intervention delivery and the structure of networks.[64–66] A recent UNAIDS policy aimed at reaching an ambitious goal: by 2020 90% of all people living with HIV will know their HIV status,

90% of all people with diagnosed HIV infection will be receiving sustained ART, and 90% of all people receiving ART will have achieved viral suppression.[67] Attainability of such goals can be evaluated either by monitoring the population close to 2020 or by using carefully designed simulation models to make early forecasts. A recent revision of forecasts and estimates shifted the 90–90–90 horizon by 10 years to 2030.[68] Eaton et al.[6] provide a summary of the models used to make predictions of policy-relevant outcomes in South Africa. Of the 12 models, 4 were microsimulation types and 8 were deterministic compartmental models. Most of the models had age and sex structures, but only microsimulation models considered sexual partnerships. Other models considered one, two, or three homogeneously mixed risk groups and for more than one risk group considered differential mixing between the groups.

Forecasts of HIV prevalence, HIV incidence, and ART coverage for South Africa based on 10 of the models in 2008 were validated using the 2012 "ground truth" household survey.[12] Although the model-based projections of overall prevalence were lower, they accurately captured decline among youth and the number of adults on ART. Despite missing some of the population estimates (e.g., differential ART coverage among men and women), the value of such models is high because they uncovered the greater need for treatment compared to the assumptions that went into them. They also identified the gaps in critical knowledge about the dynamics of HIV and necessary information that needs to be captured. Model projections can also be used to provide estimates of future costs of treatment under current and altered scenarios.

10.12 Discussion

We review major modeling methods and the use of modeling to address a number of HIV-related topics. These topics include categories of (1) estimation, (2) projections, (3) evaluation, (4) "what if" scenarios, and (5) cost-effectiveness. With the availability of multiple novel data sources and incredible computational power, simulation modeling is moving into the forefront of decision-making tools. Humans naturally think in terms of models by mentally replaying various scenarios. Computer-simulated scenarios provide an effective way to answer pressing questions where the system of interest is quite complex for humans to comprehend or requires expensive and often infeasible experiments.

By explicitly clarifying what is known and what is unknown, models reduce uncertainty. High-quality models are based on existing knowledge and data and thus provide an objective knowledge base where subjective opinions would be used otherwise.

Rigorous approaches to parameter estimation, model development, and evaluation are the key to providing assurance of quality and to making models useful. At the same time even a well-calibrated and validated model still does not guarantee precision of future prediction because of the "deep uncertainty" associated with the future. We only briefly touch on parameterization, calibration, and validation issues in this chapter, primarily because each of the topics is too broad and is the subject of a large body of research that varies by model purpose and type.

When data and knowledge are lacking the models can still provide useful guidance, because they indicate which important information components are missing and most critical. Sensitivity analysis thus serves not only the purpose of model building but also of guidance for future research.

The limitations of modeling approaches stem from the quality of the data and conceptual framework. At the same time, the quality of a model depends on its purpose. A great model designed for one purpose might be terrible for a different one. For example, a compartmental model that is good for description of a countrywide policy might be terrible when trying to forecast future incidence in a small village. It is the question *why?* that is critical and should be asked at all stages of model building, analysis, and interpretation.

Acknowledgments

Partial funding for this chapter was provided by an NIH/NIDA grant 5R01 DA025163. The author thanks William Zule (RTI International) and Anna Bershteyn (Intellectual Ventures) for invaluable comments and Michelle Myers (RTI International) for editing and formatting.

References

1. Centers for Disease Control and Prevention. How is HIV passed from one person to another?. http://www.cdc.gov/hiv/basics/transmission.html. Accessed October 17, 2016.
2. Centers for Disease Control and Prevention. HIV risk reduction tool. http://wwwn.cdc.gov/hivrisk. Accessed October 17, 2016.
3. Lightfoot M, Swendeman D, Rotheram-Borus MJ, Comulada WS, and Weiss R. Risk behaviors of youth living with HIV: Pre- and post-HAART. *Am J Health Behav.* 2005;29(2):162–171.
4. Sterman JD. Learning from evidence in a complex world. *Am J Public Health.* 2006;96(3):505–514. doi: 10.2105/AJPH.2005.066043
5. Hallett TB, Alsallaq RA, Baeten JM, et al. Will circumcision provide even more protection from HIV to women and men? New estimates of the population

impact of circumcision interventions. *Sex Transm Infect.* 2011;87(2):88–93. doi: 10.1136/sti.2010.043372

6. Eaton JW, Johnson LF, Salomon JA, et al. HIV treatment as prevention: Systematic comparison of mathematical models of the potential impact of anti-retroviral therapy on HIV incidence in South Africa. *PLoS Med.* 2012;9 (7):e1001245. doi: 10.1371/journal.pmed.1001245

7. Malcolm A, Aggleton P, Bronfman M, Galvão J, Mane P, and Verrall J. HIV-related stigmatization and discrimination: Its forms and contexts. *Crit Public Health.* 1998;8(4):347–370. doi: 10.1080/09581599808402920

8. Reyes-Estrada M, Varas-Diaz N, and Martinez-Sarson MT. Religion and HIV/AIDS stigma: Considerations for the nursing profession. *New School Psychol Bull.* 2015;12(1):48–55.

9. Kaplan EH. Needles that kill: Modeling human immunodeficiency virus trans-mission via shared drug injection equipment in shooting galleries. *Rev Infect Dis.* 1989;11(2):289–298. doi: 10.1093/clinids/11.2.289

10. Blower SM, Hartel D, Dowlatabadi H, Anderson RM, and May RM. Drugs, sex and HIV: A mathematical model for New York City. *Philos Trans R Soc Lond B Biol Sci.* 1991;331(1260):171–187. doi: 10.1098/rstb.1991.0006

11. McCormick AW, Abuelezam NN, Rhode ER, et al. Development, calibration and performance of an HIV transmission model incorporating natural history and behavioral patterns: Application in South Africa. *PLoS One.* 2014; 9(5):e98272. doi: 10.1371/journal.pone.0098272

12. Eaton JW, Bacaër N, Bershteyn A, et al. Assessment of epidemic projections using recent HIV survey data in South Africa: A validation analysis of ten mathematical models of HIV epidemiology in the antiretroviral therapy era. *Lancet Glob Health.* 2015;3(10):e598–e608. doi: 10.1016/s2214-109x(15) 00080-7

13. Bobashev GV, and Zule WA. Modeling the effect of high dead-space syringes on the human immunodeficiency virus (HIV) epidemic among injecting drug users. *Addiction.* 2010;105(8):1439–1447. doi: 10.1111/j.1360-0443.2010.02976.x

14. Vickerman P, Martin N, Turner K, and Hickman M. Can needle and syringe programmes and opiate substitution therapy achieve substantial reductions in hepatitis C virus prevalence? Model projections for different epidemic settings. *Addiction.* 2012;107(11):1984–1995. doi: 10.1111/j.1360-0443.2012.03932.x

15. Liang K-Y, Zeger SL. Longitudinal data analysis using generalized linear mod-els. *Biometrika.* 1986;73(1):13–22. doi: 10.1093/biomet/73.1.13

16. Kruse GR, Barbour R, Heimer R, et al. Drug choice, spatial distribution, HIV risk, and HIV prevalence among injection drug users in St. Petersburg, Russia. *Harm Reduct J.* 2009;6:22. doi: 10.1186/1477-7517-6-22

17. Raudenbush SW, and Bryk AS. *Hierarchical Linear Models: Applications and Data Analysis Methods. Second ed.* Newbury Park, CA: Sage; 2002.

18. Lindsay BG. *Mixture Models: Theory, Geometry, and Applications*, Vol. 5. Hayward, CA: Institute of Mathematical Statistics; 1995.

19. Hastie T, Tibsharani R, and Friedman J. *The Elements of Statistical Learning: Data Mining, Inference, and Prediction.* New York: Springer; 2009.

20. Yu HK, Kim NY, Kim SS, Chu C, and Kee MK. Forecasting the number of human immunodeficiency virus infections in the Korean population using the autoregressive integrated moving average model. *Osong Public Health Res Perspect.* 2013;4(6):358–362. doi: 10.1016/j.phrp.2013.10.009

21. Longini IM, Clark WS, Byers RH, et al. Statistical-analysis of the stages of HIV infection using a Markov model. *Stat Med.* 1989;8(7):831–843. doi: DOI 10.1002/sim.4780080708
22. Hollingsworth TD, Anderson RM, and Fraser C. HIV-1 transmission, by stage of infection. *J Infect Dis.* 2008;198(5):687–693. doi: 10.1086/590501
23. Lee S, Ko J, Tan X, Patel I, Balkrishnan R, and Chang J. Markov chain modelling analysis of HIV/AIDS progression: A race-based forecast in the United States. *Indian J Pharm Sci.* 2014;76(2):107–115.
24. Granich RM, Gilks CF, Dye C, De Cock KM, and Williams BG. Universal voluntary HIV testing with immediate antiretroviral therapy as a strategy for elimination of HIV transmission: A mathematical model. *Lancet.* 2009;373(9657):48–57. doi: 10.1016/S0140-6736(08)61697-9
25. Morris M, and Kretzschmar M. Concurrent partnerships and the spread of HIV. *AIDS.* 1997;11(5):641–648. doi: 10.1097/00002030-199705000-00012
26. Tuckwell H. *Elementary Applications of Probability Theory,* 2nd edition, Chapman and Hall, London, UK, 1995.
27. Wikipedia. System Archetype. https://en.wikipedia.org/wiki/System_archetype. Accessed October 18, 2016.
28. Subramanian S, Bobashev G, and Morris RJ. Modeling the cost-effectiveness of colorectal cancer screening: Policy guidance based on patient preferences and compliance. *Cancer Epidemiol Biomarkers Prev.* 2009;18(7):1971–1978. doi: 10.1158/1055-9965.Epi-09-0083
29. Borschev A. *The big book of simulation modeling: Multimethod modeling with AnyLogic 6.* AnyLogic North America, Chicago, IL, 2013.
30. Bershteyn A, Klein DJ, and Eckhoff PA. Age-targeted HIV treatment and primary prevention as a "ring fence" to efficiently interrupt the age patterns of transmission in generalized epidemic settings in South Africa. *Int Health.* 2016;8(4):277–285. doi: 10.1093/inthealth/ihw010
31. Bershteyn A, Klein DJ, Wenger E, and Eckhoff PA. Description of the EMOD-HIV Model v0.7. http://arxiv.org/pdf/1206.3720.pdf. Accessed October 17, 2016.
32. Harling G, Tanser F, Mutevedzi T, and Barnighausen T. Assessing the validity of respondents' reports of their partners' ages in a rural South African population-based cohort. *BMJ Open.* 2015;5(3):e005638. doi: 10.1136/bmjopen-2014-005638
33. RTI's Synthetic population viewer. http://synthpopviewer.rti.org. Accessed October 18, 2016.
34. Wikipedia. Jensen's Inequality. https://en.wikipedia.org/wiki/Jensen's_inequality. Accessed October 18, 2016.
35. Abuelezam NN, Rough K, and Seage GR, 3rd. Individual-based simulation models of HIV transmission: Reporting quality and recommendations. *PLoS One.* 2013;8(9):e75624. doi: 10.1371/journal.pone.0075624
36. Grimm V, Berger U, Bastiansen F, et al. A standard protocol for describing individual-based and agent-based models. *Ecol Model.* 2006;198(1–2):115–126. doi: 10.1016/j.ecolmodel.2006.04.023
37. Grimm V, Berger U, DeAngelis DL, Polhill JG, Giske J, and Railsback SF. The ODD protocol: A review and first update. *Ecolog Model.* 2010;221(23):2760–2768. doi: 10.1016/j.ecolmodel.2010.08.019
38. Grefenstette JJ, Brown ST, Rosenfeld R, et al. FRED (a Framework for Reconstructing Epidemic Dynamics): An open-source software system for

modeling infectious diseases and control strategies using census-based populations. *BMC Public Health.* 2013;13:940. doi: 10.1186/1471-2458-13-940

39. Lohr S. *Sampling: Design and Analysis.* Boston, MA: Brooks/Cole, Cengage Learning; 1999.

40. Boily MC, Baggaley RF, Wang L, et al. Heterosexual risk of HIV-1 infection per sexual act: Systematic review and meta-analysis of observational studies. *Lancet Infect Dis.* 2009;9(2):118–129. doi: 10.1016/S1473-3099(09)70021-0

41. Bobashev GV, Dowd W, Morris J, et al. (2016), Life trajectories of opioid users who go through recovery. In *Proceedings of the Annual Meeting of the International Society for Studies of Drug Policy (ISSDP)*; 2016.

42. Perelson AS, Ribeiro RM. Modeling the within-host dynamics of HIV infection. *BMC Biol.* 2013;11:96. doi: 10.1186/1741-7007-11-96

43. Rivadeneira PS, Moog CH, Stan GB, et al. Mathematical modeling of HIV dynamics after antiretroviral therapy initiation: A review. *Biores Open Access.* 2014;3(5):233–241. doi: 10.1089/biores.2014.0024

44. Bobashev G, Norton J, Wechsberg W, and Toussova O. Are you HIV invincible? A probabilistic study of discordant couples in the context of HIV transmission. *PLoS One.* 2014;9(5):e94799. doi: 10.1371/journal.pone.0094799

45. Patel P, Borkowf CB, Brooks JT, Lasry A, Lansky A, and Mermin J. Estimating per-act HIV transmission risk: A systematic review. *AIDS.* 2014;28(10):1509–1519. doi: 10.1097/QAD.0000000000000298

46. Bobashev GV, Morris RJ, and Zule WA. Projecting sexual and injecting HIV risks into future outcomes with agent-based modeling. In Chai S-K, Salerno JJ, Mabry PL, eds. *Advances in Social Computing, Proceedings of the Third International Conference on Social Computing, Behavioral Modeling and Prediction,* Bethesda, MD. Berlin, Heidelberg: Springer 2010:97.

47. Lasry A, Sansom SL, Wolitski RJ, et al. HIV sexual transmission risk among serodiscordant couples: Assessing the effects of combining prevention strategies. *AIDS.* 2014;28(10):1521–1529. doi: 10.1097/QAD.0000000000000307

48. Bobashev G, Zule W, and Wechsberg W. *Unobserved Risk of HIV Transmission and the Role of the Couples Intervention.* Cape Town: HIV International Forum; 2014.

49. Garnett GP, and Anderson RM. Factors controlling the spread of HIV in heterosexual communities in developing countries: Patterns of mixing between different age and sexual activity classes. *Philos Trans R Soc Lond B Biol Sci.* 1993;342(1300):137–159. doi: 10.1098/rstb.1993.0143

50. Lasry A, Sansom SL, Hicks KA, and Uzunangelov V. A model for allocating CDC's HIV prevention resources in the United States. *Health Care Manag Sci.* 2011;14(1):115–124. doi: 10.1007/s10729-010-9147-2

51. Neaigus A, Friedman SR, Goldstein M, Ildefonso G, Curtis R, and Jose B. Using dyadic data for a network analysis of HIV infection and risk behaviors among injecting drug users. *NIDA Res Monogr.* 1995;151:20–37.

52. Koopman JS, Jacquez JA, Welch GW, et al. The role of early HIV infection in the spread of HIV through populations. *J Acquir Immune Defic Syndr Hum Retrovirol.* 1997;14(3):249–258.

53. Rothenberg R. HIV transmission networks. *Curr Opin HIV AIDS.* 2009;4(4):260–265. doi: 10.1097/COH.0b013e32832c7cfc

54. Morris M, Goodreau S, and Moody J. Sexual networks, concurrency, and STD/HIV. In: Holmes KK, Sparling P, Stamm W, et al., eds. *Sexually Transmitted Diseases.* 4th ed. New York: McGraw-Hill; 2008:109–126.

55. Kretzschmar M, and Wiessing LG. Modelling the spread of HIV in social networks of injecting drug users. *AIDS.* 1998;12(7):801–811.

56. Cepeda JA, Odinokova VA, Heimer R, et al. Drug network characteristics and HIV risk among injection drug users in Russia: The roles of trust, size, and stability. *AIDS Behav.* 2011;15(5):1003–1010. doi: 10.1007/s10461-010-9816-7

57. Monteiro JF, Escudero DJ, Weinreb C, et al. Understanding the effects of different HIV transmission models in individual-based microsimulation of HIV epidemic dynamics in people who inject drugs. *Epidemiol Infect.* 2016;144(8):1683–1700. doi: 10.1017/S0950268815003180

58. Friedman SR, Curtis R, Neaigus A, Jose B, and Des Jarlais DC. *Social networks, drug injectors' lives, and HIV/AIDS.* New York: Plenum; 1999.

59. HIV Modeling Consortium. View All Models by Country. http://www. hivmodelling.org/countries/all-models. Accessed October 17, 2016.

60. Merli MG, Hertog S, Wang B, and Li J. Modelling the spread of HIV/AIDS in China: The role of sexual transmission. *Popul Stud (Camb).* 2006;60(1):1–22. doi: 10.1080/00324720500436060

61. Grassly NC, Lowndes CM, Rhodes T,Judd A, Renton A, and Garnett GP. Modelling emerging HIV epidemics: The role of injecting drug use and sexual transmission in the Russian Federation, China and India. *Inter J Drug Policy.* 2003;14:25–43.

62. Wagner BG, and Blower S. Voluntary universal testing and treatment is unlikely to lead to HIV elimination: A modeling analysis. *Nat Proceedings.* 2009;3917:1. doi: 10101/npre.2009.3917.1

63. Kretzschmar ME, van der Loeff MF, and Coutinho RA. *Elimination of HIV by test and treat: A phantom of wishful thinking? AIDS.* 2012;26(2):247–248. doi: 10.1097/ QAD.0b013e32834e1592

64. Bacaer N, Pretorius C, and Auvert B. An age-structured model for the potential impact of generalized access to antiretrovirals on the South African HIV epidemic. *Bull Math Biol.* 2010;72(8):2180–2198. doi: 10.1007/s11538-010-9535-2

65. Bendavid E, Brandeau ML, Wood R, and Owens DK. Comparative effectiveness of HIV testing and treatment in highly endemic regions. *Arch Intern Med.* 2010;170(15):1347–1354. doi: 10.1001/archinternmed.2010.249

66. UNAIDS (2014) *90-90-90. An ambitious treatment target to help end the AIDS epidemic.* http://www.unaids.org/sites/default/files/media_asset/90-90-90_en_0.pdf. Accessed February 15, 2017.

67. UNAIDS (2016) *Global AIDS Update* http://www.unaids.org/sites/default/ files/media_asset/global-AIDS-update-2016_en.pdf. Accessed February 15, 2017.

11

Review of Statistical Methods for Within-Host HIV Dynamics in AIDS Studies

Ningtao Wang

University of Texas Health Science Center, Houston, TX

Hulin Wu

University of Texas Health Science Center, Houston, TX

CONTENTS

11.1 Introduction

Highly active antiretroviral therapies (HAARTs) are currently the most effective treatment regime for HIV patients regarding suppressing HIV viral load. HIV dynamic study, in which ordinary differential equations (ODEs) play a vital quantitative role, facilitates our understanding of HIV infection pathogenesis [70,76,79,80,118]. In the 1990s, the majority of HIV dynamic ODE models, either deterministic or stochastic, focused on the interaction between CD4$^+$ T cells and virions [42,60,65,71,77,79,107,122]. With the development of polymerase chain reaction (PCR) technology that quantifies genomic viral RNA copies, HIV dynamics can be understood in a precise manner, and the host-pathogen interaction in HIV patients can be studied quantitatively using statistical methods. Nowadays, ODE models of viral dynamics provide incredible insights into the mechanisms for nonlinear interactions between virus and host cell populations and the dynamics of antiviral drug resistance.

It is very important and critical to use experimental data to estimate the model parameters, perform inference and evaluate the mathematical models using rigorous statistical methods. Some earlier reviews for these methods can be found in Wu [121] and Xiao et al. [131]. In this chapter, we give an updated review on statistical methods for ODE models for HIV dynamic data analysis and inference. We organize the rest of the chapter as follows. In Section 11.2, we give a brief review of ODE models of HIV dynamics primarily in response to antiretroviral (ARV) drug therapy. In Section 11.3, we review the model identifiability analysis methods with a focus on nonlinear ODE models for which close-form solutions are not available. In Section 11.4, we focus on the model-fitting methods that include the nonlinear least squares approaches, the nonlinear mixed-effect model approaches, and the smoothing-based approaches. In Section 11.5, we review the recent development of high-dimensional ODEs for the identification of dynamic gene regulatory network (GRN) in AIDS studies. We conclude this chapter with some discussions and future directions in Section 11.6.

11.2 Ordinary Differential Equations

11.2.1 Modeling HIV Infection

ODEs have been widely adopted in modeling dynamic systems. By considering the dynamic changes and interactions among multiple biological components, ODE models can capture the essential behavior of dynamic immune systems such as nonlinearity and delay. A substantial effort has been devoted to mathematical modeling of HIV dynamics [79], Nowak and May [70] provided an excellent and comprehensive review on earlier work on mathematical modeling of HIV infections. We start at the general dynamical features of HIV infection [100]. The model, which is widely adopted to describe the plasma viral load changes in HIV-infected individuals, has four state variables: T, the concentration of uninfected target T cells; L, the concentration of latently infected T cells; T^*, the concentration of productive infected T cells; and V, the concentration of free virus particles in the blood. The system is formulated as

$$\frac{dT}{dt} = f(T) - kTV$$

$$\frac{dL}{dt} = \eta kTV - d_L L - vL$$

$$\frac{dT^*}{dt} = (1-\eta)kTV + vL - \delta T^*$$

$$\frac{dV}{dt} = N\delta T^* - cV$$

(11.1)

Here k is the infection rate, η is the fraction of latency, v is the transition rate at which latently infected cells become virus-production active, d_L is the death rate of latently infected cells, δ is the death rate of infected cells, N is the total number of virus particles released by a productively infected cell over its life-span, and c is the clearance rate of viral particles. Furthermore, the growth rate of uninfected target T cells, $f(T)$, can take three possible forms:

$$f(T) = \begin{cases} \lambda - dT + pT\left(1 - \dfrac{T}{T_{max}}\right) & (11.2) \\[2ex] \lambda - dT + pT\left(1 - \dfrac{T+L+T^*}{T_{max}}\right) & (11.3) \\[2ex] \lambda - dT, & (11.4) \end{cases}$$

where λ denotes the rate at which new CD4$^+$ T cells are produced and d is the per capita death rate of uninfected cells. In the case (11.2), the healthy T cells are assumed to proliferate exponentially at a rate p until reaching the carrying capacity T_{max} in the absence of virus particles or infected T cells [78,79]. Perelson et al. [78] considered the case (11.3) where the proliferation of L and T^* cells were considered although their proportions are relatively small. Dropping the proliferation term leads to the case (11.4) [70].

Investigating the cases (11.2) and (11.3), Perelson et al. [78] concluded that if N is less than a critical value, say N_{crit}, the free-of-infection state will be the only steady state in the nonnegative orthant; if $N > N_{crit}$, the free-of-infection state will become unstable, but the endemic state will be either stable or unstable within a stable limit cycle. Smith and De Leenheer [100] analyzed the cases (11.2) and (11.4) without considering dynamics of latently infected T cells (i.e., $\eta = 0$). Assume f (T) to be a smooth function and there exists a positive steady state TT for the variable T such that

$$f(T) > 0, \quad 0 < T < \overline{T},$$
$$f(T) < 0, \quad T > \overline{T},$$
$$f(\overline{T}) = 0,$$
$$f'(\overline{T}) < 0.$$

Homeostasis in a healthy individual is then maintained at a steady state $\overline{T}$.

Note that the system (11.1) with the case (11.2) or (11.4) is competitive with respect to the cone

$$G = \{(T, T^*, V^*) \in \mathbb{R}^3 : T, V \geq 0, T^* \leq 0\}.$$

Thus, the solutions with initial states ordered according to the order of G (i.e., their differences are a vector in G) remain ordered for future time [99]. Smith and De Leenheer [100] conducted a global analysis of viral dynamics, by using the competitive dynamical system theory. If the basic reproduction number $R_0 < 1$, the virus will be cleared and the infection will be eradicated; if $R_0 > 1$, the virus persists in the host, and the solutions approach either a chronic steady state (11.3) or a periodic orbit (11.2). Here $R_0 = k\overline{T}(Ni)/c$, with $i = 0$ or 1.

The HIV dynamic models, with considering the time between initial infection and the production of new virus particles, are more accurate regarding the representation of the real biological processes and pharmacokinetics. Several differential models have been proposed to take into account the intracellular delay [40,54,65,68,69,116,139]. Herz et al. [42] found that including a discrete delay term would change the estimate of the viral clearance rate (c), but not the loss rate (δ) of productively infected T cells. Mittler et al. [65] obtained a different estimate of c, when assuming the intracellular delay follows a gamma distribution. Considering the imperfect drug efficacy, Nelson et al. [67] formulated a model with a discrete infection delay and a constant target cell density, and found that the estimated values of both c and δ were changed. Nelson and Perelson [69] further confirmed the delay effect on δ, which became larger comparing with the non-delay model.

It is a notable feature of delay differential equation models that the delay will generally destabilize the stable equilibrium and cause sustained oscillations through Hopf bifurcations. The studies of the within-host viral dynamics model with intracellular delay and cell division showed that sustained oscillation could occur for some realistic parameter values [15,116]. However, Li and Shu [54] eliminated the possibility of sustained oscillations, by analyzing a viral dynamic model with intracellular delay but not cell division. Let T_2 be the time between viral entry into a target cell and the production of new virus particles, and T_2 be a virus production period for new virions to be produced within and released from the infected cells. Without considering the latent-infected CD4$^+$ T cells, Zhu and Zou [139] then considered the delay differential equations

$$\frac{dT}{dt} = \lambda - dT - kTV$$

$$\frac{dT^*}{dt} = ke^{-\mu_1\tau_1}(t - t_1)^2 TV - \delta T^*, \tag{11.5}$$

$$\frac{dV}{dt} = N\delta e^{-\mu_2\tau_2}(t - \tau_2)T^* - cV$$

where μ_1 and μ_2 are their corresponding death rates. Zhu and Zou [139] obtained a "global" stability result for the infection-free equilibrium if basic reproduction number $R_0 < 1$; otherwise, infection could be locally asymptotically stable. Li and Shu [54] further studied the delay effect by analyzing model (11.5) in the absence of τ_2, and showed that R_0 completely determines the global dynamics of model (11.5). In particular, if $R_0 \leq 1$, the infection-free equilibrium is globally asymptotically stable, and hence viruses will be cleared completely; if $R_0 > 1$, the unique chronic infection equilibrium is locally asymptotically stable and acts as an attractor. It is worth mentioning that experimental data of CD4$^+$T cells *in vivo* may not well support the theoretical result of sustained oscillations [10]. Data sparsity could be a reasonable explanation, and further experimental works are badly needed to answer this question.

Antigen-specific immunity against HIV infection includes cytotoxic T cells (CTLs). Let $Z(t)$ be the concentration of CTLs. Then, without considering the latently infected cells, the model (11.1) can be modified as

$$\frac{dT}{dt} = \lambda - dT - kTV$$

$$\frac{dT^*}{dt} = kTV - \delta T^* - pT^*Z$$

$$\frac{dV}{dt} = N\delta T^* - cV \tag{11.6}$$

$$\frac{dZ}{dt} = g(T, T^*, Z) - bZ$$

where p and b are the killing and death rate of CTLs, respectively. The function $g(T, T^*, Z)$ represents the rate of antigen-specific CTL response [18,19,70,76]. Nowak and May [70] discussed the self-regulating CTL response, that is, $g(T, T^*, Z) = \rho$. Kennedy [51] and Wang et al. [114] assumed that the production rate of CTLs only depends on the concentration of the infected cells, that is, $g(T, T^*, Z) = \rho T^*$. Based on this assumption, Arnaout et al. [4] explained the biphasic decay of blood viremia in HIV patients under treatment: viral load decreases quickly while CTLs are abundant, but slowly while CTLs are rare. Nowak and Bangham [72], Liu [56], and Kajiwara and Sasaki [50] assumed that the production of CTLs also depends on the concentration of CTL themselves, leading $g(T, T^*, Z) = \rho T^*Z$, and explored the effects of between-subject variation in immune responsiveness on virus load and viral strain diversity. Culshaw et al. [16] further assumed that the production of CTLs is CD4$^+$ T-cell dependent and accordingly chose the form $g(T, T^*, Z) = \rho TT^*Z$. Assuming that the viral load is proportional to the level of infected cells since free virus is thought to be short lived in the comparison with the infected cells [4,81], Culshaw et al. [16] considered the following model

$$
\frac{dT}{dt} = \lambda - dT - kTT^*
$$

$$
\frac{dT^*}{dt} = k'TT^* - \delta T - pT^*Z,
$$

$$
\frac{dZ}{dt} = \rho TT^*Z - bZ
$$

(11.7)

where the ratio k'/k is the proportion of infected cells that survive the incubation period. Culshaw et al. [16] demonstrated the existence and the local stability of equilibria of the model (11.7). They further investigated the optimal control problem in which they maximized the benefit in terms of levels of immune cells and the systemic cost of chemotherapy.

Viral diversity is a consequence of mutations and selections [72]. A number of studies have incorporated viral diversity with HIV infection frameworks [2,70,74,100]. Nowak and Bangham [72] proposed the following model to understand the interplay between selection pressures for and against diversification,

$$
\frac{dT}{dt} = \lambda - dT - T\sum_{i=1}^{m}k_iV_i
$$

$$
\frac{dT_i^*}{dt} = k_iTV_i - \delta T_i^* - pT_i^*Z_i,
$$

$$
\frac{dV_i}{dt} = N_i\delta_i^* - cV_i
$$

$$
\frac{dZ_i}{dt} = \rho T_i^*Z_i - bZ_i
$$

(11.8)

where the index i represent the viral type. Viral mutants differ in their antigenic specificity, the rate at which they infect cells (k_i), and the rate of virus production (N_i). De Boer [17] extended model (11.8) by including a density-dependent infection term which describes the dynamics of the viral load and the immune response during acute infection. Althaus and De Boer [2] added stochastic events of viral mutation and considered the saturated interaction between infected cells and CTLs according to Michaelis–Menten kinetics. Their model of HIV/SIV infection has a broad cellular immune response targeting different viral epitopes.

11.2.2 Modeling Drug Efficacy

HAART utilizes at least three different ARV drugs, including nucleoside or nucleotide reverse transcriptase inhibitor, non-nucleoside reverse transcriptase inhibitor, and a protease inhibitor (PI). Reverse transcriptase inhibitors (RTIs) can effectively block the infection of target cells by free viruses, while PIs prevent HIV protease from cleaving the HIV polyprotein into functional units. Modeling ARV intervention can significantly facilitate our understanding of biological and clinical mechanisms.

Let η_{RTI} and η_{PI} be the efficacies of RTIs and PIs, respectively, which were assumed to be constant by Perelson and Nelson [69,79]. Based on model (11.1), the HIV viral dynamic model with HAART treatment is given as

$$
\begin{aligned}
\frac{dT}{dt} &= \lambda - dT - (1 - \eta_{RTI})kTV \\
\frac{dT^*}{dt} &= (1 - \eta_{RTI})kTV - \delta T^* \\
\frac{dV_I}{dt} &= (1 - \eta_{PI})N\delta T^* - cV \\
\frac{dV_{NI}}{dt} &= \eta_{PI}N\delta T^* - cV
\end{aligned}
\qquad (11.9)
$$

where V_I and V_{NI} are the concentration of infectious and noninfectious virus, respectively, and $V = V_I + V_{NI}$ is the total viral load. Note that the variable V_{NI} does not show up in the first three equations of (11.9), and hence the qualitative dynamics of this model is the same as that of (11.1) with the case (11.4). It is shown that the virus-free equilibrium ($E_0 = (\lambda/d, 0, 0)$) is locally asymptotically stable if $R_0 \leq 1$, while the endemic state

$$
E^* = \left(\frac{\lambda}{R_0 d}, \frac{(R_0 - 1)dc}{oN\delta(1 - \eta_{RTI})(1 - \eta_{PI})}, \frac{(R_0 - 1)d}{k(1 - \eta_{RTI})} \right)
$$

is globally asymptotically stable if $R_0 > 1$. Furthermore, R_0 is related to the threshold of drug efficacy to achieve virus eradication. For example, if we only consider RTIs, then virus can be eradicated if drug efficacy η_{RTI} is greater than the critical value $\eta_{RTI}^c = 1 - dc/(\lambda N k)$.

In practice, the drug concentration in HIV patients is not a constant, especially during the medication intervals. Once a dose is administered, drug concentration increases rapidly, reaches a peak value, and then decreases gradually [102]. We assume that drugs are taken at time t_ks and the effect of the drugs is instantaneous, which leads to a system of impulsive differential equations with a solution that is continuous for $t \neq t_\kappa$ and undergoes a sudden jump at t_κ. Let $C(t)$ be the intracellular concentration of the drug and we have

$$
\begin{aligned}
\frac{dC}{dt} &= h(t), \quad t \neq t_\kappa \\
C(t_\kappa^+) &= C(t_\kappa^-) + C^\kappa, \quad t = t_\kappa
\end{aligned}
\qquad (11.10)
$$

where $h(t)$ is the drug elimination rate and can be parameterized by either first-order elimination kinetics or the Michaelis–Menten elimination kinetics. Considering fixed doses and constant time intervals (i.e., $t_{k+1} - t_k = T$), the solution $C(t)$ is then a periodic and piecewise continuous function of time t [102,108].

The effect of antiviral treatment always changes over time, primarily due to pharmacokinetics variation, fluctuation of drug adherence, and drug resistant mutations. Without considering drug adherence and drug resistance, Gabrielsson and Weiner [33] presented a pharmacodynamic model for dose-effect relationship,

$$E = \frac{E_{max}C(t)}{C_{50} + C(t)}$$

where E_{max} is the maximal effect that can be achieved, and C_{50} is the drug concentration that corresponds to the 50% of E_{max}. Huang et al. [46], Yang and Xiao [134], and Yang et al. [135] further studied the HIV dynamic models with periodic drug efficacy. Considering the model (11.9) with ϖ-periodic drug efficacies $\eta_{RTI}(t)$ and $\eta_{PI}(t)$, Yang and Xiao [134] investigated the treatment dynamics by using the persistent theory of periodic system [5,115]. They defined a threshold parameter $r(\Theta_{M(\cdot)} (\varpi))$, which determines the extinction and persistence of the disease. They demonstrated that the disease-free equilibrium of (11.9) is globally asymptotically stable if $r(\Theta_{M(\cdot)} (\varpi)) < 1$, while the disease is persistent if $r(\Theta_{M(\cdot)} (\varpi)) > 1$.

Ding and Wu [23] and Wu et al. [125] proposed the use of the estimated viral dynamic parameters to evaluate antiviral drug efficacy, in which drug exposure and drug susceptibility were considered. Both short-term and long-term effects of antiviral therapies can be evaluated based on the viral dynamic parameters. Wu et al. [126] also related viral dynamic parameters with host factors, cellular restoration and virological endpoints for HIV-1 infected patients with combination antiretroviral therapy.

11.2.3 Modeling Drug Resistance

Although HAART has been extremely effective in suppressing the plasma viral load below the detection limit in most HIV-1-infected patients [14], the therapy often fails to eradicate virus primarily due to the emergence of drug-resistant mutants [20]. There are two possible reasons for the development of HIV drug resistance: the transmission of drug-resistant mutants to susceptible individuals, and the adaptive mutations generated during treatment [8,91]. Ribeiro and Bonhoeffer [90] analyzed both reasons and suggested that under a wide range of conditions, treatment failure is most likely due to the preexistence of drug-resistant virus before therapy. Bonhoeffer and Nowak [9] showed that, given the preexistence of drug-resistant virus, a more efficient therapy could lead to a greater initial reduction of virus load, but would also cause a faster rise of drug-resistant mutants. Huang et al. [46] and Wu et al. [124,125] considered the viral dynamic models with drug susceptibility and drug exposure.

A number of mathematical models have been developed to study the effect of ARV drugs on the evolution of drug-resistant HIV mutants. McLean and Nowak [59] examined the competition between drug-resistant and wild type, that is, drug-sensitive strains to determine which type of virus would eventually dominate the virus population during the course of Zidovudine treatment. Nowak et al. [73] considered a two-strain model and compared it with experimental data on the development of drug resistance in the nevirapine treatment. Kirschner and Webb [52] investigated drug resistance for single-drug treatments and compared the treatment outcomes at different initial CD4$^+$ T-cell levels. The effect of an immune response on the emergence of drug resistance was investigated by Wodarz and Lloyd [119] and Musekwa et al. [66]. Rong et al. [94] proposed a mathematical model including both drug-sensitive and drug-resistant strains to understand the mechanism of the emergence of drug resistance during therapy. Let $T_s(t)$ and $T_r(t)$ be the concentration of cells productively infected by drug-sensitive and drug-resistant virus, respectively, and $V_s(t)$ and $V_r(t)$ be concentration of drug-sensitive and drug-resistant virus, respectively, then the model can be formulated as

$$\frac{dT}{dt} = \lambda - dT - k_s TV_s - k_r TV_r$$

$$\frac{dT_s}{dt} = (1-u)k_s TV_s - \delta T_s$$

$$\frac{dV_s}{dt} = N_s \delta T^* - cV_s \qquad , \qquad (11.11)$$

$$\frac{dT_r}{dt} = uk_s TV_s + k_r TV_r - \delta T_r$$

$$\frac{dV_r}{dt} = N_r \delta T^* - cV_r$$

Here k_s and k_r are the rates at which uninfected cells are infected by drug-sensitive and drug-resistant virus, respectively, and N_s and N_r are the burst sizes of drug-sensitive and drug-resistant strains, respectively, u is a rate at which cells infected by the drug-sensitive virus become drug-resistant due to viral RNA mutation. Both types of infected cells are assumed to have the same death rate δ and clearance rate c. Without ARV intervention, the reproductive ratio for each strain can be derived

$$R_s = \frac{\lambda k_s N_s}{dc}$$
$$R_r = \frac{\lambda k_r N_r}{dc} .$$

The infection-free steady state is locally asymptotically stable if $R_s < 1/(1-u)$ and $R_r < 1$, and it is unstable if $R_s > 1/(1-u)$ or $R_r > 1$. The steady state with only drug-resistant virus exists if and only if $R_r > 1$. It is locally asymptotically stable if $R_s > (1-u)R_r$, and is unstable if $R_s < (1-u)R_r$. The co-existence steady state exists and is locally asymptotically stable if and only if $R_s > 1/(1-u)$ and $R_r < (1-u)R_s$.

After drug intervention, the reproductive ratios for drug-sensitive and drug-resistant strains become

$$R'_s = (1 - \in^s_{RTI})(1 - \in^s_{PI})R_s$$
$$R'_s = (1 - \in^r_{RTI})(1 - \in^r_{PI})R_r$$

Here $\in^s_{RTI}$ and $\in^r_{RTI}$ are the efficacies of RTIs for the drug-sensitive and drug-resistant strains, respectively, and $\in^s_{PI}$ and $\in^r_{PI}$ are the efficacies of PIs for the drug-sensitive and drug-resistant strains, respectively. An overall treatment effect for each strain can be defined as

$$\in^s = 1 - (1 - \in^s_{RTI})(1 - \in^s_{PI})$$
$$\in^r = 1 - (1 - \in^r_{RTI})(1 - \in^r_{PI})$$

There exist two threshold values ϵ_1 and ϵ_2 for ϵ^s such that: (i) both the drug-sensitive and drug-resistant strains coexist if $\epsilon^s < \epsilon_1$; (ii) only the drug-resistant virus will persist for $\epsilon^1 < \epsilon^s < \epsilon_2$; and (iii) both strains will be eradicated if $\epsilon^s > \epsilon_2$. This indicates that drug resistance is more likely to arise for intermediate levels of treatment efficacy, at which the reproductive ratios of both strains are close. Furthermore, a pharmacokinetics model including blood and cell compartments is implemented to estimate the drug efficacies of both strains. Simulations demonstrated that the perfect adherence to the regimen protocol will well suppress the viral load of the wild type strain while drug-resistant variants develop slowly. However, an intermediate level of adherence may result in the dominance of the drug-resistant virus.

Suboptimal adherence is associated with a high risk of developing HIV drug resistance [6,29,97,113] and is one of the major causes of treatment failure [43,75,125]. Some mathematical models have considered the effects of imperfect adherence to drug regimens [27,46,82,101,113,124]. See Heffernan and Wahl [41] for a comprehensive review. A standard definition and a reliable measure of adherence are still lacking. Wahl and Nowak [113] considered the outcome of therapy as a function of the degree of adherence to the drug regimen and determined the conditions under which a resistant strain would dominate.

The effect of drug concentrations on HIV dynamics has been modeled by a number of studies [79,122]. However, only a few of the studies have considered the interaction between drug concentrations and the dynamics of a pathogen population, which examines the necessary conditions for the emergence of drug resistance [64,102,103,104]. Let $R(t)$ denote the intracellular drug concentration that satisfies the model (11.10). Smith and Wahl [103] considered the scenario when $R(t) < R_1$, the probability that a given T cell absorbs sufficient drug to block infection is negligible for both strains; when $R_1 < R < R_2$, such probability remains negligible for drug-resistant strain, but grows monotonically with dose for the wild type; when $R > R_2$, such probability is significant for both strains, and higher for the wide type. The immune cells infected by virus are categorized depending on whether a cell has been infected or has absorbed any of the drugs. Let $T(t)$ be the population of susceptible (uninfected) CD4$^+$ T cells, T_s and T_r be the cells infected with the wild type and mutant virus, respectively. T_{Rs} is the uninfected cells which have absorbed sufficient amount of drugs so that the wild type strain is inhibited but not the mutant strain. T_{Rr} is the uninfected cells which have absorbed sufficient amount of drugs so that both strains are inhibited. Smith and Wahl [103] thus derived the model

$$\frac{dT}{dt} = \lambda - dT - k_s T V_s - k_r T V_r - \theta k_p k_R TR + m_{Rs} T_{Rs}$$

$$\frac{dT_{Rs}}{dt} = \theta k_p k_R TR - k_r T_{Rs} V_r - (d + m_{Rs}) T_{Rs} + m_{Rr} T_{Rr} - \eta k_Q T_{Rs} R$$

$$\frac{dT_{Rr}}{dt} = \eta k_Q T_{Rs} R - (d + m_{Rr}) T_{Rr}$$

$$\frac{dT_s}{dt} = k_s T V_s - d_s T_s$$

$$\frac{dT_r}{dt} = k_r T V_r + k_r T_{Rs} V_r - d_r T_r$$

$$\frac{dV_s}{dt} = \omega N_s d_s T_s - c V_s$$

$$\frac{dV_r}{dt} = \omega N_r d_r T_r - c V_r$$

$$\frac{dV_{NI}}{dt} = (1 - \omega) N_s d_s T_s + (1 - \omega) N_r d_r T_r - c V_{NI}$$

Here k_s and k_r are the rates at which drug-sensitive and drug-resistant virus infects T cells, respectively, N_s and N_r are the corresponding burst sizes, and d_s and d_r are the corresponding death rates of uninfected (infected) CD4$^+$ T cells. m_{Rs} and m_{Rr} are the drug clearance rates for intracellular compartments with an intermediate ($R_1 < R < R_2$) and high ($R > R_2$) drug concentration, respectively, and ω is the fraction of infectious virion produced by an infected T cell. Smith and Wahl [103] considered three treatment regimens: low, intermediate, and high drug levels

$$\theta = \begin{cases} 0, & \text{if } R < R_1 \\ 1/k_R, & \text{if } R_1 < R < R_2 \\ 1/k_P, & \text{if } R > R_2 \end{cases}$$

and

$$\eta = \begin{cases} 0, & \text{if } R < R_2 \\ 1, & \text{if } R > R_2 \end{cases}$$

where k_P is the rate at which the drug inhibits the wide type T cells when $R_1 < R < R_2$; k_R and k_Q are the rates at which the drug inhibits the drug-sensitive and drug-resistant T cells, respectively, when $R > R_2$. By analyzing all possible equilibria, and the stability for the three regimen, Smith and Wahl [103] concluded that drug resistance might emerge at both intermediate and high drug concentrations, whereas at low drug levels resistance would not emerge.

11.3 Model Identifiability

11.3.1 Practical Identifiability Analysis

Theoretical identifiability and practical identifiability can be examined by structure identifiability analysis and Monte Carlo simulations. Identifiability of HIV dynamic models was analyzed by earlier work of Wu et al. [120] and Miao et al. [62]. See Miao et al. [63] for a detailed review. Structure identifiability analysis assumes that both model structure and measurements are absolutely accurate, which is not valid in most biomedical research. Therefore, even when structural identifiability analysis concludes the identifiability of model parameters, the estimates of model parameters may still be unreliable. Practical identifiability analysis evaluates such reliability of parameter estimates from a statistical's point of view. In the rest of this subsection, the statistical ODE model are generally formulated as follows

$$\frac{d\mathbf{x}(t)}{dt} = \mathbf{f}(t, \mathbf{x}(t), \boldsymbol{\theta})$$
$$\mathbf{x}(0) = \mathbf{x}_0 \tag{11.12}$$
$$\mathbf{y}(t) = \mathbf{h}(\mathbf{x}(t), \mathbf{x}_0, \boldsymbol{\theta}) + \boldsymbol{\epsilon}(t)$$

where $\mathbf{x}(t)$ is the vector of state variables, and $\mathbf{y}(t)$ is the measurement vector. The parameter vector $\boldsymbol{\theta}$ is the interest of identifiability analysis. The error term $s(t)$ is usually introduced by both ODE model and measurement.

11.3.1.1 Monte Carlo Simulation

The history of Monte Carlo simulations can be traced back to Metropolis and Ulam [61]. It is widely used to assess the performance of statistical estimation methods in the statistical literature. This method obtains numeric results by using repeated random sampling, which is not only useful for practical identifiability analysis, but also helpful for statistical inference. In general, a Monte Carlo simulation procedure can be outlined as follows:

1. Determine the nominal parameter values $\boldsymbol{\theta}_0$ for simulation studies, which can be obtained by fitting the model to the experimental data if available. Otherwise it can be obtained from the literature.

2. Use the nominal parameter values to numerically solve the ODE model and obtain the solution $x(t)$ at the experimental design time points.

3. Generate N sets of simulated data from the model (11.12) with a given measurement error level.

4. Fit the ODE model to each of the N simulated data sets and obtain parameter estimates $\boldsymbol{\theta}_i$, $i = 1, 2, ..., N$.

5. Calculate the average relative estimation errors (ARE) for $\boldsymbol{\theta}$ as

$$\text{ARE} = \frac{1}{N} \sum_{i=1}^{N} \frac{\left| \boldsymbol{\theta}_0^{(k)} - \tilde{\boldsymbol{\theta}}_i^{(k)} \right|}{\left| \boldsymbol{\theta}_0^{(k)} \right|}.$$

The ARE can be used to assess whether each of the parameter estimates is acceptable or not. If the ARE of a parameter estimate is unacceptably high, we can claim that this parameter is not practically or statistically identifiable. Some parameters may not be sensitive to measurement errors and can always be well estimated, but some other parameters may be quite sensitive to measurement errors, and their AREs are large even with a small measurement error. In practice, there is no clear-cut rule of ARE to claim an "unidentifiable" parameter. Thus, the practical identifiability relies on the underlying problem and the judgment of investigators. Also notice that various statistical estimation approaches can be employed to obtain the parameter estimates, and the ARE may depend on the estimation methods.

11.3.1.2 Correlation Matrix

Monte Carlo simulation is computationally expensive since a large number of model fitting need to be performed. Rodriguez-Fernandez et al. [92,93] and Guedj et al. [36] proposed an alternative approach with less computational cost by examining the correlations between model parameters.

Assume that the parameter estimate $\hat{\boldsymbol{\theta}} = (\hat{\theta}_1, \hat{\theta}_2, ..., \hat{\theta}_p)^T$ has been obtained by fitting a model to experimental data. The correlation matrix of parameter estimates

$$\begin{pmatrix} r_{11} & r_{12} & \cdots & r_{1n} \\ r_{21} & r_{22} & \cdots & r_{2n} \\ \vdots & \vdots & \ddots & \vdots \\ r_{m1} & r_{m2} & \cdots & r_{mn} \end{pmatrix},$$

can then be derived from the Fisher information matrix [28,110], where r_{ij} is the correlation coefficient between parameter estimates $\hat{\theta}_i$ and $\hat{\theta}_j$. If the correlation coefficient r_{ij} is close to 1 or -1, parameters θ_i and θ_j are said to be practically undistinguishable. A strong correlation between two parameters indicates that one parameter strongly depends on the other one and such two parameters cannot be jointly estimated.

The derivation of correlation matrix has been provided by Rodriguez-Fernandez et al. [92]. The errors are assumed to be independent and identically distributed with $N(0,\sigma^2)$ for simplicity. Then, under a general dynamic system (11.12), the Fisher information matrix can be formulated as

$$\mathbf{I} = \sum_{i=1}^{N} \left(\frac{\partial \mathbf{y}_i}{\partial \boldsymbol{\theta}}\right)^T \boldsymbol{\Sigma}^{-1} \left(\frac{\partial \mathbf{y}_i}{\partial \boldsymbol{\theta}}\right)\Bigg|_{\boldsymbol{\theta} = \hat{\boldsymbol{\theta}}},$$

where Σ is a weight matrix of covariance. Therefore, by using Cramèr–Rao theorem, the correlation coefficient r_{ij} is

$$r_{ij} = \frac{V_{ij}}{\sqrt{V_{ii} V_{jj}}},$$

where $\mathbf{V} = \mathbf{I}^{-1}$. The correlation matrix approach requires not only the parameters but also their correlation matrix to be reliably estimated. This may be problematic for a model with most parameters unidentifiable. If any two parameters are not distinguishable, their correlation matrix estimation may be poor.

11.3.2 Sensitivity-Based Identifiability Analysis

Sensitivity analysis is often used to assess the variation of measurements induced by different model parameters. Similar to practical identifiability analysis, sensitivity-based method requires pre-specified parameter values and measurement time points; similar to structural identifiability analysis, it does not take measurement error into account. Thus, the sensitivity-based method is somewhere between the structural identifiability and practical identifiability analysis.

The sensitivity coefficient at time point $t_k (k = 1, 2, \ldots, N)$ for a given parameter vector $\boldsymbol{\theta}$ is defined as

$$s_{ij} = \frac{\partial y_i(t_k, \theta)}{\partial \theta_j}$$

where $y_i(i = 1, 2,\ldots, d)$ is the ith component of $\mathbf{y}$ and θ_j $(j = 1, 2,\ldots, q)$ is the jth component of $\boldsymbol{\theta}$. The sensitivity matrix for all time points is defined as

$$
S = \begin{pmatrix}
s_{11}(t_1) & \cdots & s_{1q}(t_1) \\
\vdots & \ddots & \vdots \\
s_{d1}(t_1) & \cdots & s_{dq}(t_1) \\
\vdots & \vdots & \vdots \\
s_{11}(t_N) & \cdots & s_{1q}(t_N) \\
\vdots & \ddots & \vdots \\
sd_1(t_N) & \cdots & s_{dq}(t_N)
\end{pmatrix},
$$

Some identifiability analysis methods have been developed based on the sensitivity matrix. Simply speaking, the larger the sensitivity coefficients are, the more notable measurements are with respect to the changes of parameters. In this sense, a parameter is unidentifiable if the measurements are not sensitive to the perturbation on this parameter. Moreover, two parameters are very likely to be indistinguishable, if there exists a strong correlation between these two parameters. Such parameter dependence can be evaluated by examining the dependence among the columns of sensitivity matrix. Typical sensitivity analysis methods includes: the correlation method [48,93,138], the principle component analysis method [21,30,49], the orthogonal method [34,136,137], and the eigenvalue method [85,86,95,109].

11.4 ODE Model Fitting Methods

11.4.1 Least Squares Approaches

In this section, we adopt the same assumption as (11.12) and formulate the statistical ODE model as

$$
\frac{d\mathbf{x}(t)}{dt} = \mathbf{f}(t, \mathbf{x}(t), \boldsymbol{\theta})
$$

$$
\mathbf{x}(0) = \mathbf{x}_0 \tag{11.13}
$$

$$
\mathbf{y}(t) = \mathbf{h}(\mathbf{x}(t), \mathbf{x}_0, \boldsymbol{\theta}) + \boldsymbol{\epsilon}(t)
$$

The parameter vector $\boldsymbol{\theta}$ is unknown and has to be estimated based on experimental data. Each component of $\boldsymbol{\theta}$ could be either constant or time varying. The error term $s(t)$ is usually introduced by both ODE model and measurement.

Standard nonlinear regression methods were widely used to fit viral dynamic models in the pioneering works [43,77,81,118]. Let $\hat{\mathbf{h}}(\theta)$ be the solution, either analytical or closed form, of $\mathbf{h}(\mathbf{x}(t), \mathbf{x}_0, \theta)$. The nonlinear least squares (NLS) estimate of θ minimizes:

$$\|\mathbf{y}(t) - \hat{\mathbf{h}}(\theta)\|_2$$

Standard inference of nonlinear regressions can be applied here [7,89,96]. Traditionally, a log-transformation of $\mathbf{y}(t)$ can be used to stabilize the variance of the error and the estimation algorithms. Recently, Xue et al. [133] extended the NLS method to estimate both constant and time-varying parameters in nonlinear ODE models. Some interesting theoretical results are obtained by considering both numerical error and measurement error in the ODE model.

11.4.2 Hierarchical Modeling Approaches

Wu et al. [123,126,122] proposed the use of nonlinear mixed-effects models for longitudinal HIV viral dynamic data first. Putter et al. [84], Han et al. [38], and Huang et al. [45,47] proposed a Bayesian modeling framework for HIV viral dynamic models. In particular, Li et al. [53] and Huang et al. [45] formulated a general framework of hierarchical ODE models for longitudinal dynamic data. Under a longitudinal data scenario, the model (11.13) can be re-written as

$$\frac{d\mathbf{x}^{(i)}(t)}{dt} = \mathbf{f}\left(t, \mathbf{x}^{(i)}(t), \theta^{(i)}\right),$$

$$\mathbf{x}^{(i)}(0) = \mathbf{x}_0^{(i)}, \tag{11.14}$$

$$\mathbf{y}^{(i)}(t_{ij}) = \mathbf{h}\left(\mathbf{x}^{(i)}(t_{ij}), \mathbf{x}_0^{(i)}, \theta^{(i)}\right) + \epsilon^{(i)}(t_{ij}), \quad j = 1, \ldots, n_i,$$

where i denotes the ith subject and j denotes the jth measurement on the ith subject. The between-subject variation of parameters can be generally specified as $\theta^{(i)} = \mathbf{g}(\theta, \mathbf{b}^{(i)})$ where θ is the population parameter, and $\mathbf{b}^{(i)}$ represents the random effect. Usually, we assume

$$\theta^{(i)} = \theta + \mathbf{b}^{(i)},$$

$$\mathbf{b}^{(i)} \sim N(\mathbf{0}, \Theta),$$

$$\epsilon^{(i)} | \mathbf{b}^{(i)} \sim N(\mathbf{0}, \textstyle\sum^{(i)}).$$

Guedj et al. [35] proposed a maximum likelihood estimation approach and investigated the statistical inference for ODE models. The corresponding full log-likelihood of the observations is

$$\ell_O = \sum_i \sum_j \log \int f(\mathbf{y}^{(i)}(t_{ij}) | \mathbf{b}^{(i)}) p(\mathbf{b}^{(i)}) d\mathbf{b}^{(i)} \tag{11.15}$$

where $f(\mathbf{y}(i) (ti_j) | \mathbf{b}(i))$ is the density of $\mathbf{y}(i) (ti_j)$ given $\mathbf{b}(i)$, and $p(\mathbf{b}(i))$ is the probability density of random effect. A Newton–Raphson algorithm, incorporated with closed-forms of both score function and Hessian matrix, was developed to obtain the full likelihood maximizer. Another promising optimization method of (11.15) is based on stochastic approximation expectation-maximization (EM) algorithm [22], which can successfully address such a log-of-integration type of objective function. Here the random effect term $\mathbf{b}(i)$ is regarded as the latent variable (or missing data) in the EM algorithm. Beside the maximum likelihood approach, the parameter estimation of mixed-effects ODE models can also be addressed by a Bayesian framework [38,117] and a two-stage smoothing-based approach [26].

11.4.3 Smoothing-Based Approaches

Varah [111] proposed a two-stage parameter estimation technique, which does not require any analytical or closed-form solutions of $\mathbf{h}$ from the ODE model (11.13). In the first stage, this method fits the measurements $\mathbf{x}$ empirically by using nonparametric smoothing methods, such as splines; and then differentiate the fitted curve to obtain the estimated derivatives, $d\hat{\mathbf{x}}/dt$. In the second stage, substituting the estimated derivatives into the ODE model, the parameter estimation problem of ODEs is then converted into a linear regression problem. The estimate of $\boldsymbol{\theta}$ in the smoothing-based method minimizes,

$$\left\| \frac{d\mathbf{x}}{dt} - \frac{d\hat{\mathbf{x}}}{dt} \right\|_2$$

instead of

$$\| \mathbf{y}(t) - \hat{\mathbf{h}}(\boldsymbol{\theta}) \|_2.$$

in the nonlinear least square approaches. This smoothing-based approach has less computational cost than other approaches, but the estimation of derivatives is usually less efficient and may lead to poor estimation of the parameters [106,111]. Liang and Wu [55] demonstrated the consistency and asymptotic normality of the estimator under some regularity conditions. Chen and Wu [11,12] extended the framework to address the time-varying parameters in the ODE models.

Instead of numerically estimating the derivatives dx/dt, Wu et al. [129] directly substitutes the estimated curve $\hat{\mathbf{x}}$ into ODE discretization algorithms, and minimizes

$$\sum_{i=1}^{n-1} \left\| \frac{\hat{\mathbf{x}}(t_{i+1}) - \hat{\mathbf{x}}(t_i)}{t_{i+1} - t_i} - F\left(t_i, \; \hat{\mathbf{x}}(t_i), \; \hat{\mathbf{x}}(t_i + 1), \; \boldsymbol{\theta}\right) \right\|_2$$

where F is determined by the discretization methods, such as Euler's method, trapezoidal rule and Runge–Kutta method.

Ramsay [88] proposed a smoothing-based approach called the principal differential analysis (PDA) to address parameter estimation problems of linear ODEs. There is always a trade-off of functions between over-smoothing and under-smoothing in such a nonparametric scenario. Varah [111] tackled this trade-off problem by interactively adjusting the number and position of knots by hand until satisfactory smoothing was obtained. Alternatively, Ramsay [88] developed a regularization method, which penalizes the second-order derivative of the curve, to determine the level of smoothness. Heckman and Ramsay [39] extended the second-order derivative penalty into a wide class of linear differential operators. Poyton et al. [83] and Varziri et al. [112] proposed an iterative procedure to improve the fitness of PDA approach. Ramsay et al. [87] proposed a popular profiling approach for ODE parameter estimation. Fang et al. [25] proposed a mixed-effects two-stage method for ODE models for longitudinal data. Ding and Wu [24] recently compared different smooth-based methods to the NLS method from a practical perspective, and proposed a new constrained local polynomial estimation approach.

All of the smoothing-based approaches require the state variables **x** to be observable and directly measured, which is sometimes difficult to be satisfied in practice. Combining structure identifiability analysis techniques with smoothing-based approaches, Wu et al. [128] proposed a pseudo-least square method to handle ODE models with partially observed state variables.

11.5 High-Dimensional ODE Modeling

Although the introduction of HAART has dramatically reduced the mortality of the HIV-infected patients, the risk of latent infection still exists among these patients. Recently, the reactivation of the latently infected cells has been discussed a promising approach to eradicating HIV [3,13,98,132]. To develop such treatment regimes, it is critical to understand the biological processes, especially the HIV dynamics at the genomic level, underlying the virus reactivation. The high-throughput technologies such as DNA microarray and RNA-Seq enable us to quantify a large number of viral RNA copies simultaneously. The high-dimensionality of such gene expression data brings new challenges in ODE modeling, including both variable selection and model fitting.

Lu et al. [57] proposed the following high-dimensional linear ODEs for the dynamic gene regulatory network (GRN) identification and applied SCAD penalization for variable selection,

$$\frac{dX_k(t)}{dt} = \sum_{j=1}^{p} \theta_{kj} X_j(t), \quad k = 1, \ldots, p,$$

where $X_\kappa(t)$ represents the gene expression level of gene κ at time t and $\theta_{\kappa j}$ quantifies the regulation from gene j onto gene κ. The stochastic approximation EM algorithm has been developed to estimate the parameters of the ODEs coupled with mixed-effects. Song et al. [105] developed a five-step pipeline to study the dynamics of GRN following a viral reactivation by using the high-dimensional linear ODEs.

Wu et al. [127] further extended the high-dimensional linear ODEs to a more general additive nonparametric ODE model for modeling nonlinear GRNs,

$$\frac{\mathrm{d}X_k(t)}{\mathrm{d}t} = \mu_k + \sum_{j=1}^{p} f_{kj}\left(X_j(t)\right), \quad k = 1, ..., p,$$

where μ_k is the baseline expression level of gene k and $f_{\kappa j}(\cdot)$ is a smooth function to quantify the nonlinear regulation from gene j onto gene κ. A two-stage smoothing-based approach has been implemented to estimate the nonlinear relationship, and an additive group LASSO penalization has been proposed for the variable selection.

11.6 Discussion

Ordinary differential equations are an important tool for quantifying the dynamic process of HIV infections. In this chapter, we reviewed ODE modeling methods for HIV dynamics, especially for understanding antiretroviral drug responses to HIV infection. We illustrated how classic ODE models were extended to account for drug efficacy and drug resistance. We then reviewed identifiability analysis and the parameter estimation methods for ODE models. In particular, we surveyed the hierarchical and mixed-effect modeling approaches for HIV dynamics, the nonlinear least square method and the smoothing-based approaches for parameter estimation, as well as the high-dimensional ODEs for HIV dynamics at the genomic level. Both practical and sensitivity-based identifiability analysis methods are discussed for ODE model diagnosis, and beneficial to parameter estimations, model simulations, and experimental designs.

It is worth of further discussion that the models in section 1.2 are mainly constructed from the simulation purpose of the true HIV dynamics. It is not easy to include every relevant biological detail in one model. These models, thus, are simplified mathematical representations of the true biological process. Besides the essential compartments, if some other biological processes are not explicitly included in one model, then this model cannot be used to understand such specific processes. For example, the models (1.5)-(1.8) do not explicitly consider the latently infected T cells, so they cannot be used to investigate the effects of latent infection; however, these models is still useful in understanding other aspects of HIV dynamics as in Perelson et al. [81]. Wu and Ding [122] suggested a modeling strategy, that is to consider all possible compartments in the model first and then simplify the model into an applicable model based on the availability of the data.

A mathematical model may not be very useful if we could not estimate its parameters and evaluate its validity based on experimental data. A major challenge of drug development for controlling viral infections is to analyze and predict the dynamics of viral load during drug therapy, and to further prevent the emergence of resistant virus. Two directions could potentially overcome such a challenge in the future precision medicine research. First, the integration of ODEs for viral dynamics with high-throughput genetic data will raise hope for effective diagnosis and treatment of infections with HIV through developing potent antiviral drugs based on individual patients' genetic makeup [44]. System mapping approaches provide a potential solution to develop statistical linkages between genetic markers and the interrelationships within ODE models [1,31,32,58,130]. Second, the integration of ODEs for viral dynamics with repeated clinical measurements will enable us to dynamically predict virus load and emergence of resistant virus during drug therapy, and lead to dynamic treatments of HIV infections. Jointly modeling of longitudinal biomarkers with ODEs and time-to-event [37] also allows us to better predict the treatment failure.

References

1. Kwangmi Ahn, Jiangtao Luo, Arthur Berg, David Keefe, and Rongling Wu. Functional mapping of drug response with pharmacodynamic-pharmacokinetic principles. *Trends in Pharmacological Sciences*, 31(7):306–311, 2010.
2. Christian L Althaus and Rob J De Boer. Dynamics of immune escape during HIV/SIV infection. *PLoS Computational Biology*, 4(7):e1000103, 2008.
3. Nancie M Archin, AL Liberty, Angela D Kashuba, Shailesh K Choudhary, JD Kuruc, AM Crooks, DC Parker, et al. Administration of vorinostat disrupts HIV-1 latency in patients on antiretroviral therapy. *Nature*, 487(7408):482–485, 2012.
4. Ramy A Arnaout, Nowak MA, Dominik Wodarz. Hiv-1 dynamics revisited: Biphasic decay by cytotoxic T lymphocyte killing? *Proceedings of the Royal Society of London B: Biological Sciences*, 267(1450):1347–1354, 2000.
5. Nicolas Bacaër. Approximation of the basic reproduction number R0 for vector-borne diseases with a periodic vector population. *Bulletin of Mathematical Biology*, 69(3):1067–1091, 2007.
6. David R Bangsberg, Sharon Perry, Edwin D Charlebois, Richard A Clark, Marjorie Roberston, Andrew R Zolopa, and Andrew Moss. Non-adherence to highly active antiretroviral therapy predicts progression to aids. *AIDS*, 15(9): 1181–1183, 2001.

7. Douglas M Bates and Donald G Watts. *Nonlinear Regression: Iterative Estimation and Linear Approximations.* Wiley Online Library, 1988.

8. SM Blower, AN Aschenbach, HB Gershengorn, and JO Kahn. Predicting the unpredictable: Transmission of drug-resistant HIV. *Nature Medicine*, 7(9):1016–1020, 2001.

9. Sebastian Bonhoeffer and Martin A Nowak. Pre-existence and emergence of drug resistance in HIV-1 infection. *Proceedings of the Royal Society of London B: Biological Sciences*, 264(1382):631–637, 1997.

10. Romulus Breban and Sally Blower. Role of parametric resonance in virological failure during HIV treatment interruption therapy. *The Lancet*, 367(9518):1285–1289, 2006.

11. Jianwei Chen and Hulin Wu. Efficient local estimation for time-varying coefficients in deterministic dynamic models with applications to HIV-1 dynamics. *Journal of the American Statistical Association*, 103(481):369–384, 2008.

12. Jianwei Chen and Hulin Wu. Estimation of time-varying parameters in deterministic dynamic models. *Statistica Sinica*, 18(3):987–1006, 2008.

13. Tae-Wook Chun, Lieven Stuyver, Stephanie B Mizell, Linda A Ehler, Jo Ann M Mican, Michael Baseler, Alun L Lloyd, et al. Presence of an inducible HIV-1 latent reservoir during highly active antiretroviral therapy. *Proceedings of the National Academy of Sciences*, 94(24):13193–13197, 1997.

14. Ann C Collier, Robert W Coombs, David A Schoenfeld, Roland L Bassett, Joseph Timpone, Alice Baruch, Michelle Jones, et al. Treatment of human immunodeficiency virus infection with saquinavir, zidovudine, and zalcitabine. *New England Journal of Medicine*, 334(16):1011–1018, 1996.

15. Rebecca V Culshaw and Shigui Ruan. A delay-differential equation model of HIV infection of CD4$^+$ T-cells. *Mathematical Biosciences*, 165(1):27–39, 2000.

16. Rebecca V Culshaw, Shigui Ruan, and Raymond J Spiteri. Optimal HIV treatment by maximising immune response. *Journal of Mathematical Biology*, 48(5): 545–562, 2004.

17. Rob J De Boer. Understanding the failure of CD8+ T-cell vaccination against simian/human immunodeficiency virus. *Journal of Virology*, 81(6):2838–2848, 2007.

18. Rob J De Boer and Alan S Perelson. Towards a general function describing T cell proliferation. *Journal of Theoretical Biology*, 175(4):567–576, 1995.

19. Rob J De Boer and Alan S Perelson. Target cell limited and immune control models of HIV infection: A comparison. *Journal of Theoretical Biology*, 190(3):201–214, 1998.

20. Steven G Deeks. Treatment of antiretroviral-drug-resistant HIV-1 infection. *The Lancet*, 362(9400):2002–2011, 2003.

21. D Degenring, C Froemel, G Dikta, and R Takors. Sensitivity analysis for the reduction of complex metabolism models. *Journal of Process Control*, 14(7):729–745, 2004.

22. Bernard Delyon, Marc Lavielle, and Eric Moulines. Convergence of a stochastic approximation version of the em algorithm. *Annals of Statistics*, 27:94–128, 1999.

23. AA Ding and H Wu. Assessing antiviral potency of anti-HIV therapies in vivo by comparing viral decay rates in viral dynamic models. *Biostatistics*, 2:13–29, 2001.

24. AA Ding and H Wu. Estimation of ODE parameters using constrained local polynomial regression. *Statistica Sinica*, 24:1613–1631, 2014.

25. H Fang, Y Wu, and L Zhu. A two-stage estimation method for random coefficient differential equation models with application to longitudinal HIV dynamic data. *Statistica Sinica*, 21:1145–1170, 2011.

26. Yun Fang, Hulin Wu, and Li-Xing Zhu. A two-stage estimation method for random coefficient differential equation models with application to longitudinal HIV dynamic data. *Statistica Sinica*, 21(3):1145, 2011.

27. NM Ferguson, CA Donnelly, J Hooper, AC Ghani, C Fraser, LM Bartley, RA Rode, et al. Adherence to antiretroviral therapy and its impact on clinical outcome in HIV-infected patients. *Journal of the Royal Society Interface*, 2(4):349–363, 2005.

28. B Roy Frieden. *Science from Fisher Information: A Unification*. Cambridge University Press, 2004.

29. Gerald H Friedland and Ann Williams. Attaining higher goals in HIV treatment: The central importance of adherence. *AIDS (London, England)*, 13:S61–72, 1999.

30. C Froemel. Parameterreduktion in stoff wechselmodellen mit methoden der statistik. Master's thesis. Fachhochschule Aachen, Aachen, 2003.

31. Guifang Fu, Jiangtao Luo, Arthur Berg, Zhong Wang, Jiahan Li, Kiranmoy Das, Runze Li, and Rongling Wu. A dynamic model for functional mapping of biological rhythms. *Journal of Biological Dynamics*, 5(1):84–101, 2011.

32. Guifang Fu, Zhong Wang, Jiahan Li, and Rongling Wu. A mathematical framework for functional mapping of complex phenotypes using delay differential equations. *Journal of Theoretical Biology*, 289:206–216, 2011.

33. Johan Gabrielsson and Daniel Weiner. *Pharmacokinetic and Pharmacodynamic Data Analysis: Concepts and Applications*, volume 2. CRC Press, 2001.

34. Kapil G Gadkar, Rudiyanto Gunawan, and Francis J Doyle. Iterative approach to model identification of biological networks. *BMC Bioinformatics*, 6(1):155, 2005.

35. Jérémie Guedj, Rodolphe Thiébaut, and Daniel Commenges. Maximum likelihood estimation in dynamical models of HIV. *Biometrics*, 63(4):1198–1206, 2007.

36. Jérémie Guedj, Rodolphe Thiébaut, and Daniel Commenges. Practical identifiability of HIV dynamics models. *Bulletin of Mathematical Biology*, 69(8):2493–2513, 2007.

37. Jeremie Guedj, Rodolphe Thiébaut, and Daniel Commenges. Joint modeling of the clinical progression and of the biomarkers' dynamics using a mechanistic model. *Biometrics*, 67(1):59–66, 2011.

38. Cong Han, Kathryn Chaloner, and AA Perelson. Bayesian analysis of a population HIV dynamic model. In *Case Studies in Bayesian Statistics*, Pages 223–238. Springer, New York; 1999, 2002.

39. Nancy E Heckman and James O Ramsay. Penalized regression with model-based penalties. *Canadian Journal of Statistics*, 28(2):241–258, 2000.

40. Jane M Heffernan and Lindi M Wahl. Monte Carlo estimates of natural variation in HIV infection. *Journal of Theoretical Biology*, 236(2):137–153, 2005.

41. Jane M Heffernan and Lindi M Wahl. Treatment interruptions and resistance: A review. In *Deterministic and Stochastic Models of AIDS and HIV with Intervention*, Pages 423–456. World Scientific, 2005.

42. Andreas VM Herz, Sebastian Bonhoeffer, Roy M Anderson, Robert M May, and Martin A Nowak. Viral dynamics in vivo: Limitations on estimates of intracellular delay and virus decay. *Proceedings of the National Academy of Sciences*, 93 (14):7247–7251, 1996.

43. David D Ho, Avidan U Neumann, Alan S Perelson, Wen Chen, John M Leonard, and Martin Markowitz. Rapid turnover of plasma virions and CD4 lymphocytes in HIV-1 infection. *Nature*, 373(6510):123–126, 1995.

44. Wei Hou, Yihan Sui, Zhong Wang, Yaqun Wang, Ningtao Wang, Jingyuan Liu, Yao Li, et al. Systems mapping of HIV-1 infection. *BMC Genetics*, 13(1):91, 2012.

45. Yangxin Huang, Dacheng Liu, and Hulin Wu. Hierarchical Bayesian methods for estimation of parameters in a longitudinal HIV dynamic system. *Biometrics*, 62(2):413–423, 2006.

46. Yangxin Huang, Susan L Rosenkranz, and Hulin Wu. Modeling HIV dynamics and antiviral response with consideration of time-varying drug exposures, adherence and phenotypic sensitivity. *Mathematical Biosciences*, 184(2):165–186, 2003.

47. Yangxin Huang and Hulin Wu. A Bayesian approach for estimating antiviral efficacy in HIV dynamic models. *Journal of Applied Statistics*, 33:155–174, 2006.

48. John A Jacquez and Peter Greif. Numerical parameter identifiability and estimability: Integrating identifiability, estimability, and optimal sampling design. *Mathematical Biosciences*, 77(1):201–227, 1985.

49. Ian T Jolliffe. Discarding variables in a principal component analysis. I: Artificial data. *Applied Statistics*, 21:160–173, 1972.

50. Tsuyoshi Kajiwara and Toru Sasaki. A note on the stability analysis of pathogen-immune interaction dynamics. *Discrete and Continuous Dynamical Systems Series B*, 4:615–622, 2004.

51. James Kennedy. Particle swarm optimization. In *Encyclopedia of Machine Learning*, Pages 760–766. Springer, 2010.

52. Denise E Kirschner and GF Webb. Understanding drug resistance for monotherapy treatment of HIV infection. *Bulletin of Mathematical Biology*, 59(4):763–785, 1997.

53. Lang Li, Morton B Brown, Kyung-Hoon Lee, and Suneel Gupta. Estimation and inference for a spline-enhanced population pharmacokinetic model. *Biometrics*, 58(3):601–611, 2002.

54. Michael Y Li and Hongying Shu. Global dynamics of an in-host viral model with intracellular delay. *Bulletin of Mathematical Biology*, 72(6):1492–1505, 2010.

55. Hua Liang and Hulin Wu. Parameter estimation for differential equation models using a framework of measurement error in regression models. *Journal of the American Statistical Association*, 103(484):1570–1583, 2008.

56. Wei-min Liu. Nonlinear oscillations in models of immune responses to persistent viruses. *Theoretical Population Biology*, 52(3):224–230, 1997.

57. Tao Lu, Hua Liang, Hongzhe Li, and Hulin Wu. High-dimensional odes coupled with mixed-effects modeling techniques for dynamic gene regulatory network identification. *Journal of the American Statistical Association*, 106(496):1242–1258, 2011.

58. Jiangtao Luo, William W Hager, and Rongling Wu. A differential equation model for functional mapping of a virus-cell dynamic system. *Journal of Mathematical Biology*, 61(1):1–15, 2010.

59. Angela R McLean and Martin A Nowak. Competition between zidovudine-sensitive and zidovudine-resistant strains of HIV. *AIDS*, 6(1):71–80, 1992.

60. Stephen J Merrill. Modeling the interaction of HIV with cells of the immune system. In *Mathematical and Statistical Approaches to AIDS Epidemiology*, Pages 371–385. Springer, 1989.

61. Nicholas Metropolis and Stanislaw Ulam. The Monte Carlo method. *Journal of the American Statistical Association*, 44(247):335–341, 1949.

62. C Miao, H Dykes, L Demeter, and H Wu. Differential equation modeling of HIV viral fitness experiments: Model identification, model selection, and multi-model inference. *Biometrics*, 65:292–300, 2009.
63. Hongyu Miao, Xiaohua Xia, Alan S Perelson, and Hulin Wu. On identifiability of nonlinear ode models and applications in viral dynamics. *SIAM Review*, 53(1): 3–39, 2011.
64. Rachelle E Miron and Robert J Smith. Modelling imperfect adherence to HIV induction therapy. *BMC Infectious Diseases*, 10(1):1–16, 2010.
65. John E Mittler, Bernhard Sulzer, Avidan U Neumann, and Alan S Perelson. Influence of delayed viral production on viral dynamics in HIV-1 infected patients. *Mathematical Biosciences*, 152(2):143–163, 1998.
66. Senelani D Musekwa, Tinevimbo Shiri, and Winston Garira. A two-strain HIV-1 mathematical model to assess the effects of chemotherapy on disease parameters. *Mathematical Biosciences and Engineering*, 2(4):811–832, 2005.
67. Patrick W Nelson, John E Mittler, and Alan S Perelson. Effect of drug efficacy and the eclipse phase of the viral life cycle on estimates of HIV viral dynamic parameters. *JAIDS Journal of Acquired Immune Deficiency Syndromes*, 26(5):405–412, 2001.
68. Patrick W Nelson, James D Murray, and Alan S Perelson. A model of HIV-1 pathogenesis that includes an intracellular delay. *Mathematical Biosciences*, 163 (2):201–215, 2000.
69. Patrick W Nelson and Alan S Perelson. Mathematical analysis of delay differential equation models of HIV-1 infection. *Mathematical Biosciences*, 179(1):73–94, 2002.
70. Martin Nowak and Robert M May. *Virus Dynamics: Mathematical Principles of Immunology and Virology: Mathematical Principles of Immunology and Virology.* Oxford University Press, 2000.
71. Martin A Nowak, Roy M Anderson, Angela R McLean, TF Wolfs, Jaap Goudsmit, and Robert M May. Antigenic diversity thresholds and the development of aids. *Science*, 254(5034):963–969, 1991.
72. Martin A Nowak and Charles RM Bangham. Population dynamics of immune responses to persistent viruses. *Science*, 272(5258):74–79, 1996.
73. Martin A Nowak, Sebastian Bonhoeffer, George M Shaw, and Robert M May. Anti-viral drug treatment: Dynamics of resistance in free virus and infected cell populations. *Journal of Theoretical Biology*, 184(2):203–217, 1997.
74. Martin A Nowak, Robert M May, Rodney E Phillips, Sarah Rowland-Jones, David G Lalloo, Steven McAdam, et al. Antigenic oscillations and shifting immunodominance in HIV-1 infections. *Nature*, 375(6532):606–611, 1995.
75. David L Paterson, Susan Swindells, Jeffrey Mohr, Michelle Brester, Emanuel N Vergis, Cheryl Squier, Marilyn M Wagener, and Nina Singh. Adherence to protease inhibitor therapy and outcomes in patients with HIV infection. *Annals of Internal Medicine*, 133(1):21–30, 2000.
76. Alan S Perelson. Modelling viral and immune system dynamics. *Nature Reviews Immunology*, 2(1):28–36, 2002.
77. Alan S Perelson, Paulina Essunger, Yunzhen Cao, Mika Vesanen, Arlene Hurley, Kalle Saksela, Martin Markowitz, and David D Ho. Decay characteristics of HIV-1-infected compartments during combination therapy. *Nature*, 387:188–191, 1997.
78. Alan S Perelson, Denise E Kirschner, and Rob De Boer. Dynamics of HIV infection of CD4$^+$ T cells. *Mathematical Biosciences*, 114(1):81–125, 1993.

79. Alan S Perelson and Patrick W Nelson. Mathematical analysis of HIV-1 dynamics in vivo. *SIAM Review*, 41(1):3–44, 1999.

80. Alan S Perelson and Patrick W Nelson. Modeling viral infections. *Proceedings of Symposia in Applied Mathematics*, 59:139–172, 2002.

81. Alan S Perelson, Avidan U Neumann, Martin Markowitz, John M Leonard, and David D Ho. HIV-1 dynamics in vivo: Virion clearance rate, infected cell lifespan, and viral generation time. *Science*, 271(5255):1582–1586, 1996.

82. Andrew N Phillips, Michael Youle, Margaret Johnson, and Clive Loveday. Use of a stochastic model to develop understanding of the impact of different patterns of antiretroviral drug use on resistance development. *AIDS*, 15(17):2211–2220, 2001.

83. AA Poyton, M Saeed Varziri, Kimberley McAuley, PJ McLellan, and James O Ramsay. Parameter estimation in continuous-time dynamic models using principal differential analysis. *Computers & Chemical Engineering*, 30(4): 698–708, 2006.

84. H Putter, SH Heisterkamp, JMA Lange, and F De Wolf. A Bayesian approach to parameter estimation in HIV dynamical models. *Statistics in Medicine*, 21:2199–2214, 2002.

85. T Quaiser, W Marquardt, and M Mönnigmann. Local identifiability analysis of large signaling pathway models. *Proceedings of FOSBE 2007*, Pages 465–470, 2007.

86. Tom Quaiser and Martin Mönnigmann. Systematic identifiability testing for unambiguous mechanistic modeling-application to jak-stat, map kinase, and nf-κb signaling pathway models. *BMC Systems Biology*, 3(1):50, 2009.

87. James Ramsay, Giles Hooker, David Campbell, and Jiguo Cao. Parameter estimation for differential equations: A generalized smoothing approach. *Journal of the Royal Statistical Society-B*, 69:741–796, 2007.

88. James O Ramsay. Principal differential analysis. In *Encyclopedia of Statistical Sciences*, 1996.

89. David A Ratkowsky. *Nonlinear Regression Modeling*. 1970.

90. Ruy M Ribeiro and Sebastian Bonhoeffer. Production of resistant HIV mutants during antiretroviral therapy. *Proceedings of the National Academy of Sciences*, 97 (14):7681–7686, 2000.

91. Ruy M Ribeiro, Sebastian Bonhoeffer, and Martin A Nowak. The frequency of resistant mutant virus before antiviral therapy. *AIDS*, 12(5):461–465, 1998.

92. Maria Rodriguez-Fernandez, Jose A Egea, and Julio R Banga. Novel metaheuristic for parameter estimation in nonlinear dynamic biological systems. *BMC Bioinformatics*, 7(1):483, 2006.

93. Maria Rodriguez-Fernandez, Pedro Mendes, and Julio R Banga. A hybrid approach for efficient and robust parameter estimation in biochemical pathways. *Biosystems*, 83(2):248–265, 2006.

94. Libin Rong, Zhilan Feng, and Alan S Perelson. Emergence of HIV-1 drug resistance during antiretroviral treatment. *Bulletin of Mathematical Biology*, 69(6):2027–2060, 2007.

95. Klaus Schittkowski. Experimental design tools for ordinary and algebraic differential equations. *Industrial & Engineering Chemistry Research*, 46(26):9137–9147, 2007.

96. George Arthur Frederick Seber and Christopher John Wild. *Nonlinear Regression*. Wiley, New York, 1989.

97. Ajay K Sethi, David D Celentano, Stephen J Gange, Richard D Moore, and Joel E Gallant. Association between adherence to antiretroviral therapy and human immunodeficiency virus drug resistance. *Clinical Infectious Diseases*, 37(8): 1112–1118, 2003.

98. Kotaro Shirakawa, Leonard Chavez, Shweta Hakre, Vincenzo Calvanese, and Eric Verdin. Reactivation of latent HIV by histone deacetylase inhibitors. *Trends in Microbiology*, 21(6):277–285, 2013.

99. Hal L Smith. *Monotone Dynamical Systems: An Introduction to the Theory of Competitive and Cooperative Systems*. Number 41. American Mathematical Soc, 2008.

100. Hal L Smith and Patrick De Leenheer. Virus dynamics: A global analysis. *SIAM Journal on Applied Mathematics*, 63(4):1313–1327, 2003.

101. RJ Smith. Adherence to antiretroviral HIV drugs: How many doses can you miss before resistance emerges? *Proceedings of the Royal Society of London B: Biological Sciences*, 273(1586):617–624, 2006.

102. RJ Smith and LM Wahl. Distinct effects of protease and reverse transcriptase inhibition in an immunological model of HIV-1 infection with impulsive drug effects. *Bulletin of Mathematical Biology*, 66(5):1259–1283, 2004.

103. RJ Smith and LM Wahl. Drug resistance in an immunological model of HIV-1 infection with impulsive drug effects. *Bulletin of Mathematical Biology*, 67(4): 783–813, 2005.

104. Robert J Smith and Bhagwan D Aggarwala. Can the viral reservoir of latently infected $CD4^+$ T cells be eradicated with antiretroviral HIV drugs? *Journal of Mathematical Biology*, 59(5):697–715, 2009.

105. Jaejoon Song, Michelle Carey, Hongjian Zhu, Juan C Ramirez Idarraga, and Hulin Wu. Identifying the dynamic gene regulatory network during latent HIV-1 reactivation using high-dimensional ordinary differential equations. *International Journal of Computational Biology and Drug Design*, 2017. Accepted.

106. J Swartz and H Bremermann. Discussion of parameter estimation in biological modelling: Algorithms for estimation and evaluation of the estimates. *Journal of Mathematical Biology*, 1(3):241–257, 1975.

107. Wai-Yuan Tan and Hulin Wu. Stochastic modeling of the dynamics of $CD4^+$ T-cell infection by HIV and some Monte Carlo studies. *Mathematical Biosciences*, 147(2):173–205, 1998.

108. Sanyi Tang and Yanni Xiao. One-compartment model with Michaelis-Menten elimination kinetics and therapeutic window: An analytical approach. *Journal of Pharmacokinetics and Pharmacodynamics*, 34(6):807–827, 2007.

109. Sandor Vajda, Herschel Rabitz, Eric Walter, and Yves Lecourtier. Qualitative and quantitative identifiability analysis of nonlinear chemical kinetic models. *Chemical Engineering Communications*, 83(1):191–219, 1989.

110. Harry L Van Trees. *Detection, Estimation, and Modulation Theory*. Wiley, 2004.

111. JM Varah. A spline least squares method for numerical parameter estimation in differential equations. *SIAM Journal on Scientific and Statistical Computing*, 3(1): 28–46, 1982.

112. MS Varziri, AA Poyton, KB McAuley, PJ McLellan, and JO Ramsay. Selecting optimal weighting factors in iPDA for parameter estimation in continuous-time dynamic models. *Computers & Chemical Engineering*, 32(12):3011–3022, 2008.

113. Lindi M Wahl and Martin A Nowak. Adherence and drug resistance: Predictions for therapy outcome. *Proceedings of the Royal Society of London B: Biological Sciences*, 267(1445):835–843, 2000.

114. Kaifa Wang, Wendi Wang, and Xianning Liu. Global stability in a viral infection model with lytic and nonlytic immune responses. *Computers & Mathematics with Applications*, 51(9):1593–1610, 2006.
115. Wendi Wang and Xiao-Qiang Zhao. Threshold dynamics for compartmental epidemic models in periodic environments. *Journal of Dynamics and Differential Equations*, 20(3):699–717, 2008.
116. Yan Wang, Yicang Zhou, Jianhong Wu, and Jane Heffernan. Oscillatory viral dynamics in a delayed HIV pathogenesis model. *Mathematical Biosciences*, 219 (2):104–112, 2009.
117. Yi Wang, Kent M Eskridge, and Shunpu Zhang. Semiparametric mixed-effects analysis of pk/pd models using differential equations. *Journal of Pharmacokinetics and Pharmacodynamics*, 35(4):443–463, 2008.
118. Xiping Wei, Sajal K Ghosh, Maria E Taylor, Victoria A Johnson, Emilio A Emini, Paul Deutsch, Jeffrey D Lifson, et al. Viral dynamics in human immunodeficiency virus type 1 infection. *Nature*, 373(6510):117–122, 1995.
119. Dominik Wodarz and Alun L Lloyd. Immune responses and the emergence of drug-resistant virus strains in vivo. *Proceedings of the Royal Society of London-B*, 271(1544):1101–1110, 2004.
120. H Wu, H Zhu, H Miao, and AS Perelson. Parameter identifiability and estimation of HIV/AIDS dynamic models. *Bulletin of Mathematical Biology*, 70(3):785–799, 2008.
121. Hulin Wu. Statistical methods for HIV dynamic studies in aids clinical trials. *Statistical Methods in Medical Research*, 14:171–192, 2005.
122. Hulin Wu and A Adam Ding. Population HIV-1 dynamics in vivo: Applicable models and inferential tools for virological data from aids clinical trials. *Biometrics*, 55(2):410–418, 1999.
123. Hulin Wu, Adam Ding, and V DeGruttola. Estimation of HIV dynamic parameters. *Statistics in Medicine*, 17:2463–2485, 1998.
124. Hulin Wu, Yangxin Huang, Edward P Acosta, Jeong-Gun Park, Song Yu, Susan L Rosenkranz, Daniel R Kuritzkes, Joseph J Eron, Alan S Perelson, and John G Gerber. Pharmacodynamics of antiretroviral agents in HIV-1 infected patients: Using viral dynamic models that incorporate drug susceptibility and adherence. *Journal of Pharmacokinetics and Pharmacodynamics*, 33(4):399–419, 2006.
125. Hulin Wu, Yangxin Huang, Edward P Acosta, Susan L Rosenkranz, Daniel R Kuritzkes, Joseph J Eron, Alan S Perelson, and John G Gerber. Modeling long-term HIV dynamics and antiretroviral response: Effects of drug potency, pharmacokinetics, adherence, and drug resistance. *JAIDS Journal of Acquired Immune Deficiency Syndromes*, 39(3):272–283, 2005.
126. Hulin Wu, DR Kuritzkes, and DR McClernon et al. Characterization of viral dynamics in human immunodeficiency virus type 1-infected patients treated with combination antiretroviral therapy: Relationships to host factors, cellular restoration and virological endpoints. *Journal of Infectious Diseases*, 179(4):799–807, 1999.
127. Hulin Wu, Tao Lu, Hongqi Xue, and Hua Liang. Sparse additive ordinary differential equations for dynamic gene regulatory network modeling. *Journal of the American Statistical Association*, 109(506):700–716, 2014.
128. Hulin Wu, Hongyu Miao, Hongqi Xue, David J Topham, and Martin Zand. Quantifying immune response to influenza virus infection via multivariate nonlinear ode models with partially observed state variables and time-varying parameters. *Statistics in Biosciences*, 7(1):147–166, 2015.

129. Hulin Wu, Hongqi Xue, and Arun Kumar. Numerical discretization-based estimation methods for ordinary differential equation models via penalized spline smoothing with applications in biomedical research. *Biometrics*, 68(2):344–352, 2012.
130. Rongling Wu, Jiguo Cao, Zhongwen Huang, Zhong Wang, Junyi Gai, and Eduardo Vallejos. Systems mapping: How to improve the genetic mapping of complex traits through design principles of biological systems. *BMC Systems Biology*, 5(1):1, 2011.
131. H Xiao, Y Miao, S Tang, and H Wu. Modeling antiretroviral drug responses for HIV-1 infected patients using differential equation models. *Advanced Drug Delivery Reviews*, 65:940–953, 2013.
132. Sifei Xing, Cynthia K Bullen, Neeta S Shroff, Liang Shan, Hung-Chih Yang, Jordyn L Manucci, Shridhar Bhat, et al. Disulfiram reactivates latent HIV-1 in a BCL-2-transduced primary CD4+ T cell model without inducing global T cell activation. *Journal of Virology*, 85(12):6060–6064, 2011.
133. H Xue, H Miao, and H Wu. Sieve estimation of constant and time-varying coefficients in nonlinear ordinary differential equation models by considering both numerical error and measurement error. *Annals of Statistics*, 38(4):2351–2387, 2010.
134. Youping Yang and Yanni Xiao. Threshold dynamics for an HIV model in periodic environments. *Journal of Mathematical Analysis and Applications*, 361(1): 59–68, 2010.
135. Youping Yang, Yanni Xiao, Ning Wang, and Jianhong Wu. Optimal control of drug therapy: Melding pharmacokinetics with viral dynamics. *Biosystems*, 107 (3):174–185, 2012.
136. K Zhen Yao, Benjamin M Shaw, Bo Kou, Kim B McAuley, and DW Bacon. Modeling ethylene/butene copolymerization with multi-site catalysts: Parameter estimability and experimental design. *Polymer Reaction Engineering*, 11(3):563–588, 2003.
137. Hong Yue, Martin Brown, Joshua Knowles, Hong Wang, David S Broomhead, and Douglas B Kell. Insights into the behaviour of systems biology models from dynamic sensitivity and identifiability analysis: A case study of an nf-κb signalling pathway. *Molecular BioSystems*, 2(12):640–649, 2006.
138. Daniel E Zak, Gregory E Gonye, James S Schwaber, and Francis J Doyle. Importance of input perturbations and stochastic gene expression in the reverse engineering of genetic regulatory networks: Insights from an identifiability analysis of an in silico network. *Genome Research*, 13(11):2396–2405, 2003.
139. Huiyan Zhu and Xingfu Zou. Impact of delays in cell infection and virus production on HIV-1 dynamics. *Mathematical Medicine and Biology*, 25(2):99–112, 2008.

12

Precision in the Specification of Ordinary Differential Equations and Parameter Estimation in Modeling Biological Processes

Sarah E. Holte

Fred Hutchinson Cancer Research Center, Seattle, WA

Yajun Mei

Georgia Institute of Technology, Atlanta, GA

CONTENTS

12.1 Introduction

In recent years, the use of differential equations to describe the dynamics of within-host viral infections, most frequently HIV-1 or Hepatitis B or C dynamics, has become quite common. The pioneering work described in [1,2,3,4] provided estimates of both the HIV-1 viral clearance rate, c, and infected cell turnover rate, δ, and revealed that while it often takes years for HIV-1 infection to progress to AIDS, the virus is replicating rapidly and continuously throughout these years of apparent latent infection. In addition, at least two compartments of viral-producing cells that decay at different rates were identified. Estimates of infected cell decay and viral clearance rates dramatically changed the understanding of HIV replication, etiology, and pathogenesis. Since that time, models of this type have been used extensively to describe and predict both *in vivo* viral and/or immune system dynamics and the transmission of HIV throughout a population. However, there are both mathematical and statistical challenges associated with models of this type, and the goal of this chapter is to describe some of these as well as offer possible solutions or options. In particular statistical aspects associated with parameter estimation, model comparison and study design will be described. Although the models developed by Perelson et al. [3,4] are relatively simple and were developed nearly 20 years ago, these models will be used in this chapter to demonstrate concepts in a relatively simple setting. In the first section, a statistical approach for model comparison is described using the model developed in [4] as the null hypothesis model for formal statistical comparison to an alternative model. In the next section, the concept of the mathematical sensitivity matrix and its relationship to the Fisher information matrix (FIM) will be described, and will be used to demonstrate how to evaluate parameter identifiability in ordinary differential equation (ODE) models. The next section demonstrates how to determine what types of additional data are required to address the problem of nonidentifiable parameters in ODE models. Examples are provided to demonstrate these concepts. The chapter ends with some recommendations.

Throughout the remainder of this chapter, the term "compartments" refers to the time-varying states in a system of ODEs and the term "parameters" refers to the constants (either known or unknown) in the vector field which defines the specific system of ODEs. The following notation will be used. The m states of an ODE with time t as independent variable will be described by $\mathbf{X}(t) = (X_1(t), \ldots, X_m(t))$ with a (possibly unknown) parameter vector $\Theta = (\theta_1, \cdots, \theta_p)$ and vector field, f, which describes the system. The general system of ODEs is described as:

$$\frac{d\mathbf{X}}{dt} = f(\mathbf{X}, \Theta) \quad \mathbf{X}(0) = \mathbf{X}_0 \tag{12.1}$$

Given the true states $\mathbf{X}(t)$, one then observes noisy data from one or more of the states

$$\mathbf{Y}(t_j) = \mathbf{X}(t_j) + \varepsilon(t_j), \tag{12.2}$$

for $j = 1, 2, \ldots, n$, where $\varepsilon(tj)$ is the measurement error assumed to be independently and identically distributed with zero mean.

12.2 Model Mis-Specification and Statistical Model Comparison

Highly active antiretroviral therapy (HAART) has produced dramatic reduction of viral loads in HIV-1-infected children and adults. Soon after HAART was introduced, estimates of decay rates of viral RNA and infected cell populations were obtained using mathematical models [1–4], and estimates of the time on treatment required to eradicate viral infection were made. Many researchers have used these models to measure the biphasic decline of HIV-1-infected cell compartments in adults [5–7] and children [8,9] and discuss the possibility of viral eradication after 2 or more years of therapy. However, it is now obvious that even after many years of successful treatment, ongoing viral replication persists in at least one population of CD4+ T cells in peripheral blood [10,11]. In addition, interruption of therapy is generally associated with rapid rebound of virus [6,12,13], indicating that viral infection has not been eradicated as predicted. Finally, intermittent episodes of detectable viremia, or "blips" in viral load are sometimes observed in patients who otherwise have been successfully treated with HAART to establish viral loads below the level of detection. Thus, it has become clear that HIV continues to replicate in most individuals long after the times initially estimated for eradication based on the biphasic model developed by Perelson [4]. Since that time, much has been learned about the reservoirs responsible for this persistent infection. These include reactivation of replication competent provirus in latently infected cells which has been shown to persist long after virus is successfully suppressed [10,11,14–16], failing efficacy of the treatment regimen, and possibly most important, hidden reservoirs of productively infected cells in various compartments other than peripheral blood mononuclear cells. Most of these hypotheses assume that the original models developed by Ho, Wei, and Perelson [1–4] are correct, and the reason eradication was not achieved is that additional sources of viral replication were overlooked. In order to accommodate longer and longer periods of viral persistence, many researchers continue to add additional linear (on the log scale) compartments with differing constant decay rates. Indeed, previous estimates of time to eradication of infected cells were based on the assumption that the per capita rates of decay were constant over time. However, it seems unlikely that a single, constant decay rate for an infected cell population is maintained throughout the time course used in estimates of eradication of infected cell populations, especially when no aspects of the immune response or homeostasis are included in the model. In this section, a model which contains "density-dependent" per capita decay rates for HIV-infected cells is considered as an alternative to the Perelson biphasic decay model and is formulated and compared to the Perelson model via statistical inference; treating the

Perelson model as the "null hypothesis." Additional details on the approach can be found in [17].

Assuming constant per capita decay rates, the decline (or growth) of a population is exponential, and depends on the size of the population in a linear way, that is, the decay in the population is proportional (via a constant) to the size of the population, and can be described with linear differential equations. In a density-dependent decay model, this proportionality is variable: the per capita decay rate depends on the size of the population, resulting in a model described by nonlinear differential equations which governs the population dynamics. Population dynamics models of this type are often used in population biology [18] as an alternative to long-term exponential growth or decay: density dependent homeostatic mechanisms are described for lymphocyte populations in mice [19] and humans [12,20,21]; time-dependent decay of a single infected cell compartment was suggested as a possible alternative explanation for the biphasic decay pattern observed in HIV-1 decline by [8] and [22].

In order to assess the accuracy of the assumption of simple exponential decay of infected cell populations, a parameterized model for HIV-1 plasma RNA decline after HAART was developed [17]. In this model, a single parameter can be tested with statistical methods to determine if density-dependent decay is a factor in the biphasic pattern that has been observed in HIV-1 RNA decay after treatment. Incorporating the density-dependent decay mechanism for both the short-lived and long-lived infected cells described in [4] can dramatically alter conclusions about the rate at which infected cells are decaying and the associated estimates of time to eradication of both short-lived and long-lived infected cells. This model also has parameters which can be tested to determine if, in addition to density-dependent decay, more than one population of infected cells is contributing to the overall population of viral RNA. The possibility that only one population of infected cells is contributing to the total viral load in the presence of density-dependent decay was suggested in [8] and [22], that is, that what has previously been described as biphasic decay is the result of density-dependent decay of this single population.

It should be noted that the alternative model evaluated is designed to test the assumption of simple exponential decay of infected cell populations, and does not specify the mechanisms; possible mechanisms include differential activity by the immune system or natural cellular homeostasis responsible for this nonlinear decay. Data used for analysis was collected from HIV-1-infected children initiating treatment with HAART consisting of at least three agents, at least one of which was a protease inhibitor. Blood samples were taken prior to starting therapy and at multiple time points afterwards, with data collected so that both first- and second-phase decay could be estimated. Adherence to the prescribed drug regimen was assessed by direct observation and parent interviews. These data have been presented previously [9,17] where additional details on study design and methods are provided.

The following model for decay of HIV-1 RNA after initiation of HAART is used to test the assumption of constant log linear decay of infected cell compartments. Here, X represents the population of short-lived infected cells, Y the population of long-lived infected cells, and V the population of HIV-1 RNA.

$$\frac{dX}{dt} = -\delta X^r \tag{12.3}$$

$$\frac{dY}{dt} = -\mu Y^r \tag{12.4}$$

$$\frac{dV}{dt} = p_x X + p_y Y - cV \tag{12.5}$$

These equations extend the model described in [4] by allowing for density-dependent decay of infected cell populations. Note that the right-hand sides of Equations 12.3 and 12.4 can be written as $(\delta X^{r-1})\,X$ and $(\mu Y^{r-1})\,Y$, respectively, so that the per capita decay rate for the short-lived infected cells is δX^{r-1} and for long-lived infected cells is μY^{r-1}. If r is not equal to one, the per capita decay rate of these two populations depends on the density of the decaying population. Note that if the parameter r is equal to one, this model reduces to the model presented in [4] which is referred to as the constant decay model for viral decay after initiation of HAART. The parameter p_x represents the contribution to the viral RNA population from short-lived infected cells and p_y represents the contribution to the viral RNA population from long-lived infected cells. To test whether or not density-dependent decay is a factor in the decline of the infected cell populations X and Y, the primary hypothesis of interest is $H0 : r = 1$. Other relevant estimates and tests are whether $p_x = 0$ and $p_y = 0$, that is, whether at least two populations of infected cells contribute to the total viral load, and whether $\delta = 0$ and $\mu = 0$, that is, whether there is significant decay in the infected cell populations which are producing viral RNA in the presence of density-dependent decay.

To obtain the model solutions for plasma viremia, short- and long-lived infected cells, we solved Equations 12.3 and 12.4 under the assumption that $r \neq 1$ to obtain

$$X(t) = [\delta * (r-1) * t + x_0^{1-r}]^{\frac{1}{1-r}}$$
$$Y(t) = [\mu * (r-1) * t + y_0^{1-r}]^{\frac{1}{1-r}} \tag{12.6}$$

and substituted these solutions into Equation 12.5 to obtain

$$\frac{dV}{dt} = p_x[\delta * (r-1) * t + x_0^{1-r}]^{\frac{1}{1-r}} + p_y[\mu * (r-1) * t + y_0^{1-r}]^{\frac{1}{1-r}} - cV \qquad (12.7)$$

If $r = 1$ the solutions to Equations 12.3 and 12.4 are simple first-order exponential decay curves and the model is identical to the one presented in [4]. Equation 12.6 describes the model-predicted densities of short-lived infected and long-lived infected cells after drug therapy and the solution of Equation 12.7 describes the model-predicted plasma viremia density after drug therapy. We used numerical solutions to Equation 12.7 in the Marquart nonlinear least squares algorithm to estimate δ, μ, r, p_x, and p_y. All analyses allowed used observed initial viral load, and both infected cell populations for each child; assuming that, conditional on initial viral load and infected cell compartments, the viral load trajectories are independent and conducted various diagnostics to verify this assumption. Profile bootstrap methods were used to calculate the 95% confidence intervals for the parameters of interest. Additional details on methods for parameters estimation and inference, as well as other details of the study design and methods can be found on [9,17].

The estimates of time to eradication of the short-lived infected and long-lived infected cell populations under the density-dependent decay model were obtained by using Equation 12.6 with the estimated parameters to determine the time required for the initial populations to decay to one infected cell. For the constant decay model, we used first-order exponential trajectories for the infected cell populations.

Data from all six children were used to fit both the density-dependent and constant models. The estimates of δ, μ, r, p_x, and p_y from the density-dependent and constant decay models and associated 95% confidence intervals are shown in Table 12.1. For all but one child (Child 4), the confidence interval for the estimate of the parameter r does not contain one, indicating that density-dependent decay plays a role in the decline of infected cell populations after initiation of treatment in this data set. In other words, the assumption of simple exponential decay for both short- and long-lived infected cells is violated for the data we analyzed. Also p_x and p_y, the viral production rates for short-lived and long-lived infected cells, are both significantly different than zero, indicating that at least two populations of infected cells are contributing to the viral pool in the presence of density-dependent decay. Finally, our estimates of both δ and μ, the decay coefficients for the short-lived and long-lived infected cell populations, are significantly different than zero for all but one child using the constant decay model. In contrast, the estimated coefficient, μ, is not significantly different than zero for five of the six children using the density-dependent model, suggesting that there may be no overall decline in the long-lived infected cell compartment. Both the estimated density-dependent and constant decay model trajectories along with the observed plasma viremia data are shown in Figure 12.1. Projections based on the constant and density-dependent decay models for time to viral eradication (viral load <1 copy) are shown

TABLE 12.1

Parameter Estimates from Constant and Density-Dependent Decay Models with 95% Parametric Bootstrap Confidence Intervals

Child	Density-Dependent Decay				
	δ	μ	p_x	p_y	r
1	0.0172	0.00243	80.3	7.81	0.21
	(0.00037 to 186)	(−0.0001 to 0.0265)	(79.4 to 2,993,371)	(0.00287 to 305)	(0.01 to 0.56)
2	0.236	0.00672	146	1.02	0.08
	(0.00156 to 0.682)	(0.00002 to 0.0160)	(128 to 959)	(0.361 to 3.14)	(0.02 to 0.50)
3	0.00616	−0.00001	484	0.76	0.43
	(0.00160 to 0.193)	(−0.00022 to 0.00618)	(402 to 2038)	(0.00001 to 22.2)	(0.17 to 0.67)
4	0.0106	0.00023	202	1.16	0.31
	(0.00006 to 0.257)	(−0.00 to 0.0112)	(0.837 to 4898)	(0.02 to 3.15)	(−0.00246 to 0.59)
5	0.00356	−0.00003	520	0.0671	0.34
	(0.00138 to 0.0132)	(−0.00008 to 0.00028)	(457 to 1380)	(0.00099 to 0.77)	(0.24 to 0.45)
6	0.252	0.0265	816	163	0.13
	(0.00320 to 158)	(0.00001 to 0.0860)	(588 to 5,382,581)	(1.09 to 1733)	(0.01 to 0.55)

(Continued)

TABLE 12.1 *(Continued)*

Parameter Estimates from Constant and Density-Dependent Decay Models with 95% Parametric Bootstrap Confidence Intervals

| Child | | Constant Decay | | | |
	δ	μ	p_x	p_y	r
1	0.273	0.032	67.1	8.60	†
	(0.214 to 0.972)	(0.0131 to 0.0487)	(66.5 to 212)	(1.96 to 28.8)	
2	0.797	0.020	141	0.941	†
	(0.638 to 1.22)	(0.0150 to 0.0257)	(113 to 495)	(0.520 to 1.70)	
3	0.318	0.001	54.9	1.26	†
	(* to 0.723)	(−0.0253 to 0.0467)	(* to 218)	(0.417 to 9.95)	
4	0.123	0.010	2.48	0.525	†
	(0.0437 to 0.394)	(0.00486 to 0.0139)	(0.694 to 44.6)	(0.171 to 1.02)	
5	0.135	0.006	137	0.669	†
	(0.130 to 0.199)	(0.00127 to 0.0105)	(* to 310)	(0.301 to 1.84)	
6	1.28	0.095	798	114	†
	(0.857 to 3.87)	(0.0575 to 0.132)	(554 to 2368)	(39.8 to 333)	

* The corresponding value is a negative value that does not have any biological meaning and one can replace it by "0" if needed.

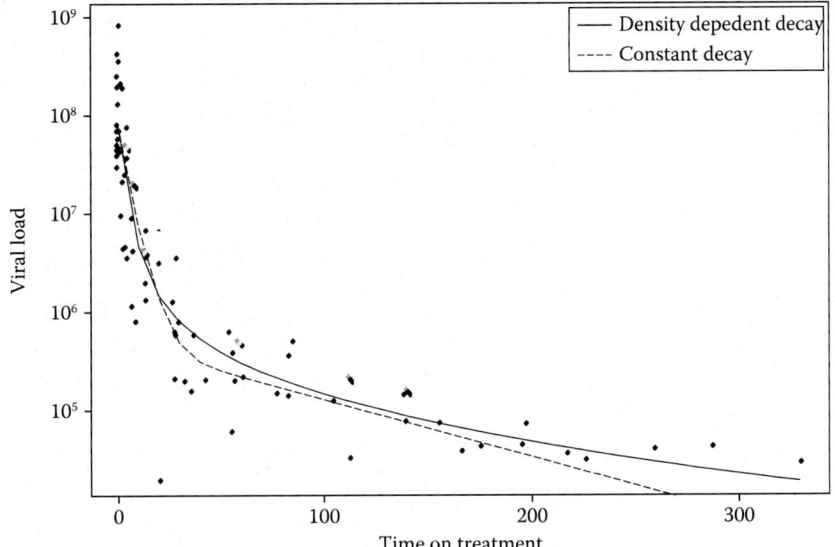

FIGURE 12.1
Total body plasma HIV-1 RNA by days since start of treatment for children with fitted trajectories from the density-dependent and constant decay models. Solid lines indicate fitted model trajectories from the density-dependent decay model, and dashed lines indicate fitted model trajectories from the constant decay model.

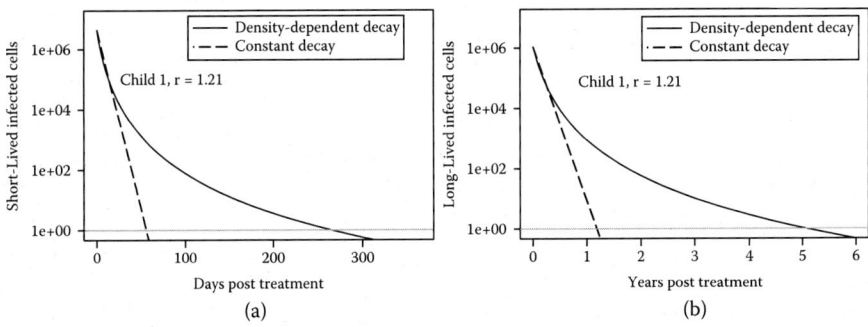

FIGURE 12.2
Projected short-lived (a) and long-lived (b) infected cell populations for Child 1. Solid lines indicate fitted model trajectories from the density-dependent decay model, and dashed lines indicate fitted model trajectories from the constant decay model.

in Figure 12.2a and b for Child 1. The estimated time to eradication of short-lived cells for that child under the constant decay model was 56 days while that time was 271 days based on the density-dependent decay model. For the long-lived infected cell population, the estimated time to eradication based on the constant decay model was 1.2 years. In contrast, that estimates as 5.2 years based on the density-dependent decay model.

The statistical analysis presented here rejects the constant decay model for infected cells developed by Perelson in [4] in favor of the density-dependent decay model for this data set. The qualitative conclusions are quite different. In the constant decay model, both short- and long-lived infected cells are predicted to be eradicated within a few years. In the density-dependent decay model, the decay parameter for long-lived infected cells is not significantly different than zero for five out of the six children evaluated so that the long-lived cell population may not be eradicated at all. If that population is decaying, the estimate of time to eradication is significantly longer, in some cases by many years, than the original estimates obtained by Perelson.

This example is provided in order to emphasize the need to carefully evaluate assumptions and compare models with formal statistical procedures. Like all statistical analysis, it is not the case that we conclude the density-dependent decay model is the correct model; in fact, it almost certainly is not. However, we are able to reject the Perelson constant decay model in favor of the density-dependent decay model indicating that additional work with careful attention to model assumptions is needed in order to build and validate a model before using it to make predictions.

12.3 Model Parameter Identifiability and Study Design

Although the work in [1,2] had enormous impact on identifying the rapid dynamics of within-host viral dynamics, 68% confidence intervals were reported in [1] for the cell-free viral RNA clearance rate, c, since 95% intervals were too large to be meaningful. This suggested that "information" about the parameter c is very limited based on the observations of viral load used to estimate that parameter. In other words, observed viral load is not "sensitive" to the viral clearance parameter, c, in the model used in that work.

Similarly, Lewin et al. [23] used measurements of hepatitis B viral load after treatment with potent antiviral therapy and a mathematical model that included parameters for the death rate of infected cells, δ, the clearance of free virion, c, and two parameters, ε and η, representing drug efficacy at different points in the viral replication cycle to evaluate complex decay profiles after treatment for hepatitis B infection. In that work, they were unable to estimate the efficacy parameter, η, which represents the efficacy of drug therapy in preventing new cells from becoming infected. They conducted their estimation of the remaining three parameters by setting $\eta = 0.5$ and repeating the analysis with $\eta = 0$ and $\eta = 1$. They found very little difference in the resulting estimates of c, δ, and ε in all three analyses, suggesting that hepatitis B viral load is not "sensitive" to the parameter η in the model used in their work.

This inability to accurately estimate certain parameters is well known in a variety of fields. In numerical linear algebra, when not all parameters can be estimated from the available data the model is referred to as "ill-posed" (if no unique solution exists) or "ill-conditioned" (if solutions are unstable) [24]. In the study of differential equations, parameters are referred to as "sloppy" or "stiff," depending on whether their uncertainty is large or require small step sizes to be accurately estimated from the data, respectively; see, for example, [25,26,27]. In statistics, the parameters which cannot be estimated from the available data are referred to as being nonidentifiable.

In the mathematical differential equations literature, sensitivity analysis is a widely used approach to provide guidance on which observations and at what time points measurements should be obtained in order to provide the most precise estimates of individual model parameters. Specifically, sensitivity analysis evaluates which compartments in a system of ODE's are *sensitive* to changes in a specific parameter in the system by calculating the rate of change of the compartment with respect to the parameter (over time), thereby providing information about times at which compartments are most sensitive (i.e., vary the most with respect to) a specific parameter in the system. Unfortunately, sensitivity analysis is a univariate method, and it is not clear how to evaluate sensitivity when one wants to estimate two or more parameters simultaneously, for example, estimation of HIV or hepatitis B viral clearance and infected cell decay parameters.

A powerful statistical tool for simultaneous parameter estimation is the FIM, which has been well described in the statistical literature. However, the properties of ODE system are not widely studied in the statistical literature, while the mathematical literature generally does not focus on the concepts of identifiability and inference for ODE parameter estimates. Fortunately, there is a simple relationship between sensitivity analysis and the FIM. This insight allows matrix characteristics of the FIM to be explored by evaluating the corresponding characteristics of the simpler matrix derived from sensitivity analysis, which will be referred to as the sensitivity matrix. As a consequence, a combination of sensitivity analysis and the FIM can be used to determine how data should be collected in order to ensure the stable estimation of specific parameters in systems of ODEs. That is, these two tools can be used in combination for study design by identifying which model compartments, and at which time points within these compartments, observations should be measured in order to precisely estimate parameters of interest.

12.3.1 The Sensitivity Matrix

In the differential equations literature, traditional sensitivity analysis involves analysis of the derivative of $\mathbf{X}(t)$ with respect to a single parameter θ over time. Specifically, the sensitivity function, $\dfrac{\partial \mathbf{X}}{\partial \theta}(t)$, quantifies the effect of variations of the parameter θ on the time course of model outcome(s). In addition to other useful properties, the sensitivity functions provide information about time points at which measurements from compartments or states described by the differential equations are most informative for the estimation of the specific parameter θ, since it identifies time points at which measurements are most "sensitive" to the specific parameter θ.

The sensitivity function(s) for a system of differential equations with respect to a single parameter, θ, can be calculated by noting that the sensitivity function $\frac{\partial \mathbf{X}}{\partial \theta}(t)$ satisfies the differential equation

$$\frac{d}{dt}\left(\frac{\partial \mathbf{X}}{\partial \theta}\right) = \left(\frac{\partial f}{\partial \mathbf{X}}\right)\left(\mathbf{X}(t,\theta);\theta\right)\frac{\partial \mathbf{X}}{\partial \theta} + \frac{\partial f}{\partial \theta}\left(\mathbf{X}(t,\theta);\theta\right).$$

This allows one to numerically calculate the sensitivity function $\frac{\partial \mathbf{X}}{\partial \theta}(t)$ as the solution to this differential equation even if there are no closed forms for $\mathbf{X}(t)$.

For ease of notation throughout the rest of this subsection and the following two subsections, it is assumed that $\mathbf{X}$ refers to a single state system from which observations Y are obtained. The extension to the case where data are collected from multiple states is straight forward and follows the ideas described here with somewhat more complicated notation. This will be revisited in Section 12.3.4 where adding data from additional compartments to improve parameter identifiability and estimation precision is described.

When there are multiple parameters $\Theta = (\theta_1, \ldots, \theta_p)$ to be estimated and the compartment $\mathbf{X}(t)$ is observed at time $t = t_1, \ldots, t_n$, the sensitivity matrix is defined as:

$$J(\Theta) = \begin{pmatrix} \dfrac{\partial \mathbf{X}(t_1,\Theta)}{\partial \theta_1} & \cdots & \dfrac{\partial \mathbf{X}(t_n,\Theta)}{\partial \theta_1} \\ & \cdots & \\ \dfrac{\partial \mathbf{X}(t_1,\Theta)}{\partial \theta_p} & \cdots & \dfrac{\partial \mathbf{X}(t_1,\Theta)}{\partial \theta_p} \end{pmatrix}, \qquad (12.8)$$

which is a $p \times n$ matrix ($p \times (m \times n)$ matrix when data is observed from all the m states of the system) of time-varying functions. Note that each row of $J(\Theta)$ includes the values of the sensitivity function $\frac{\partial \mathbf{X}(t,\Theta)}{\partial \theta_i}$ at observed time $t = t_1, \ldots, t_n$. Hence, by looking at each row of $J(\Theta)$ separately, one will know when is the most informative time to sample from the compartment $\mathbf{X}$, described by that row in order to estimate a specific parameter, θ_i individually.

Unfortunately, in practice, one usually needs to estimate the unknown parameters $\Theta = (\theta_1, \ldots, \theta_p)$ simultaneously. In this case, it will not be suitable to look at the sensitivity functions $\frac{\partial \mathbf{X}(t,\Theta)}{\partial \theta_i}$ (other than to eliminate parameters that cannot be estimated from data from a specific compartment) because this will not explain how the model variations would affect the simultaneous estimation of parameters. Without additional tools, it is unclear how to use the sensitivity matrix $J(\Theta)$ to evaluate which of a collection of parameters can be estimated simultaneously given the available data, or to design the time points at which measurements are most informative for simultaneously estimating multiple parameters Θ.

12.3.2 The FIM

The FIM is well known in statistics and can be combined with sensitivity analysis to provide a deep understanding of the simultaneous estimation of multiple parameters. Based on the observed value Y_i's, the least square estimates (LSE) of $\Theta = (\theta_1, \ldots, \theta_p)$ is defined to be

$$\hat{\Theta} = \arg \min_{\Theta} \sum_{j=1}^{n} \left(Y_j - \mathbf{X}(t_j, \Theta) \right)^2,$$

The LSE estimate $\hat{\Theta}$ is the maximum likelihood estimate (MLE) if the error terms $\varepsilon(t_j)$ in (12.2) are independent and identically distributed as $N(0, \sigma^2)$. Under this setting, the log-likelihood function is given by

$$\log L(\Theta) = -\frac{1}{2\sigma^2} \sum_{j=1}^{n} \left(Y_j - \mathbf{X}(t_j, \Theta) \right)^2 - \log(\sqrt{2\pi}\sigma)^n,$$

and the corresponding score function by

$$\frac{\partial \log L(\Theta)}{\partial \Theta} = \frac{1}{\sigma^2} \sum_{j=1}^{n} \left(Y_j - \mathbf{X}(t_j, \Theta) \right) \frac{\partial \mathbf{X}(t_j, \Theta)}{\partial \Theta}.$$

If $Y_j - \mathbf{X}(t_j, \Theta)$ is a real-valued random variable and $\frac{\partial \mathbf{X}(t_j, \Theta)}{\partial \Theta}$ is a $p \times 1$ vector, the FIM is given by

$$I(\Theta) = E\left(\left(\frac{\partial \log L(\Theta)}{\partial \Theta} \right) \left(\frac{\partial \log L(\Theta)}{\partial \Theta} \right)^T \right) = \frac{1}{\sigma^2} \sum_{j=1}^{n} \left(\frac{\partial \mathbf{X}(t_j, \Theta)}{\partial \Theta} \right) \left(\frac{\partial \mathbf{X}(t_j, \Theta)}{\partial \Theta} \right)^T.$$

$$(12.9)$$

By the Cramer–Rao inequality, for any unbiased estimator $\hat{\Theta} = \hat{\theta}_1, \ldots, \hat{\theta}_p$ of $\Theta = (\theta_1, \ldots, \theta_p)$,

$$\text{Var}(\hat{\Theta}) = [I(\Theta)]^{-1}$$

is positive semidefinite. If the lower bound is sharp, then in order to minimize $\text{Var}(\hat{\theta}_1), \ldots, \text{Var}(\hat{\theta}_p)$, we need to minimize all diagonal elements of the matrix $[I(\Theta)]^{-1}$.

12.3.3 Combining the Sensitivity Matrix and FIM

To establish the relationship between FIM $I(\Theta)$ in (12.9) and sensitivity matrix $J(\Theta)$ in (12.8), define a $p \times 1$ vector

$$v_j = \frac{\partial \mathbf{X}(t_j, \Theta)}{\partial \Theta}. \tag{12.10}$$

Then, the sensitivity matrix $J(\Theta)$ in (12.8) can be rewritten as

$$J(\Theta) = (v_1, v_2, \ldots, v_n)$$

where the vectors v_j form the columns of $J(\Theta)$. Similarly, the FIM $I(\Theta)$ in (12.9) can be rewritten as

$$\mathcal{I}(\Theta) = \frac{1}{\sigma^2} \sum_{j=1}^{n} v_j v_j^T.$$

Hence, we have

$$\mathcal{I}(\Theta) = \frac{1}{\sigma^2} J(\Theta)(J\Theta))^T.$$

Based on this relationship, it is easy to derive

- $\mathcal{I}(\Theta)$ in invertible (i.e., $rank(I(\Theta)) = p$) if and only if $rank(J(\Theta)) = p$.
- The smallest eigenvalue of $I(\Theta)$ is proportional to

$$\min_{u \in \mathbb{R}^p : \|u\| = 1} \| (J(\Theta))^T u \|^2 = \min_{u \in \mathbb{R}^p : \|u\| = 1} \sum_{j=1}^{n} (v_j^T u)^2.$$

Therefore, in order to evaluate parameter identifiability and obtain the most precise estimates of the parameters Θ, one should collect measurements at times $t_1, t_2, \ldots, t_n$ such that

$$\min_{u \in \mathbb{R}^p : \|u\| = 1} \left[\sum_{i=1}^{n} (v_i^T u)^2 \right] \text{ is maximized,} \tag{12.11}$$

where v_i is defined in (12.10).

12.3.4 Study Design: Impact of New Compartment or Time Points

As pointed out by Wu et al. [28] for the models described in [3], the information contained in the total viral load measurements V, is not sufficient for identifying both the viral clearance rate c and infected cell turnover rate δ. However, knowing the concentration of infectious virions V_I provides sufficient additional information to identify all parameters. To understand this, the FIM again provides insight on how additional measurements from a new compartment can provide the sufficient information. This example will be explored in further detail in Section 12.4.2.

In general, assume that measurements of $Y = X(t, \Theta) + \varepsilon$ from a single compartment of a system of ODEs are observed with the goal of estimating a collection of parameters Θ in the ODE model. Define $p \times 1$ vectors, v_j, as described in (12.10) and the $p \times n$ sensitivity matrix $J_1(\Theta) = (v_1, v_2, \ldots, v_n)$. The $p \times p$ FIM is

$$\mathcal{I}_1(\Theta) = \frac{1}{\sigma^2} \sum_{j=1}^{n} v_j v_j^T = \frac{1}{\sigma^2} J_1(\Theta)(J_1(\Theta))^T.$$

As noted in Section 12.3.3, the smallest eigenvalue of $\mathcal{I}_1(\Theta)$ is proportional to

$$\min_{u \in \mathbb{R}^p : \|u\| = 1} \| (J_1(\Theta))^T u \|^2 = \min_{u \in \mathbb{R}^p : \|u\| = 1} \sum_{j=1}^{n} (v_j^T u)^2.$$

Hence, if $v_1, \ldots, v_n$ are nearly linearly dependent, then the smallest eigenvalue of $\mathcal{I}_1(\Theta)$ may be close to zero (so $\mathcal{I}_1(\Theta)$ may be poorly conditioned), and thus the diagonal elements of $\mathcal{I}_1^{-1}(\Theta)$ could be very large, so that the variance of the estimates of Θ are very large.

Now, suppose we take observations from new compartment $Y^*(t) = X^*(t, \Theta) + \varepsilon^*(t)$. Define

$$v_j^* = \frac{\partial X^*(t_j, \Theta)}{\partial \Theta}, \quad j = 1, 2, \ldots, n_1$$

Then, adding observations from the new compartment $Y^*(t)$ will lead to new sensitivity matrix

$$J_2(\Theta) = (v_1, v_2, \ldots, v_n, v_1^*, v_2^*, \ldots, v_{n_1}^*), \tag{12.12}$$

and $p \times (n + n_1)$ matrix, and leads to new FIM

$$\mathcal{I}_2(\Theta) = \frac{1}{\sigma^2} \left(\sum_{j=1}^{n} v_j v_j^T + \sum_{j=1}^{n_1} v_j^* v_j^{*T} \right) = \frac{1}{\sigma^2} J_2(\Theta)(J_2(\Theta))^T. \tag{12.13}$$

If the span of the v_j^*'s is orthogonal or nearly orthogonal to the span of the original v_j's, then the smallest eigenvalues of $\mathcal{I}_2(\Theta)$ can be significantly larger than that of $\mathcal{I}_1(\Theta)$, implying that adding observations from the new compartment X^* as demonstrated in (12.12) and (12.13) can significantly improve the estimate of Θ. The sensitivity matrices for each compartment of the system of ODEs can be evaluated as guides to determine which states or compartments are sensitive to the parameter(s) of interest.

12.4 Examples

This section contains examples on the combined use of sensitivity analysis and the FIM in order to determine which parameters can be estimated from a given set of data or to design studies to ensure that all parameters will be identifiable. Both examples demonstrate how to use sensitivity analysis to determine which additional compartments should be used to generate observations for analysis in order to eliminate problems of lack of identifiability and improve precision when parameters are poorly estimated.

12.4.1 Model Parameter Identifiability: Lumped Parameters

As a simple example to illustrate the use of sensitivity analysis and the FIM to evaluate parameter identifiability, suppose the observations

$$Y(t) = X(t) + \varepsilon,$$

where $X(t) = X(t, g(\theta 1, \theta 2), \theta 3, \ldots, \theta p)$, where the function g does not depend on t, $\theta_3, \ldots, \theta_p$. The question is whether we can estimate the lumped parameters $\theta 1, \theta 2$ based on the observations Y. Intuition suggests that the answer is no, but it is useful to formalize this using the FIM and sensitivity matrix. In this case, note that

$$\frac{\partial X}{\partial \theta_i} = \frac{\partial X}{\partial g} \frac{\partial g}{\partial \theta_i}, \quad for\ i = 1, 2.$$

Thus, for the sensitivity matrix $J(\Theta)$ in (12.8), its first two rows are linearly dependent, and $rank(J(\Theta)) < p$. Hence, the FIM $I(\Theta)$ in (12.9) has rank less than p and so is not invertible.

This implies that we cannot estimate $\theta_1, \theta_2, \ldots, \theta_p$ simultaneously based on the observed values Y.

12.4.2 Models for Viral Decay of HIV after Treatment

As described above, 68% confidence intervals were reported in [3] for the cell-free viral RNA clearance rate, c, since 95% intervals were too large to be meaningful. This suggested that "information" about the parameter c is very limited based on the observations of viral load used to estimate that parameter. In [3], the following system of differential equation are used to describe viral decay after treatment. Before treatment,

$$\frac{dT^*}{dt} = kTV - \delta T^*$$

$$\frac{dV}{dt} = N\delta T^* - cV,$$

(12.14)

where T^* is the infected cells and V is the viral RNA. The parameter k denotes the viral infectivity, T the uninfected target cells, N the burst size, and c the viral clearance rate. After the treatment,

$$\frac{dT^*}{dt} = kTV_1 - \delta T^*$$

$$\frac{dV_I}{dt} = -cV_I \qquad (12.15)$$

$$\frac{dV_{NI}}{dt} = N\delta T^* - cV_{NI},$$

where V_I and V_{NI} denote the infectious and noninfectious viral RNA, respectively.

It is assumed that the system is at quasi-steady state before the treatment and the parameter T, the uninfected target cells, remains constant at T_0. In other words, the initial values for the system (12.15) are given by $T^*(0) = T_0^*$, $V_I(0) = V_0$, and $V_{NI}(0) = 0$, where (T_0^*, V_0) are the values for the steady state of the system (12.14).

When measured in a clinical setting, the observed viral load data are a combination of infectious and noninfectious viral load, so that $V(t) = V_I(t) + V_{NI}(t)$ provides the model for the mean structure of the observed data, $\{v_0, \ldots, v_n\}$, at sampling times $\{t_0, \ldots, t_n\}$ for a single patient. A standard approach to estimating c and δ from the observed data is to use nonlinear least squares.

Specifically, the solution $V(t) = V_I(t) + V_{NI}(t)$ to (12.15) can be obtained with either analytic or numerical techniques, and c and δ can be estimated by minimizing

$$\sum_{j=1}^{n} \left(\log(v_j) - \log(V(t_j, c, \delta)) \right)^2 \qquad (12.16)$$

with respect to c and δ. In this case, log transformation serves to satisfy the assumption that viral load measurements follow a log-normal distribution so that (12.16) is the maximum likelihood estimator for c and δ.

In order to evaluate the precision of joint estimation of c and δ from data on total viral load, we simulated data from each of the three compartments V_{NI}, V_I, and T^* using $c = 3$ and $\delta = 0.5$ in the model described in [3] and (12.15). Figure 12.3 shows the simulated data with the estimated values $\hat{c} = 3.586$ and $\hat{\delta} = 0.456$, based on nonlinear least squares (12.16), and the corresponding model solution for total viral load, $V(t) = V_I(t) + V_{NI}(t)$.

In Figure 12.4, the contours of the likelihood surfaces or cost function for joint estimation of c and δ based on the simulated total viral load (infectious plus noninfectious) data are shown. These contours indicate that data on total viral load are sufficient for estimating the infected cell turnover rate δ but will not provide reasonable precision for estimation of viral clearance rate c, as indicated by the curved "ridge" in the c-axis of the joint estimation surface.

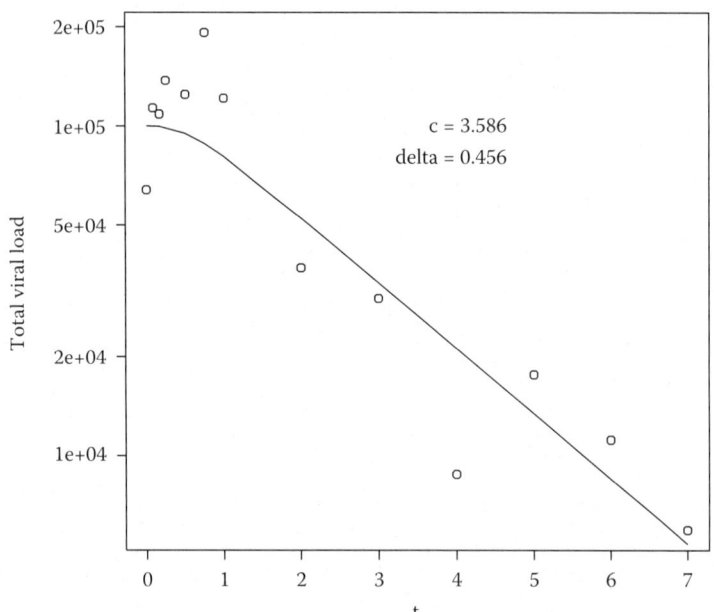

FIGURE 12.3
Data simulated with mean specified by total viral load ($V_{NI}(t) + V_I(t)$).

While the parameter c can be estimated from total viral load, this "ridge" indicates that estimation is not likely to be very precise. Simulated data with additional time points did not significantly change the properties of the likelihood surface for joint estimation of c and δ (data not shown), indicating that the addition of data on total viral load at additional time points will not provide substantially more precise estimates for the parameter c.

In order to evaluate why data on total viral load is not sufficient for estimating the viral clearance rate c based on the model (12.14), we calculated the sensitivity functions for total viral load $V(t) = V_I(t) + V_{NI}(t)$ as defined by (12.14) with respect to c and δ, and V_c and V_δ, respectively. The results are shown in Figure 12.5. Figure 12.5a shows why precise estimation of the parameter c from total viral load is difficult. While not truly nonidentifiable, the sensitivity equation, V_c, is quite flat, although not exactly zero, indicating that while c is technically identifiable from total viral load, that compartment is not very sensitive to small changes in c so that precise estimation of c from data on total viral load cannot be achieved with much precision. Conversely, Figure 12.5b shows the sensitivity of total viral load to the parameter δ, $V_\delta(t)$. Total viral load is much more sensitive to small changes in δ, and so δ can be estimated with reasonable precision from total viral load.

When estimating parameters in a system of ODEs, collecting data at additional time points from a single state is only one option for adding data to

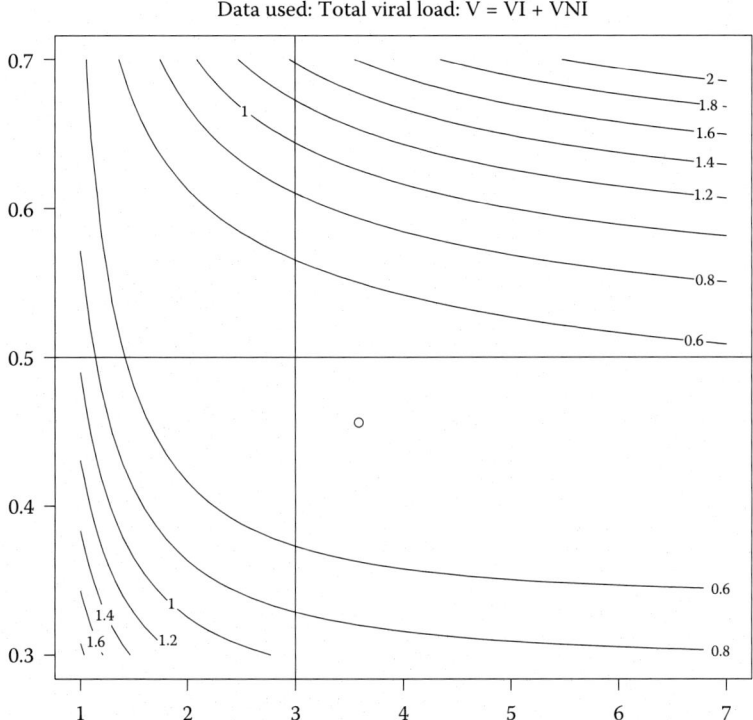

FIGURE 12.4
Contours of the likelihood function for joint estimation of c and δ based on observed simulated viral load.

improve precision of parameter estimates. Collecting data from other states represented in the system is another option, which is considered here. Sensitivity analysis can guide the choice of which compartment to sample, as well as the times at which data should be sampled. Sensitivity analysis of the infected cell compartment, $T^*(t)$, has properties similar to the total viral load. That is, based on the model (12.14), $T^*(t)$ is not sensitive to c but is sensitive to δ (analysis not shown). However, in Figure 12.5c and d, we show the sensitivity of infectious viral load with respect to viral clearance rate c and infectious viral load with respect to the parameter δ, respectively. Figure 12.5c suggests that observing data on infectious viral load will significantly improve precision in the estimation of the viral clearance parameter c. Figure 12.5d confirms that the infectious cell clearance rate, δ, is not identifiable from data on infectious viral load, which is obvious since the model for infectious viral load, $V_I(t) = V_0 e^{-ct}$, does not depend on the parameter δ.

Based on the sensitivity analysis, we expect that using observed data on both the total viral load and infectious viral load in combination with nonlinear regression and model equations for $V(t)$ and $V_I(t)$ will improve precision

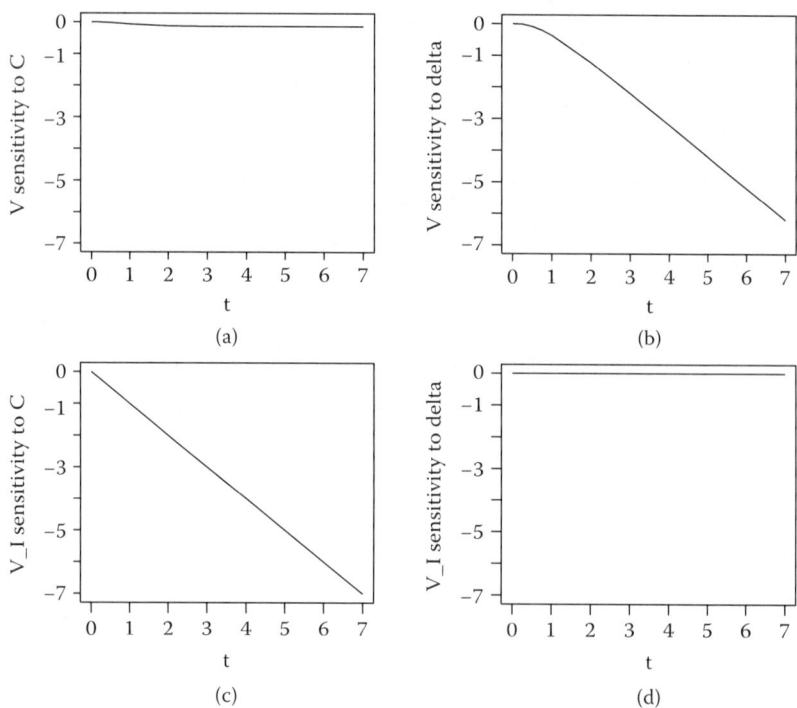

FIGURE 12.5

Sensitivity equation (a) V_C, (b) V_δ, (c) V_{I_c}, and (d) V_{I_δ}.

in estimates of the viral clearance parameters c. When using data from more than one compartment, nonlinear regression is conducted in a manner similar to the procedure used for a single compartment, for example, minimizing (12.16) over c and δ. When data from more than one compartment is available for parameter estimation, minimization of

$$\sum_{j=1}^{n}\left[\left(\log(v_j)-\log\left(V(t_j,c,\delta)\right)\right)^2/\sigma_V + \left(\log(v_{I_j})-\log\left(V_I(t_j,c,\delta)\right)\right)^2/\sigma_{V_I}\right]$$

with respect to c and δ provides the MLEs for these parameters, assuming a log-normal distribution for both total viral load and infectious viral load with measurement errors σV and σV_I, respectively.

Figure 12.6 shows contours of the likelihood surface for joint estimation of c and δ (based on simulated data) using data from: (a) the total (infectious + noninfectious) viral load compartments $V(t) = V_I(t) + V_{NI}(t)$ and (b) total *and* the infectious viral load compartments $V_I(t)$. Note the difference in the change in scale on the horizontal axis for the parameter c. As expected, based on the sensitivity analysis, adding data from the infectious viral load

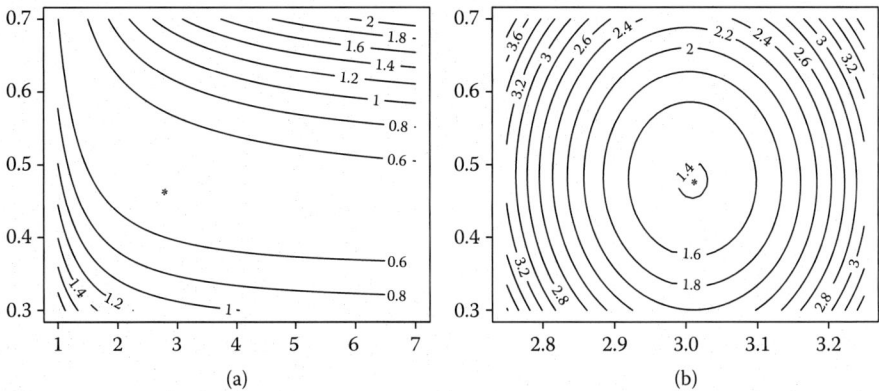

FIGURE 12.6
Contours of the likelihood function for joint estimation of c and δ based on observed (a) total viral load and infected cells and (b) total viral load and infectious viral load. Estimates of c and δ are shown with *.

compartment dramatically improves the precision in estimation of the viral clearance rate c (Figure 12.5b). Contours of the likelihood surface for estimation of c and δ using simulated data from the infected cell compartment and total viral load were examined and do not improve precision in estimation of c (results not shown). While the infectious viral load compartment carries most of the "information" on the parameter c for the model (12.14), the infected cell turnover rate δ is not identifiable from infectious viral load alone, and so, observation on either total viral load or infected cell densities is needed in combination with measurements of infectious viral load to estimate both c and δ with reasonable precision.

A complete description of the expected variance from Fisher information for joint estimation of c and δ from individual and combination of compartments is shown in Table 12.2.

TABLE 12.2

Expected Variance from Fisher Information
for Joint Estimation of c and δ

	c	δ
V only	1.94	0.05
V_I only	0.01	NA
V and T^*	0.3	0.01
V and V_I	0.01	0.0002
T^* only	0.65	0.02

12.5 Discussion

As described in the introduction, mathematical models have had tremendous impact on the field of HIV and viral dynamics in helping to understand the etiology of the disease and response to treatment. ODE models have been used extensively to evaluate a variety of aspects related to viral and immune-response dynamics. They have also been applied to predict the spread of epidemics of infectious diseases, and in some cases have been relatively successful, provided the time period of evaluation is short. ODE models, however, can be extremely sensitive to the assumptions and so careful attention to the mathematical details is required in interpreting their predictions. In a recent high-profile example, mathematical models incorrectly predicted the magnitude of the 2014/15 Ebola epidemic [29]. Similarly, recent conclusions about a hidden reservoir in the lymph system that prevents viral eradication were put forth in terms of a highly complex ODE model [30], yet no aspects of immune response were included and all compartments assumed constant decay, both of which can drastically alter the dynamics. Models of these types are common, but too often little attention is given to validating model assumptions and the various aspects of parameter estimation.

This chapter has emphasized the need for careful evaluation of any ODE model since the predictions of these models can be very sensitive to the underlying assumptions. Statistical testing and model validation are important prior to making conclusions about the dynamics being modeled. Here, we demonstrated how a very slight change to a model's form—for example, changes in parameter values resulting in a change in the form of the model, or the compartments measured—can result in dramatically altered predictions. In our example, when a constant decay rate is replaced by a density-dependent decay rate, the predicted time to eradication of infected cells is vastly changed. The statistical analysis conducted rejected the constant decay rate model in favor of the density-dependent decay rate model in the data analyzed. It has recently been shown that many other factors (not modeled here) contribute to the inability of potent therapy to eradicate infection and, indeed, this example is not intended to provide an accurate model for time to viral eradication. Rather, it demonstrates the type of investigation, including the formal statistical testing of one model against another, which is needed when using mathematical models to describe any phenomena.

This chapter also discusses the concept of parameter identifiability and its relationship to model-state sensitivity to parameters. The primary conclusion is that for a given structure of an ODE system, it may not be possible to estimate a particular parameter even while fully observing data from that state. Or, a particular parameter may be estimated with very poor precision using observations from a given state. In the former case, no number of additional observation will allow the estimation of that parameter; in order to obtain an estimate, data from additional states of the system must be obtained. In the latter case, additional observations from the particular state may aid precision, but observations from other states can dramatically improve the precision of the estimate.

In summary, understanding the sensitivity and validity of model specification is a crucial component in the application of dynamical systems to population-based studies. In this direction, there are many opportunities to improve the performance of ODE models in the areas of viral dynamics and epidemiological transmission dynamics. The development of new methods as well as the rigorous application of tools from other disciplines will improve our statistical understanding of parameter estimates, their inference, and potentially even estimation and inference for the entire functional form that defines an ODE model.

References

1. David D Ho, Avidan U Neumann, Alan S Perelson, Wen Chen, John M Leonard, Martin Markowitz, et al. Rapid turnover of plasma virions and CD4 lymphocytes in HIV-1 infection. *Nature* **373** (1995), no. 6510, 123–126.
2. Xiping Wei, Sajal K Ghosh, Maria E Taylor, Victoria A Johnson, Emilio A Emini, Paul Deutsch, et al. Viral dynamics in human immunodeficiency virus type 1 infection. *Nature* **373** (1995), no. 6510, 117–122.
3. Alan S Perelson, Avidan U Neumann, Martin Markowitz, John M Leonard, and David D Ho. HIV-1 dynamics in vivo: Virion clearance rate, infected cell lifespan, and viral generation time. *Science* **271** (1996), no. 5255, 1582–1586.
4. Alan S Perelson, Paulina Essunger, Yunzhen Cao, Mika Vesanen, Arlene Hurley, Kalle Saksela, et al. Decay characteristics of HIV-1-infected compartments during combination therapy. *Nature* **387** (1997), 188–191.
5. Daan W Notermans, Jaap Goudsmit, Sven A Danner, Frank de Wolf, Alan S Perelson, and John Mittler. Rate of HIV-1 decline following antiretroviral therapy is related to viral load at baseline and drug regimen. *AIDS* **12** (1998), no. 12, 1483–1490.
6. Avidan U Neumann, Roland Tubiana, Vincent Calvez, Catherine Robert, Tai-Sheng Li, Henri Agut, et al. HIV-1 rebound during interruption of highly active antiretroviral therapy has no deleterious effect on reinitiated treatment. *AIDS* **13** (1999), no. 6, 677–683.
7. Hulin Wu, Daniel R Kuritzkes, Daniel R McClernon, Harold Kessler, Elizabeth Connick, Alan Landay, et al. Characterization of viral dynamics in human immunodeficiency virus type 1-infected patients treated with combination antiretroviral therapy: Relationships to host factors, cellular restoration, and virologic end points. *Journal of Infectious Diseases* **179** (1999), no. 4, 799–807.
8. Katherine Luzuriaga, Hulin Wu, Margaret McManus, Paula Britto, William Borkowsky, Sandra Burchett, et al. Dynamics of human immunodeficiency virus type 1 replication in vertically infected infants. *Journal of Virology* **73** (1999), no. 1, 362–367.

9. Ann J Melvin, Allen G Rodrigo, Kathleen M Mohan, Paul A Lewis, Laura Manns-Arcuino, Robert W Coombs, et al. HIV-1 dynamics in children. *JAIDS Journal of Acquired Immune Deficiency Syndromes* **20** (1999), no. 5, 468–473.

10. Linqi Zhang, Bharat Ramratnam, Klara Tenner-Racz, Yuxian He, Mika Vesanen, Sharon Lewin, et al. Quantifying residual HIV-1 replication in patients receiving combination antiretroviral therapy. *New England Journal of Medicine* **340** (1999), no. 21, 1605–1613.

11. Bharat Ramratnam, John E Mittler, Linqi Zhang, Daniel Boden, Arlene Hurley, Fang Fang, et al. The decay of the latent reservoir of replication-competent HIV-1 is inversely correlated with the extent of residual viral replication during prolonged anti-retroviral therapy. *Nature Medicine* **6** (2000), no. 1, 82–85.

12. Richard T Davey, Niranjan Bhat, Christian Yoder, Tae-Wook Chun, Julia A Metcalf, Robin Dewar, et al. HIV-1 and T cell dynamics after interruption of highly active antiretroviral therapy (HAART) in patients with a history of sustained viral suppression. *Proceedings of the National Academy of Sciences* **96** (1999), no. 26, 15109–15114.

13. Felipe García, Montserrat Plana, Carmen Vidal, Anna Cruceta, Giuseppe Pantaleo, Tomás Pumarola, et al. Dynamics of viral load rebound and immunological changes after stopping effective antiretroviral therapy. *AIDS* **13** (1999), no. 11, F79–F86.

14. Manohar R Furtado, Duncan S Callaway, John P Phair, Kevin J Kunstman, Jennifer L Stanton, Catherine A Macken, et al. Persistence of HIV-1 transcription in peripheral-blood mononuclear cells in patients receiving potent antiretroviral therapy. *New England Journal of Medicine* **340** (1999), no. 21, 1614–1622.

15. Tae-Wook Chun and Anthony S Fauci. Latent reservoirs of HIV: Obstacles to the eradication of virus. *Proceedings of the National Academy of Sciences* **96** (1999), no. 20, 10958–10961.

16. Diana Finzi, Joel Blankson, Janet D Siliciano, Joseph B Margolick, Karen Chadwick, Theodore Pierson, et al. Latent infection of CD4+ T cells provides a mechanism for lifelong persistence of HIV-1, even in patients on effective combination therapy. *Nature Medicine* **5** (1999), no. 5, 512–517.

17. Sarah E Holte, Ann J Melvin, James I Mullins, Nicole H Tobin, and Lisa M Frenkel. Density-dependent decay in HIV-1 dynamics. *JAIDS Journal of Acquired Immune Deficiency Syndromes* **41** (2006), no. 3, 266–276.

18. Frank Charles Hoppensteadt. *Mathematical Methods of Population Biology.* vol. **4**. Cambridge University Press, Cambridge, 1982.

19. Corinne Tanchot and Benedita Rocha. The peripheral T cell repertoire: Independent homeo-static regulation of virgin and activated CD8+ T cell pools. *European Journal of Immunology* **25** (1995), no. 8, 2127–2136.

20. AT Haase. Population biology of HIV-1 infection: Viral and CD4+ T cell demographics and dynamics in lymphatic tissues. *Annual Review of Immunology* **17** (1999), no. 1, 625–656.

21. Richard D Hockett, J Michael Kilby, Cynthia A Derdeyn, Michael S Saag, Michael Sillers, Kathleen Squires, et al. Constant mean viral copy number per infected cell in tissues regardless of high, low, or undetectable plasma HIV RNA. *The Journal of Experimental Medicine* **189** (1999), no. 10, 1545–1554.

22. Ramy A Arnaout, Nowak Martin A, and Dominik Wodarz. HIV-1 dynamics revisited: Biphasic decay by cytotoxic T lymphocyte killing? *Proceedings of the Royal Society of London B: Biological Sciences* **267** (2000), no. 1450, 1347–1354.

23. Sharon R Lewin, Ruy M Ribeiro, Tomos Walters, George K Lau, Scott Bowden, Stephen Locarnini, et al. Analysis of hepatitis B viral load decline under potent therapy: Complex decay profiles observed. *Hepatology* **34** (2001), no. 5, 1012–1020.

24. Lloyd N Trefethen and David Bau III. *Numerical Linear Algebra.* vol. **50**. SIAM, Philadelphia, PA, 1997.

25. Mark K Transtrum, Benjamin B Machta, Kevin S Brown, Bryan C Daniels, Christopher R Myers, and James P Sethna. Perspective: Sloppiness and emergent theories in physics, biology, and beyond. *The Journal of Chemical Physics* **143** (2015), no. 1, 010901.

26. G Wanner and E Hairer. *Solving Ordinary Differential Equations II.* vol. **1**. Springer-Verlag, Berlin, 1991.

27. Marc Nico Spijker. Stiffness in numerical initial-value problems. *Journal of Computational and Applied Mathematics* **72** (1996), no. 2, 393–406.

28. Hulin Wu, A Adam Ding, and Victor De Gruttola. Estimation of HIV dynamic parameters. *Statistics in Medicine* **17** (1998), no. 21, 2463–2485.

29. Declan Butler. Models overestimate ebola cases. *Nature* **515** (2014), no. 7525, 18–18.

30. Ramon Lorenzo-Redondo, Helen R Fryer, Trevor Bedford, Eun-Young Kim, John Archer, Sergei L Kosakovsky Pond, et al. Persistent HIV-1 replication maintains the tissue reservoir during therapy. *Nature* **530** (2016), no. 7588, 51–56.

Index

H

HAART, *see* Highly active antiretroviral therapy
Hazard ratio, 67
Heavily treatment-experienced patients, 7
Hepatitis C (HCV) testing, 88
Hierarchical Dirichlet process models, 143–147
Highly active antiretroviral therapy (HAART), 4, 74, 259
HIV, *see* Human immunodeficiency virus
HIV-1 vaccine clinical trials, sample size for, 17–39
  cell-mediated immune responses, 19
  data safety monitoring procedure, 29
  example, 26–29
  maximum error margin allowed, 21
  power analysis, 20
  precision analysis, 21–22
  procedure for sample size estimation, 23–25
  sample size determination, 20–25
  sensitivity analysis, 25–26
  Thai efficacy trial, 19
Human immunodeficiency virus (HIV), 3, 54
  broadly neutralizing antibodies against, 165–166
  non-inferiority trials, *see* Statistical issues in HIV non-inferiority trials
  ribonucleic acid (HIV RNA) copy numbers, 110

I

ICS assay, *see* Intracellular cytokine staining assay
Immunizations, operation of, 161
Immunoglobulin variable-region gene (IgVRG) repertoire and its analysis, 157–178
  affinity maturation, 161
  allelic exclusion, 160
  analysis, 167–174
  antibody combinatorial diversity, 161

Artemis complex, 161
B-cell biology, 159–163
broadly neutralizing antibodies against HIV, 165–166
centrocytes, 162
class switch recombination, 162
clonal kinship, 173
clonal partitioning, 173–174
clone, 162
cognate T cells, 161
complementarity determining regions, 159
dark zone, 162
follicular dendritic cells, 162
germinal centers, 162
IgVRG repertoire sequencing, 164–165
immunizations, operation of, 162
junctional diversity, 161
kappa light chain genes, 160
lambda light chain genes, 160
light zone, 162
massive parallel sequencing, 164
next-generation sequencing, 164
secondary lymphoid tissues, 160
sequencing by synthesis, 164
software availability, 174
somatic hypermutation, 162
stochastic generative models for VDJ recombination and affinity maturation, 168–171
Infinite mixture models, 141
Instrumental variables (IV) approach, 12
Integrity, 53
Intent-to-treat (ITT) approach, 11
Intracellular cytokine staining (ICS) assay, 147
Inverse probability of sampling weights, generalizing evidence from HIV trials using, 63–86
  analysis, 77–78
  applications, 74–81
  assumptions and notation, 67–68
  background, 64–65
  cohort and trial data, 74–77
  external validity, 64
  hazard ratio, 67
  inference about population treatment effects, 69–71